Stroke and Ageing

Guest Editors

Dominique A. Cadilhac
Olivia Brancatisano
Tharshanah Thayabaranathan

MDPI

Basel • Beijing • Wuhan • Barcelona • Belgrade • Novi Sad • Cluj • Manchester

Guest Editors

Dominique A. Cadilhac
Department of Medicine
School of Clinical Sciences at
Monash Health
Monash University
Clayton
Australia

Olivia Brancatisano
Department of Medicine
School of Clinical Sciences at
Monash Health
Monash University
Clayton
Australia

Tharshanah Thayabaranathan
Department of Medicine
School of Clinical Sciences at
Monash Health
Monash University
Clayton
Australia

Editorial Office
MDPI AG
Grosspeteranlage 5
4052 Basel, Switzerland

This is a reprint of the Special Issue, published open access by the journal *Healthcare* (ISSN 2227-9032), freely accessible at: https://www.mdpi.com/journal/healthcare/special_issues/C61S236O3G.

For citation purposes, cite each article independently as indicated on the article page online and as indicated below:

Lastname, A.A.; Lastname, B.B. Article Title. *Journal Name* **Year**, *Volume Number*, Page Range.

ISBN 978-3-7258-4481-4 (Hbk)
ISBN 978-3-7258-4482-1 (PDF)
https://doi.org/10.3390/books978-3-7258-4482-1

Contents

healthcare

MDPI

Editorial

Advancing Comprehensive Stroke Care—From Acute Recovery to Long-Term Wellbeing

Tharshanah Thayabaranathan [1,*] and Dominique A. Cadilhac [1,2]

[1] Stroke and Ageing Research Group, Department of Medicine, School of Clinical Sciences at Monash Health, Monash University, Clayton, VIC 3168, Australia; dominique.cadilhac@monash.edu

[2] Stroke Group, Florey Institute of Neuroscience and Mental Health, University of Melbourne, Heidelberg, VIC 3084, Australia

* Correspondence: tharshanah.thayabaranathan@monash.edu; Tel.: +613-7511-1968

Introduction

Stroke is one of the most complex diseases of our time; it impacts individuals across many facets of functioning, depending on the areas of the brain that have been damaged. Despite substantial advances in acute management, the global burden of stroke is increasing, especially in low- and middle-income countries (LMICs), where stroke occurs at younger ages and leads to more years lived with disability [1,2]. It has been estimated that nearly 89% of stroke-related disability-adjusted life years (DALYs) now occur in LMICs [1,2]. This disproportionate burden in LMICs contrasts with high-income countries, which increasingly face challenges related to ageing populations [3]. Consequently, there is an urgent need to prevent stroke, and to also embrace the full spectrum of treatment and recovery care including rehabilitation, avoiding complications, and providing support for mental health. Since stroke can often be fatal or increase the risk of death, appropriate palliative care support is also a priority.

The Special Issue "Stroke and Ageing" brings together ten articles from different regions that cover the spectrum of advancing practice to meet healthcare needs after stroke. Each article contributes to the growing body of evidence supporting an integrated, person-centred, and lifespan-oriented approach to stroke care. Drawing on insights from Australia, China, South Korea, and the United Kingdom, the articles reflect diverse healthcare contexts and patient populations and are listed below:

1. Lee, J.H. Analysis of Grip Strength Thresholds for Stroke Management and Prevention in South Korean Older Adults. *Healthcare* **2025**, *13*, 781.
2. Carey, L.M.; Cahill, L.S.; Blennerhassett, J.M.; Nilsson, M.; Lannin, N.A.; Thijs, V.; Hillier, S.; Cadilhac, D.A.; Donnan, G.A.; Morris, M.E.; et al. A Network of Sites and Upskilled Therapists to Deliver Best-Practice Stroke Rehabilitation of the Arm: Protocol for a Knowledge Translation Study. *Healthcare* **2023**, *11*, 3080.
3. Marsden, D.L.; Boyle, K.; Birnie, J.; Buzio, A.; Dizon, J.; Dunne, J.; Greensill, S.; Hill, K.; Lever, S.; Minett, F.; et al. Improving Practice for Urinary Continence Care on Adult Acute Medical and Rehabilitation Wards: A Multi-Site, Co-Created Implementation Study. *Healthcare* **2023**, *11*, 1241.
4. Lightbody, C.E.; Patel, K.; Holland, E.-J.; Sutton, C.J.; Brown, C.; Tishkovskaya, S.V.; Bowen, A.; Read, J.; Thomas, S.; Roberts, T.; et al. Accelerating the Delivery of Psychological Therapies After Stroke: A Feasibility Stepped-Wedge Cluster Randomised Controlled Trial. *Healthcare* **2025**, *13*, 824824.

5. Baker, C.; Thomas, S.; Tjokrowijoto, P.; Ryan, B.; Kneebone, I.; Stolwyk, R. Aphasia Depression and Psychological Therapy (ADaPT): Perspectives of People with Post-Stroke Aphasia on Participating in a Modified Cognitive Behavioral Therapy. *Healthcare* **2024**, *12*, 771.
6. Hunter, S.; Vogel, K.; O'Leary, S.; Blennerhassett, J.M. Evaluating Feasibility of a Secondary Stroke Prevention Program. *Healthcare* **2023**, *11*, 2673.
7. Rehman, S.; Barker, S.; Jose, K.; Callisaya, M.; Castley, H.; Schultz, M.G.; Moore, M.N.; Simpson, D.B.; Peterson, G.M.; Gall, S. Co-Designed Cardiac Rehabilitation for the Secondary Prevention of Stroke (CARESS): A Pilot Program Evaluation. *Healthcare* **2024**, *12*, 776.
8. Wang, X.; Jiang, H.; Zhao, Z.; Kevine, N.T.; An, B.; Ping, Z.; Lin, B.; Zhang, Z. Mediation Role of Behavioral Decision-Making Between Self-Efficacy and Self-Management Among Elderly Stroke Survivors in China: Cross-Sectional Study. *Healthcare* **2025**, *13*, 704.
9. Wong, D.; Sanders, L.M.; Beauchamp, A.; Formby, C.; Smith, E.E.; Hansen, C.; McKinley, K.; De Jongh, K.; Borschmann, K. "When the Word Is too Big, It's Just too Hard": Stroke Survivors' Perspectives About Health Literacy and Delivery of Health Information. *Healthcare* **2025**, *13*, 541.
10. Lightbody, C.E.; Gordon, C.; Burton, C.; Davidson, C.; Jenkinson, D.; Patel, A.S.; Petrie, F.J.; Rouncefield-Swales, A.; Sprigg, N.; Stewart, K.; et al. Prepare: Improving End-of-Life Care Practice in Stroke Care: Insights from a National Survey and Semi-Structured Interviews. *Healthcare* **2025**, *13*, 848.

The article by Lee illustrates the use of cross-sectional, national survey data to identify sex-specific thresholds for absolute and relative grip strength as predictors of stroke risk in older Korean adults (article 1). The findings from the study may support the potential use of grip strength as a simple, scalable tool for stroke risk stratification. However, validation in longitudinal cohort studies is needed. The other nine articles cover four main themes: *physical rehabilitation, psychological health, secondary prevention,* and *end-of-life care* for people with stroke. Collectively, these articles underscore a common conclusion that stroke care must encompass long-term functional recovery, quality of life, and overall wellbeing across the remaining lifespan. A summary of the four main themes covered in this Special Issue is provided in the next sections.

1. Physical Rehabilitation

Rehabilitation is the single most effective intervention for improving quality of life after stroke. However, it is estimated that only 30–50% of patients receive guideline-recommended physical rehabilitation, often due to geographic, financial, or staffing constraints [4,5].

The authors of two implementation studies included in this issue provide examples of approaches to improve access to evidence-based rehabilitation after stroke. Carey et al. present their protocol for an innovative, multicentre knowledge translation project to increase access to upper limb rehabilitation by upskilling and credentialing occupational therapists or physiotherapists and using a network model to increase reach across Australia (article 2). Grounded in implementation science theory, their project is designed to ensure therapists know what should be delivered while establishing a model of care to promote consistent adoption in real-world settings. The target population are those with loss of body sensation, which can affect one in two people after stroke [6]. This example illustrates to readers how to design studies to increase the adoption of new, effective models of care and the importance of establishing partnerships with consumers, policy-makers, clinicians, healthcare organisations, and researchers.

In the article by Marsden et al., the focus is on improving the detection and management of urinary incontinence in acute hospitals and in-patient rehabilitation settings (article 3).

Urinary incontinence is a common complication after stroke, affecting more than half of stroke patients within the first month, 38% at one year, and 17% in the long term [7]. The authors of this multi-site, pre–post intervention study aimed to increase the adoption of a co-designed urinary continence care intervention known as SCAMP. Conducted in 15 wards among 12 Australian hospitals, the knowledge translation intervention significantly improved assessment and care planning for patients with incontinence; overall, the odds of receiving assessments and management plans for urinary incontinence increased 4-fold. Given the psychological, physical, and social distress associated with incontinence [7], the study contributes meaningfully to supporting patient dignity and autonomy. The research provides another example of the importance of co-design, whereby project leads and implementation champions (mainly nurses), clinical experts in continence care, and researchers ensured clinical relevance to the settings for adoption. The use of implementation science theory is also exemplified for readers.

Globally, as noted by Feigin et al. and the World Health Organization, rehabilitation must become a 'universal health service' accessible to all, not just those with private insurance or urban access [8,9]. The articles by Carey et al. and Marsden et al. provide foundational models and adaptable implementation frameworks designed for scalability across diverse healthcare systems.

2. Psychological Health

Psychological distress, including depression, anxiety, and emotional dysregulation, affects up to 60% of survivors of stroke, yet it is one of the most under-addressed aspects of post-stroke care [10,11]. In this Special Issue, there are two complementary studies providing insights on novel approaches to addressing psychological problems after stroke.

Lightbody et al. (the ADOPTS trial) conducted a feasibility stepped-wedge randomised controlled trial co-designed to embed psychological support pathways within four English National Health Service (NHS) stroke units (article 4). Their approach included mood screening algorithms, staff training, supervision structures, and integration with an existing programme, NHS Talking Therapies. The intervention was found to improve staff confidence, and the authors were also able to illustrate how psychological care can be systematised and scaled. An important lesson was to allow sufficient time for staff training, since time to release clinical staff for training can be challenging.

Baker et al. conducted qualitative interviews with survivors of stroke who also had aphasia, a communication disorder that can result in being excluded from mental health services (article 5). Their evaluation of ADaPT, a modified Cognitive–Behavioural Therapy programme tailored through visual supports and simplified language, revealed benefits to participants in mood regulation, communication, and self-acceptance. The programme was delivered through both telehealth and in-person modes, allowing for flexibility in delivery and accessibility.

The World Stroke Organization (WSO) and authors such as Ignacio et al. have emphasised that post-stroke depression remains a leading determinant of poor recovery, reintegration, and survival [2,11]. To address this, psychological interventions must be inclusive, proactive, and embedded within early discharge and long-term follow-up care.

3. Secondary Prevention

Globally, over 25% of strokes are recurrent, and nearly 80% of these could be prevented through risk factor modification [1,12]. Recurrent strokes are associated with greater severity and higher mortality rates compared to first-ever stroke events [13]. There is an urgent need to provide support for people after stroke to avoid another event through the use of medications, e.g., to lower blood pressure, and lifestyle behaviour change, such as improving diet and increasing exercise. Patient adherence to lifelong prevention strategies remains a major challenge. For example, 21% of survivors of stroke discontinue their blood pressure-lowering medications within the first year [14]. In this Special Issue, we include two articles with a focus on new programmes to increase support for secondary stroke prevention.

Hunter et al. piloted a 12-week secondary prevention programme combining supervised exercise, education, and telehealth coaching (article 6). Their results, obtained from 37 participants as part of a non-randomised feasibility study, provided evidence of improvements in modifiable risk factors and physical fitness. The intervention was highly acceptable; almost all 'felt safe to exercise' and 'would recommend the programme to others'.

In the second non-randomised feasibility (pilot) trial by Rehman et al., the intervention was based on adapting a cardiac rehabilitation programme available in Australia. The programme was co-designed for survivors of stroke as a community-based model (article 7). The 10 participants improved their functional capacity and reported less fatigue, with strong indications of behavioural engagement. The authors noted various implementation challenges, including the division of care between state and federally funded programmes and services within the Australian context.

Overall, these studies align with the growing global movement towards providing comprehensive, community-delivered secondary prevention. The WSO and the World Heart Federation have each called for an integration of stroke and cardiac prevention models and for using shared infrastructure and health coaches, especially in rural and resource-constrained settings [15,16]. Another essential feature is the need to tailor and individualise programmes to ensure greater success.

An important aspect for adopting and changing behaviour includes a person's self-efficacy and ability to self-manage their condition [17]. In the article by Wang et al., behavioural decision-making was found to mediate the relationship between self-efficacy (the ability to organise and execute action processes to achieve behavioural goals) and self-management (article 8). This research was undertaken with 291 elderly survivors of stroke from Henan Province, China. This suggests that simply providing education to patients after a stroke is not enough. Health professionals must also help patients develop the cognitive and behavioural skills needed to apply knowledge, assess risks, and sustain healthy behaviours that support recovery.

An essential component to support self-efficacy and self-management is understanding levels of health literacy as part of providing health education. In this Special Issue, Wong et al. discuss health literacy among people with stroke to illustrate the need for clinicians to tailor information and not make assumptions about patients' prior knowledge (article 9). Using the Ophelia framework [18], they demonstrated that survivors with low health literacy would be less likely to understand their stroke, follow prevention advice, or feel confident in their care. The authors call for universal precautions in stroke communication and emphasise that every patient needs information tailored to their literacy and cognitive level, which is especially pertinent in multicultural and ageing societies.

4. End-of-Life Care

In many health systems, end-of-life care for stroke is under-resourced, under-researched, and inconsistently implemented. The study by Lightbody et al. offers a rare window into this domain through a UK-wide survey and interviews with multidisciplinary staff (article 10). Their findings are sobering: despite high stroke-related mortality and known prognostic uncertainty, only a minority of stroke units use stroke-specific tools to guide end-of-life decisions. The variability in practice was exacerbated by a lack of training and integration with palliative care services. These challenges reflect global trends. In LMICs, limited access to specialist care and cultural taboos around death further compound the problem. The solution, as Lightbody and colleagues argue, lies in pragmatic changes: stroke-adapted guidance, shared decision-making tools, training for all staff, and stronger integration with supportive care pathways.

Across the ten studies included in this Special Issue, four key principles emerge. First, a lifespan approach recognises stroke as a chronic condition requiring continuous support across physical, communication, sensory, incontinence, and psychological domains. Second, there is a strong focus on real-world implementation, with pragmatic designs such as stepped-wedge trials and co-design methods emphasising feasibility and sustainability. Third, a commitment to equity and inclusion is evident, with tailored interventions for people with aphasia, culturally diverse groups, and rural populations. Finally, the studies highlight the value of interdisciplinary collaboration, with examples such as integrated psychological support, multidisciplinary continence care, and telehealth coaching. Together, these principles underscore a shift toward holistic, patient-centred stroke care.

Summary

Stroke is not solely a medical condition—it is a complex societal challenge. Its impact extends beyond mortality, encompassing lost productivity, increased care needs, and a long-term dependence on health and social systems. The ten studies presented in this Special Issue make it clear that the solutions may be within reach. We now possess the tools, knowledge, and evidence base required to transform stroke care. What remains is a collective will to act—to implement these strategies at scale, to embed them into systems, and to sustain them over time.

As editors of this Special Issue, we commend the authors for their scholarly rigour and for providing research that has clinical relevance and will lead to greater inclusion and accessibility to evidence-based programmes that support long-term wellbeing. The articles in this Special Issue represent a range of research methods, including co-design, use of implementation science theory, and feasibility trials, contributing to the growing need to find solutions that require complex system thinking and evaluation.

Author Contributions: T.T. drafted the manuscript and incorporated feedback. D.A.C. provided overall guidance on the article's structure, drafted parts of the manuscript, and provided critical review. All authors have read and agreed to the published version of the manuscript.

Funding: This research received no external funding.

Acknowledgments: We express our deep appreciation to the contributing authors, reviewers, and the journal editorial team. We extend our gratitude to stroke survivors and their support networks, whose lived experiences provide essential insights that shape and advance the science of neurorehabilitation and recovery. We also sincerely thank Olivia Brancatisano for her support as a co-guest editor for this Special Issue.

Conflicts of Interest: D.A.C. reports grants from Boehringer Ingelheim, Amazon Web Services, Stroke Foundation, and Moleac unrelated to this article. D.A.C. is also a co-author for two papers published in this Special Issue. T.T. declares no conflict of interest.

References

1. Feigin, V.L.; Stark, B.A.; Johnson, C.O.; Roth, G.A.; Bisignano, C.; Abady, G.G.; Abbasifard, M.; Abbasi-Kangevari, M.; Abd-Allah, F.; Abedi, V.; et al. Global, regional, and national burden of stroke and its risk factors, 1990–2019: A systematic analysis for the Global Burden of Disease Study 2019. *Lancet Neurol.* **2021**, *20*, 795–820. [CrossRef] [PubMed]
2. Feigin, V.L.; Brainin, M.; Norrving, B.; Martins, S.; Sacco, R.L.; Hacke, W.; Fisher, M.; Pandian, J.; Lindsay, P. World Stroke Organization (WSO): Global Stroke Fact Sheet 2022. *Int. J. Stroke* **2022**, *17*, 18–29. [CrossRef] [PubMed]
3. Thayabaranathan, T.; Kim, J.; Cadilhac, D.A.; Thrift, A.G.; Donnan, G.A.; Howard, G.; Howard, V.J.; Rothwell, P.M.; Feigin, V.; Norrving, B.; et al. Global stroke statistics 2022. *Int. J. Stroke* **2022**, *17*, 946–956. [CrossRef] [PubMed]

4. Winstein, C.J.; Stein, J.; Arena, R.; Bates, B.; Cherney, L.R.; Cramer, S.C.; Deruyter, F.; Eng, J.J.; Fisher, B.; Harvey, R.L.; et al. Guidelines for Adult Stroke Rehabilitation and Recovery: A Guideline for Healthcare Professionals From the American Heart Association/American Stroke Association. *Stroke* **2016**, *47*, e98–e169. [CrossRef] [PubMed]
5. Cieza, A.; Causey, K.; Kamenov, K.; Hanson, S.W.; Chatterji, S.; Vos, T. Global estimates of the need for rehabilitation based on the Global Burden of Disease study 2019: A systematic analysis for the Global Burden of Disease Study 2019. *Lancet* **2020**, *396*, 2006–2017. [CrossRef] [PubMed]
6. Kessner, S.S.; Schlemm, E.; Cheng, B.; Bingel, U.; Fiehler, J.; Gerloff, C.; Thomalla, G. Somatosensory Deficits After Ischemic Stroke. *Stroke* **2019**, *50*, 1116–1123. [CrossRef] [PubMed]
7. Gordon, C.; Davidson, C.E.; Roffe, C.; Clegg, A.; Booth, J.; Lightbody, C.E.; Harris, C.; Sohani, A.; Watkins, C. Evaluating methods of detecting and determining the type of urinary incontinence in adults after stroke: A systematic review. *Neurourol. Urodyn.* **2024**, *43*, 364–381. [CrossRef] [PubMed]
8. Feigin, V.L.; Vos, T.; Nichols, E.; Owolabi, M.O.; Carroll, W.M.; Dichgans, M.; Deuschl, G.; Parmar, P.; Brainin, M.; Murray, C. The global burden of neurological disorders: Translating evidence into policy. *Lancet Neurol.* **2020**, *19*, 255–265. [CrossRef] [PubMed]
9. World Health Organization. *Rehabilitation in Health Systems*; World Health Organization: Geneva, Switzerland, 2017. Available online: https://www.who.int/publications/i/item/9789241549974 (accessed on 9 May 2025).
10. Khazaal, W.; Taliani, M.; Boutros, C.; Abou-Abbas, L.; Hosseini, H.; Salameh, P.; Sadier, N.S. Psychological Complications at 3 Months Following Stroke: Prevalence and Correlates Among Stroke Survivors in Lebanon. *Front. Psychol.* **2021**, *12*, 663267. [CrossRef] [PubMed]
11. Ignacio, K.H.D.; Muir, R.T.; Diestro, J.D.B.; Singh, N.; Yu, M.H.L.L.; Omari, O.E.; Abdalrahman, R.; Barker-Collo, S.L.; Hackett, M.L.; Dukelow, S.P.; et al. Prevalence of depression and anxiety symptoms after stroke in young adults: A systematic review and meta-analysis. *J. Stroke Cerebrovasc. Dis.* **2024**, *33*, 107732. [CrossRef] [PubMed]
12. Stroke Foundation. *National Stroke Audit—Rehabilitation Services Report 2020*; Stroke Foundation: Melbourne, Australia, 2020. Available online: https://informme.org.au/media/drtlcbvp/rehab_strokeservicesreport_2020.pdf (accessed on 9 May 2025).
13. Appelros, P.; Nydevik, I.; Viitanen, M. Poor Outcome After First-Ever Stroke. *Stroke* **2003**, *34*, 122–126. [CrossRef] [PubMed]
14. Dalli, L.L.; Kim, J.; Thrift, A.G.; Andrew, N.E.; Sanfilippo, F.M.; Lopez, D.; Grimley, R.; Lannin, N.A.; Wong, L.; Lindley, R.I.; et al. Patterns of Use and Discontinuation of Secondary Prevention Medications After Stroke. *Neurology* **2021**, *96*, e30–e41. [CrossRef] [PubMed]
15. World Stroke Organization. *Advocacy Priorities: Driving Sustainable Action for Circulatory Health*; WSO: Geneva, Switzerland, 2021. Available online: https://www.world-stroke.org/assets/downloads/Advocacy_priorities_online.pdf (accessed on 9 May 2025).
16. World Heart Federation. *World Heart Vision 2030: Driving Policy Change*; WHF: Geneva, Switzerland, 2021. Available online: https://world-heart-federation.org/about-whf/ (accessed on 9 May 2025).
17. Lynch, E.A.; Nesbitt, K.; Gulyani, A.; Chan, R.J.; Bidargaddi, N.; Cadilhac, D.; Bonevski, B.; Jones, F.; Allan, L.P.; Godecke, E.; et al. Do self-management interventions improve self-efficacy and health-related quality of life after stroke? A systematic review. *Int. J. Stroke* **2025**, 17474930251340286. [CrossRef] [PubMed]
18. Osborne, R.H.; Elmer, S.; Hawkins, M.; Cheng, C. *The Ophelia Manual. The Optimising Health Literacy and Access (Ophelia) Process to Plan and Implement National Health Literacy Demonstration Projects. Ophelia Framework*; Centre for Global Health and Equity, School of Health Sciences, Swinburne University of Technology: Melbourne, VIC, Australia, 2021. Available online: https://healthliteracydevelopment.com (accessed on 9 May 2025).

healthcare

MDPI

Article

Analysis of Grip Strength Thresholds for Stroke Management and Prevention in South Korean Older Adults

Jong Hyeon Lee

Department of Sport Industry Studies, Yonsei University, Seoul 03722, Republic of Korea; leejh01@yonsei.ac.kr

Abstract: Background/Objectives: Muscle weakness in older adults is associated with cardiovascular disease and all-cause mortality. However, its association with stroke prevalence remains underexplored. This study aimed to analyze the absolute grip strength (AGS) and weight-adjusted relative grip strength (RGS) thresholds for stroke prediction in South Korean older adults and to assess their sex-specific predictive ability. Methods: Data from 5185 older adults (2231 men; 2954 women) from the Korea National Health and Nutrition Examination Survey (KNHNES, 2014–2018) were analyzed using complex sampling methods. Receiver operating characteristic (ROC) curve analysis was performed to determine AGS and RGS thresholds and predictive performance, while multivariate logistic regression was used to adjust for confounders and to assess independent effects. Results: In older men, both the AGS and RGS demonstrated significant predictive ability for stroke, with AUCs of 0.637 and 0.623, respectively. In women, the AGS (AUC: 0.608) and RGS (AUC: 0.615) were predictive; however, only the RGS was significant for stroke management (odds ratio (OR): 3.026; 95% confidence interval (CI), 1.541–5.943). In men, AGS (OR: 3.544, 95% CI, 2.094–5.998) and RGS (OR: 2.585, 95% CI, 1.529–4.369) were significant. The stroke prediction thresholds were AGS 28.55 kg and RGS 0.47 for men and RGS 0.36 for women. Conclusions: The AGS and RGS provide practical indicators for stroke risk prediction based on sex-specific differences, highlighting their potential for public health and clinical applications. Future studies should investigate the stroke type, severity, and additional functional fitness indices.

Keywords: stroke; absolute grip strength; relative grip strength; older adults; KNHNES

1. Introduction

Stroke is a neurological injury caused by the sudden disruption of blood flow to the brain, resulting in symptoms such as muscle weakness, speech and vision impairment, and loss of coordination, emphasizing the need for early diagnosis and prevention [1,2]. Globally, approximately 12.2 million cases of stroke occur annually, and one in four people over the age of 25 years experiences a stroke during their lifetime. Stroke is recognized as a serious public health problem and is the second leading cause of death worldwide [3]. It is also a major cause of death in Korea, with over 600,000 cases occurring annually [4], and the mortality rate within one year after stroke is reported to be 20.1% as of 2022, at 18.5% in men and 22.1% in women [5]. As of 2022, the number of stroke cases in South Korea was reported to be 110,574 (61,988 men and 48,586 women). Also, the prevalence of stroke among Korean older adults is approximately 7.5%, which is more than four times higher than that observed in younger adults [5].

Mobility has been emphasized in rehabilitation sites for recovery from gait disturbances caused by stroke symptoms. However, muscle weakness due to sarcopenia and decreased neuromuscular control ability in older adults leads to reduced physical activity. This decline, combined with changes in blood flow dynamics, impairs venous return, slows the recovery rate during rest, and increases the risk of stroke due to cerebrovascular dysfunction caused by thrombosis [6]. Muscles, as key metabolic organs, can weaken due to muscle loss, disrupting blood sugar and lipid metabolism, and increasing stroke risk. Stroke-induced upper motor neuron damage exacerbates muscle dysfunction, leading to reduced muscle fiber size, motor unit loss, altered recruitment rates, and reduced walking speed and endurance [7]. Therefore, the need for an exercise program that not only improves muscle mass and strength but also complements traditional function-oriented interventions has been emphasized, as evidence suggests that stroke recovery is facilitated by enhancing muscle strength [8]. Therefore, identifying the muscle strength level through one-repetition maximum (1RM) measurement before starting strength training is generally emphasized; however, in the case of neurological damage due to stroke, muscle endurance at the submaximal level is more closely related to functional recovery in daily life than one-time maximal muscle strength [9–12]. Consequently, exercise intensity of an effective muscle strength improvement program is 70% of the maximal muscle strength [13], and 1RM measurement can be dangerous and unnecessary waste in the rehabilitation of stroke patients [8]. Grip strength (GS) is easy to measure, reflects overall muscle strength in older adults, and effectively predicts stroke risk, making it valuable for stroke prevention and rehabilitation [14]. Large-scale cohort studies, such as the China Health and Retirement Longitudinal Study (CHARLS), have demonstrated that changes in GS over time are associated with stroke incidence, reinforcing its role in stroke prevention [15]. Additionally, while the Jamar dynamometer is a standard tool for GS assessment, evidence suggests that electronic dynamometers provide comparable accuracy at a lower cost, making them a practical alternative for large-scale applications [16]. The importance of measurement is further highlighted, as it has been revealed that when GS is weak, essential daily movements such as getting up from a chair, walking, and climbing stairs are critically limited [17,18]. Stronger GS in stroke patients is linked to earlier hospital discharge [19,20] and better daily function, showing high correlations with the Frenchay Arm Test ($r = 0.91$), Motor Club Assessment ($r = 0.86$), and Peg Test ($r = 0.79$). Grip strength training also enhances cognitive function by improving the efficiency of the white matter network in stroke patients [21]. These findings suggest that GS may be an effective method for the prevention and treatment of stroke.

Although GS is most widely associated with all-cause mortality [22–25], several thresholds of GS have been reported to predict diseases, with values of 28 kg for men and 18 kg for women suggested as the criteria for determining sarcopenia in Asians [26]. For diabetes, the threshold is 28.3 kg for men and 23.4 kg for women, regardless of race [14]. Similar figures have been reported for older adults; to safely lift an object weighing more than 10 kg without injury, a grip strength of more than 28.5 kg for men and 18.5 kg for women is required [27].

Thus, the core mechanisms of post-stroke recovery and the effects of muscle strength intervention, as assessed by GS, have been presented [17,28]; however, the muscle strength threshold for early and specific prevention and management of stroke has not been investigated to date. In addition, muscle strength has been suggested to be related to cardiovascular mortality rather than disease prevention; therefore, physical fitness values, including muscle strength, that prevent disease occurrence itself rather than death, should be suggested for early disease prediction to prevent the occurrence of fatal conditions. Therefore, deriving thresholds for both absolute grip strength (AGS) and relative grip strength (RGS) is essential to optimize tailored prevention and rehabilitation programs, accounting for sex differences in physique and muscle strength distribution among older adults. AGS is measured in kilograms using a dynamometer, and relative grip strength, RGS, is calculated by dividing AGS by body weight or body mass index (BMI). RGS is commonly used to minimize the confounding effect of body weight when examining the relationship between grip strength and disease prevalence [29].

While previous studies, such as Liu et al. (2021) [15], have established the link between low GS and increased stroke risk in the Chinese population, our study further distinguishes between AGS and RGS in predicting stroke risk among South Korean older adults. Additionally, we incorporate key metabolic risk factors such as hypertension, dyslipidemia, and diabetes mellitus to strengthen our predictive model. This study aims to identify AGS and RSG thresholds for stroke prevention and management using data from the Korea National Health and Nutrition Examination Survey (KNHNES) [30], a nationally representative dataset of older adults in South Korea, to evaluate the classification performance of AGS and RGS in stroke prediction, explore their clinical applicability, and assess the potential preventive impact of maintaining GS above the identified thresholds. Also, our research considers the longitudinal implications of grip strength changes and their potential interactions with metabolic risk factors, which may further refine stroke prediction models. These findings will provide evidence to guide public health policies that address sex differences in stroke risk and support programs aimed at preventing muscle strength decline in older adults.

2. Materials and Methods

2.1. Data Acquisition and Participants

This study used data from the KNHNES, conducted by the Korea Centers for Disease Control and Prevention. Raw data from 2014 to 2018, with GS data, were used after submitting the plan and purpose of this study and receiving approval. In this study, older adults were defined as those aged 65 years or older, and the age group was set as the subpopulation. In this study, 5185 participants (2231 men and 2954 women) with both stroke and GS indicators were analyzed.

2.2. Research Variables

2.2.1. Stroke Prevalence

In this study, to identify the prevalence of stroke in older adults, a binary variable was reconstructed for participants who had been diagnosed with stroke, currently had stroke, were receiving stroke treatment, or were experiencing stroke–stroke sequelae. If none of the above applied, the participants were classified as having no stroke.

2.2.2. Grip Strength

In this study, GS (kg) data were collected from the KNHNES (2014–2018), with measurements performed thrice for each hand (left and right) using a digital grip dynamometer (TTK 5401, Takei, Japan) following standardized procedures. Participants were instructed to sit upright with their elbows flexed at 90 degrees, their forearms in a neutral position, and their wrists slightly extended (0–30 degrees). They were asked to squeeze the dynamometer with maximum effort for a few seconds without any additional body movement. Trained examiners conducted all assessments to ensure measurement, accuracy, and consistency. Individuals unable to undergo GS measurement due to conditions such as arm, hand, or thumb loss or fracture; hand paralysis; use of a cast or bandage on the hand or wrist; history of wrist surgery or arthritis within the past three months; or recent hand pain, stiffness, or worsening symptoms were excluded from the measurements. The highest value among the six measurements was considered as the AGS. Additionally, the RGS was calculated as the AGS divided by body weight.

2.2.3. Covariates

Age, household income, marital status, and educational level were adjusted to analyze the relationship between GS and stroke in older adults. In addition, health behavioral variables such as alcohol consumption, smoking, obesity, and strength training practice were adjusted. Also, our analysis controlled metabolic conditions such as physician-diagnosed hypertension, dyslipidemia, and diabetes mellitus, as these factors have been previously identified as significant contributors to stroke risk [31]. While heart failure and atrial fibrillation [32] were not included due to dataset limitations, we acknowledge their potential relevance and suggest future research explore their role in grip strength-related stroke prediction. Household income was classified into four quartiles. Education level was reclassified as "elementary school" for Seodang/Chinese schools, no school, and elementary schools; middle school and high school items were used as they were; and for 2/3-year college, 4-year college, and graduate school or higher, a variable item was reclassified as "college or higher". Alcohol consumption was measured using annual drinking frequency data, and variables were constructed with the items "Never drank in the past year", "Once a week or less", "2–3 times a week", and "4 or more times a week". Smoking data were reconstructed as binary variables in which data on current smoking status were surveyed, with items such as currently smoking or occasionally smoking as "smoking", in the past but currently quitting, and never smoking as "non-smoking". Obesity was assessed using body mass index (BMI) data, and pregnant women were excluded from the analysis. BMI classifications were as follows: underweight (less than 18.5 kg/m^2), normal weight (18.5–24.9 kg/m^2), and obese (25 kg/m^2 or higher). Strength training practice was categorized as a binary variable: individuals who did not engage in strength training were classified as "no practice", while those who performed strength training at least once per week were classified as "practice".

2.3. Data Analysis

To determine the AGS and RGS cutoff values for stroke prevention, sex-stratified receiver operating characteristic (ROC) curve analysis was conducted, with the area under the curve (AUC) evaluated under a null hypothesis value of 0.5. The highest Youden index was used to define the cutoff thresholds [33], and the stroke prediction accuracy was assessed using a confusion matrix to calculate sensitivity, specificity, positive predictive value (PPV), negative predictive value (NPV), and accuracy [34]. A complex sample analysis method was used to represent the older South Koreans. Variance estimation strata (kstrata) and cluster variables (psu) were set, and integrated weights were calculated based on the survey sample size for each year (2014: wt_ivex × 7550/39,199; 2015: wt_ivex × 7380/39,199; 2016: wt_ivex × 8150/39,199; 2017: wt_ivex × 8127/39,199; 2018: wt_ivex × 7992/39,199). Participants aged 65 years or older were analyzed as a subpopulation, with sex-specific filters created to minimize bias in population estimation. Data analyses reflected the estimated population size using the finite-population correction method. Descriptive statistics (mean and standard error (SE)) and cross-tabulation were performed to analyze the demographic and GS distributions by sex, with independence tests for categorical variable differences. Stroke risk was analyzed by dividing the participants into weak and strong GS groups based on the thresholds. Adjusted odds ratios (aOR) and 95% confidence intervals (CIs) were derived using a complex sample logistic regression model with four adjustment levels: Model 1 (age, income, and education), Model 2 (Model 1 + alcohol consumption, smoking, hypertension, diabetes, and dyslipidemia), and Model 3 (Model 2 + strength training practice). All analyses were performed using SPSS ver. 27.0, with statistical significance set at $p < 0.05$.

2.4. Ethics Statement

This study utilized KNHNES open-source, anonymized personal data. Since the KNHNES is conducted directly by the state for public welfare in accordance with Article 2, Paragraph 1, of the Bioethics Act and Article 2, Paragraph 2, Subparagraph 1, of the Enforcement Decree of the same Act, it can be conducted without review by the Research Ethics Review Committee. Nevertheless, we disclose that the data for the 6th period, 2014 and 2015, were collected after review (Approval Number: 2013-12EXP-03-5C). In addition, the data for the 7th period (2016, 2017, 2018) were collected without review, according to the opinion of the Research Ethics Review Committee of the Korea Disease Control and Prevention Agency. Informed consent was obtained from all participants at the time of data collection, and all data collection and analysis procedures were conducted in compliance with the research ethics guidelines of the Declaration of Helsinki.

3. Results

3.1. ROC Curve Analysis of Grip Strength for Stroke Management

The results of the ROC curve analysis were used to determine the AGS and RGS thresholds for stroke prevention, and are shown in Table 1. For older men, the AGS had an AUC of 0.637 (95% CI, 0.591–0.684) and an accuracy of 0.74, while the RGS had an AUC of 0.623 (95% CI, 0.574–0.672) and an accuracy of 0.65. For older women, the AGS had an AUC of 0.608 (95% CI, 0.557–0.659) and an accuracy of 0.69, while the RGS had an AUC of 0.615 (95% CI, 0.556–0.664) and an accuracy of 0.49. Detailed results are presented in Table 1.

Table 1. ROC curve analysis of absolute grip strength and relative grip strength for stroke prediction.

		AUC	95% CI	Cut off (kg)	Sensitivity	Specificity	PPV	NPV	Accuracy
Men	AGS	0.637	0.591–0.684	28.55 ***	0.759	0.469	0.12	0.95	0.74
	RGS	0.623	0.574–0.672	0.47 ***	0.658	0.565	0.10	0.95	0.65
Women	AGS	0.608	0.557–0.659	17.25 ***	0.704	0.493	0.08	0.96	0.69
	RGS	0.615	0.556–0.664	0.36 ***	0.481	0.721	0.07	0.97	0.49

AUC: area under ROC curve; CI: confidence interval; PPV: positive predictive value; NPV: negative predictive value; AGS: absolute grip strength; RGS: relative grip strength. *** $p < 0.001$.

3.2. Participant Characteristics

Descriptive statistics for age, AGS, and RGS values of older adults and the distribution according to the calculated GS thresholds are shown in Table 2.

Table 2. Descriptive analysis and frequency distribution of participants' age and grip strength.

Men			Women		
Age (year)	72.33 ± 0.128		Age (year)	73.38 ± 0.116	
AGS (kg)	33.071 ± 0.185		AGS (kg)	19.503 ± 0.134	
RGS (kg)	0.512 ± 0.003		RGS (kg)	0.350 ± 0.002	
	n	B		n	B
AGS < 28.55 kg	550	473,807	AGS < 17.25 kg	824	789,010
AGS ≥ 28.55 kg	1589	1,446,953	AGS ≥ 17.25 kg	1873	1,686,428
RGS < 0.47 kg	764	654,058	RGS < 0.36 kg	1425	1,316,331
RGS ≥ 0.47 kg	1374	1,265,504	RGS ≥ 0.36 kg	1270	1,157,139

AGS: absolute grip strength; RGS: relative grip strength; n: unweighted frequency; B: estimated population size.

The results for the prevalence of stroke and other adjusted variables are shown in Table 3.

Table 3. Participant characteristics by stroke prevalence and adjusted variables.

Variables	Men			Women				
	n	B	%	n	B	%	x^2	p
No stroke	2076	1,863,169	42.0	2804	2,574,921	58.0	9.544	0.008
Stroke	155	143,747	50.9	150	138,518	49.1		
Household income: 1Q	261	243,127	51.0	246	233,971	49.0	80.611	0.000
2Q	374	348,722	48.7	386	366,786	51.3		
3Q	663	590,363	47.1	745	661,834	52.9		
4Q	915	801,723	36.1	1558	1,416,140	66.5		
Married	2212	19,920,213	42.5	2935	2,697,069	57.5	0.374	0.568
Not married	19	14,903	47.7	19	16,369	52.3		
Elementary school	683	595,548	25.8	1872	1,709,850	76.4	654.672	0.000
Middle school	451	402,845	51.7	425	375,786	48.3		
High school	546	479,857	61.6	316	299,020	38.4		
College or higher	406	383,932	71.7	153	151,233	28.3		
No hypertension	1034	934,806	44.9	1218	1,146,452	55.1	9.967	0.008
Hypertension	1182	1,058,571	40.5	1717	1,552,700	59.5		
No dyslipidemia	1686	1,520,699	48.1	1764	1,638,152	51.9	139.587	0.000
Dyslipidemia	529	472,019	30.8	1171	1,061,000	69.2		
No diabetes	1707	1,553,779	42.6	2290	2,095,785	57.4	0.026	0.897
Diabetes	508	438,939	42.3	643	598,528	57.7		
No alcohol consumption	548	478,407	42.9	683	637,452	57.1	415.341	0.000
Once a week or less	763	682,570	44.9	948	836,444	55.1		
2–3 times a week	337	412,395	77.3	91	91,798	22.7		
4 times a week or more	359	336,924	88.7	55	55,529	11.3		
No smoking	1787	1,596,397	38.3	2810	2,570,487	61.7	407.538	0.000
Smoking	400	367,397	86.9	63	55,600	13.1		
Normal weight	1044	930,407	45.9	1189	1,094,519	54.1	4.759	0.168
Underweight	70	64,815	46.7	72	73,994	53.3		
Obese	659	607,614	42.5	910	822,744	57.5		
No strength training	1484	1,311,133	36.4	2503	2,289,759	63.6	305.324	0.000
Strength training practice	604	554,118	68.4	274	256,368	31.6		

n: unweighted frequency; B: estimated population size; %: rates by stroke prevalence; Q: quartile.

The diagnosis rate for stroke tended to be significantly higher in men than in women ($x^2 = 9.544$, $p = 0.008$). In addition, there were significant differences by sex in household income ($x^2 = 80.611$, $p = 0.000$), education level ($x^2 = 654.672$, $p < 0.000$), hypertension ($x^2 = 9.967$, $p = 0.008$), dyslipidemia diagnosis ($x^2 = 129.587$, $p = 0.000$), alcohol consumption ($x^2 = 415.341$, $p < 0.000$), smoking ($x^2 = 407.538$, $p = 0.000$), and strength training practice ($x^2 = 305.324$, $p = 0.000$).

3.3. Difference in Stroke Prevalence by Grip Strength Level

In Model 3, which included all adjusted variables, older men with AGS below the threshold showed a significantly higher stroke prevalence risk (354.4%, 95% CI: 2.094–5.998, $p = 0.000$), and those with RGS below the threshold also showed a significantly higher risk (258.5%; 95% CI 1.529–4.369; $p = 0.000$) compared to those above the threshold. Similarly, for older women, those with RGS below the threshold had a significantly higher stroke prevalence risk (302.6%; 95% CI 1.541–5.943; $p = 0.001$). However, the association between the AGS and stroke prevalence in older women was not statistically significant after adjustment in Model 3. The detailed results are presented in Table 4.

Table 4. Analysis of the relationship between older adults' handgrip strength and stroke prevalence.

Sex	Model		OR	95% CI	*p*
Men	Unadjusted	AGS (kg)	3.642 ***	2.471–5.367	0.000
		RGS (kg)	2.624 ***	1.770–3.889	0.000
Women		AGS (kg)	1.831 **	1.202–2.790	0.005
		RGS (kg)	2.336 ***	1.478–3.693	0.000
Men	Model 1	AGS (kg)	3.431 ***	2.168–5.428	0.000
		RGS (kg)	2.241 ***	1.461–3.436	0.000
Women		AGS (kg)	1.767 *	1.139–2.740	0.011
		RGS (kg)	2.497 ***	1.523–4.092	0.000
Men	Model 2	AGS (kg)	3.600 ***	2.121–6.112	0.000
		RGS (kg)	2.627 ***	1.556–4.436	0.000
Women		AGS (kg)	1.972	0.926–4.197	0.078
		RGS (kg)	3.104 **	1.569–6.140	0.001
Men	Model 3	AGS (kg)	3.544 ***	2.094–5.998	0.000
		RGS (kg)	2.585 ***	1.529–4.369	0.000
Women		AGS (kg)	1.899	0.890–4.055	0.097
		RGS (kg)	3.026 **	1.541–5.943	0.001

OR, odds ratio; CI, confidence interval; Model 1: adjusted for age, household income, marital status, and educational level; Model 2: Model 1 + alcohol consumption, smoking, diagnosed hypertension, diabetes, and dyslipidemia; Model 3: Model 2 + strength training practice; AGS, absolute grip strength; RGS, relative grip strength * $p < 0.05$; ** $p < 0.01$; *** $p < 0.001$.

4. Discussion

This study is the first to present the AGS and RGS thresholds for stroke prediction in older adults in South Korea, using large-scale open-source data, with sex-specific differentiation. By analyzing the KNHANES data, we identified grip strength thresholds for stroke risk and offer a reference for strength-training goals in stroke prevention and management.

The AUC of the older adults' GS threshold derived in this study was 0.608–0.637, which is generally considered fair, and is similar to those previously reported for cardiovascular disease and mortality (AUC: 0.65–0.75) [35], metabolic syndrome (AUC: 0.65–0.71) [36], frailty (AUC: 0.6–0.7) [14], and all-cause mortality (AUC: 0.66–0.72) [35]. However, these studies generally considered multiple diseases in an integrated manner and were not predictive studies for any single specific disease. Stroke is a major cause of death worldwide, with fatal sequelae, and is a serious public health concern, especially in older age groups [37]. Therefore, the classification performance evaluation results of this study are significant for clinical evaluation and establishment of prevention strategies for stroke risk and its clinical significance. In addition, compared to Liu et al. (2021) [15], who reported an HR of 1.89

for weak GS in predicting stroke, our study found similar trends, though our AUC values indicate only fair discrimination. While AGS and RGS provide additional insights into stroke risk, their predictive performance should be interpreted in the context of established stroke risk models such as the Framingham Stroke Risk Score [38]. Combining grip strength with these models may enhance their predictive accuracy and clinical applicability.

Among the derived GS thresholds, the AGS for men was 28.55 kg and for women was 17.2 kg, which is similar to the AGS thresholds for cardiovascular and metabolic diseases for men (26–30 kg) and for women (16–20 kg) [35], and the thresholds for all-cause mortality of 26–28 kg for men and 15–18 kg for women [39]. In particular, RGS assessment is needed to supplement the risk that is difficult to capture with the AGS alone in older adults with high body weight. The threshold related to cardiovascular disease and all-cause mortality was 0.45–0.55 for men and 0.35–0.45 for women [35], and the Asian Working Group for Sarcopenia (AWGS) suggested a threshold of 0.40 for men and 0.30 for women in the diagnosis of sarcopenia [26]. This study suggests that the management of RGS may be more essential for managing stroke, as higher values of 0.47 for men and 0.36 for women were presented.

The sensitivity of AGS for men was 75.9%, demonstrating a strong performance in identifying stroke patients, whereas the RGS exhibited higher specificity (56.5%) than the AGS, indicating its usefulness in identifying individuals without stroke risk. Among older women, the AGS sensitivity was 70.4% and the RGS specificity was higher at 72.1%, suggesting better predictive accuracy for the AGS in identifying stroke risk. Although the PPV for all GS measures was below 12%, limiting their accuracy in predicting actual stroke cases, the NPV exceeded 95%, indicating a high predictive performance for the non-occurrence of strokes. This suggests that grip strength testing could serve as a key determinant in identifying individuals at low stroke risk, potentially reducing the need for additional assessments. Therefore, the AGS is considered a suitable early screening tool for stroke because of its high sensitivity and overall accuracy, whereas the RGS, with its relatively high specificity, serves as a complementary measure. Therefore, evaluating both the AGS and RGS is recommended to enhance the prediction of stroke risk in older adults.

In addition, this study attempted to increase the explanatory power of the results by adding the results of the multivariate logistic regression analysis adjusted for sociodemographic factors, health behaviors, comorbidities, and strength training practice to the results of the ROC curve analysis. The analysis results showed that the AGS in men had a relatively superior predictive performance to the RGS, with a higher AUC, and its OR was also higher than that of the RGS (3.544 vs. 2.585). This suggests that although RGS is important in stroke management, AGS is a relatively more powerful variable and was statistically significant in the fully adjusted Model 3. In contrast, in women, RSG showed a higher predictive performance relative to body weight. In Model 3, AGS did not statistically significantly predict stroke, whereas RGS was identified as a significant variable, revealing the possibility that assessing muscle strength relative to body weight may be more useful for predicting stroke in older women. These results suggest that GS weakness evaluated in a multivariate model should be utilized as a useful risk factor, although it does not have high predictive performance as a single variable for stroke prediction. However, the wide confidence intervals observed for RGS suggest potential heterogeneity within our dataset, which may be influenced by variations in muscle mass distribution, lifestyle factors, and unmeasured confounders. Future studies should aim to include larger sample sizes and more diverse populations to enhance the robustness of grip strength-based stroke prediction models.

This study highlights the need to consider sex-specific utilization of grip strength indicators in older adults. Among older men, higher muscle mass relative to body weight supports the predictive utility of both the AGS and RGS for stroke risk, with the AGS showing a stronger predictive power. This may be attributed to the closer association between absolute muscle mass and the risks of stroke, cardiovascular diseases, and all-cause mortality in men; therefore, weakened muscle contraction and relaxation due to sarcopenia may exacerbate endothelial dysfunction, increase vascular inflammation and stress, and impair peripheral circulation, particularly in the brain, making older men more vulnerable to these mechanisms [40–43]. In contrast, older women generally exhibit lower muscle mass and higher body fat, with RGS identified as a significant predictor of chronic conditions such as diabetes and stroke [44–46]. This study also found that RGS was a relevant variable for predicting stroke in older women. Notably, the rate of strength training participation among older women was significantly lower than that among men, suggesting a greater reliance on aerobic activities such as walking rather than high-intensity or resistance exercises [47]. To improve stroke prevention in women, interventions should focus on increasing lean mass through strength training, while avoiding excessive restrictions on carbohydrates and proteins that may impair muscle maintenance. As maximal strength gains from resistance training show no sex differences [48], future research should explore social factors, body image perceptions, and attitudes toward exercise that influence strength training participation to inform public health policies.

A rapid decrease in vascular elasticity is one of the representative mechanisms of aging, which causes poor blood flow to the brain, and the resulting decrease in functional physical strength leads to a rapid decrease in muscle strength, thus increasing the risk of stroke [49]. Therefore, regular strength training can be a preventive measure, because it lowers systemic inflammation and improves blood circulation [50]. Lower extremity strength plays a major role in improving cerebral blood flow and maintaining peripheral vascular function. Because the vicious cycle of sarcopenia resulting from stroke is likely to be repeated [50,51], the importance of maintaining muscle strength and checking GS is further emphasized [52]. Therefore, evaluating the effectiveness of a strength improvement program by considering the AGS and RGS thresholds of older men and the RGS of older women may be useful in stroke prevention. However, while GS is a valuable biomarker for stroke risk, it should be considered in conjunction with metabolic conditions such as hypertension, dyslipidemia, and diabetes mellitus. Its role as a functional indicator complements traditional cardiovascular risk assessments and may enhance risk stratification in clinical and public health settings.

This study had several limitations. First, because of its cross-sectional design using large open-source data, causality between grip strength and stroke could not be established. Our study does not account for longitudinal changes in grip strength, which may play a crucial role in stroke risk prediction. Future research should incorporate longitudinal data to evaluate how changes in grip strength over time influence stroke incidence and severity. Additionally, it did not differentiate between ischemic stroke-induced hemiparesis, which can cause severe asymmetry in grip strength, and hemorrhagic stroke and its functional deficits [53,54]. This relationship may vary according to stroke phase, and future studies should explore nonlinear associations. Also, future research should differentiate between ischemic and hemorrhagic stroke subtypes, as these conditions may have distinct pathophysiological mechanisms that influence the role of muscle strength in stroke risk. Second, the low positive predictive value of the AGS and RGS stroke prediction cut-offs warrants caution in their interpretation. For better stroke management and identification, specialized stroke diagnostic tools such as the Cincinnati prehospital stroke scale (CPSS) [55] and LA Prehospital Stroke Scale [56] may be used. Third, this study did not include other muscle-strength-related measures. Although GS is a common proxy, future research should consider functional fitness measures such as calf circumference, and the strength, assistance with walking, rising from a chair, climbing stairs, and falls (SARC-F) questionnaire to identify sarcopenia-related patient outcomes [57]; adding these tests' thresholds and their association with stroke risk could further enhance predictive accuracy. Fourth, handedness and inter-hand strength differences were not specifically analyzed in this study. Since the highest GS value among both hands was used as AGS, potential effects of hand dominance and stroke-induced asymmetry were not accounted for. However, a previous study [15] has also adopted the approach of selecting the highest value from the dominant hand only, whereas our study followed the Hong et al. (2021) [58] method, which considers the maximum value among six trials from both hands to ensure a more comprehensive assessment of grip strength. Future studies should investigate how handedness and stroke laterality influence GS-based stroke risk prediction. In addition, future studies could apply propensity score matching to address the imbalance between patients with stroke and controls. Although this study aimed to provide a practical and intuitive indicator for stroke risk prediction based on GS thresholds, without additional statistical adjustments, its significance remains unclear. Finally, the data were limited to South Korea; therefore, applying the findings to the global older adult populations may be challenging. Future cross-national and racial comparative studies are required.

5. Conclusions

The significant cut-off values for stroke risk management in older adults in South Korea were determined as an AGS of 28.55 kg and RGS of 0.47 for men, and an RGS of 0.36 for women. Based on these thresholds, a multivariate model adjusted for demographic variables, comorbidities, health behaviors, and strength training showed significant prediction of stroke risk, excluding AGS in women. However, because of the relatively low AUC and PPV, these grip strength thresholds should be used primarily as tools for early prevention rather than for definitive stroke diagnosis in community health centers, hospitals, and nursing facilities. Regular measurement of both AGS and RGS can help identify high-risk older adults with values below the threshold, allowing for early intervention and preventive measures. Future studies should explore the integration of GS into established stroke risk models and investigate its predictive utility in different population subgroups. Additionally, examining the interaction between grip strength and other functional fitness measures may provide a more comprehensive understanding of its role in stroke prevention and management.

This study confirmed that AGS in older men and RGS in older women are more strongly associated with stroke risk. To maximize stroke prevention, older men should focus on strength-building exercises, while women should benefit from weight management, and strength training, within a comprehensive program.

Funding: This work was supported by the Yonsei University Research Fund (Post Doc. Researcher Supporting Program) of 2025 (project no.: 2025-12-0043) and the National Research Foundation of Korea (NRF) grant funded by the Korean government for the Global Humanities and Social Sciences Convergence Research Program (project no.: 2025-11-0087, title: Development and Evaluation of a Korean Evidence-Based Salutogenic Intervention Program for Cancer Survivors).

Institutional Review Board Statement: This study utilized anonymized KNHNES data and was exempt from Research Ethics Review Committee approval as per the Bioethics Act. Data for the sixth period (2014–2015) were approved (Approval Number: 2013-12EXP-03-5C), whereas data for the seventh period (2016–2018) were collected without review based on the committee's guidance. All the procedures adhered to the principles of the Declaration of Helsinki.

Informed Consent Statement: Informed consent was obtained from all participants at the time of data collection by the Korea Disease Control and Prevention Agency.

Data Availability Statement: The data supporting the findings of this study are available from the Korea National Health and Nutrition Examination Survey (KNHNES). For further details, please contact the corresponding author.

Acknowledgments: The authors would like to express their gratitude to the professors, clinicians, and researchers from Yonsei University who provided invaluable guidance and support for the epidemiological study of grip strength and stroke.

Conflicts of Interest: The author declares no conflicts of interest.

Abbreviations

The following abbreviations are used in this manuscript:

1RM	One repetition maximum
GS	Grip strength
AGS	Absolute grip strength
RGS	Relative grip strength
ROC	Receiver operating characteristics
AUC	Area under the curve
OR	Odd ratio
CI	Confidence interval
CPSS	Cincinnati Pre-hospital Stroke Scale

References

1. Barthels, D.; Das, H. Current advances in ischemic stroke research and therapies. *Biochim. Biophys. Acta Mol. Basis Dis.* **2020**, *1866*, 165260. [CrossRef] [PubMed]
2. Potter, T.B.H.; Tannous, J.; Vahidy, F.S. A contemporary review of epidemiology, risk factors, etiology, and outcomes of premature stroke. *Curr. Atheroscler. Rep.* **2022**, *24*, 939–948. [CrossRef] [PubMed]
3. GBD 2019 Stroke Collaborators. Global, regional, and national burden of stroke and its risk factors, 1990–2019: A systematic analysis for the Global Burden of Disease Study 2019. *Lancet Neurol.* **2021**, *20*, 795–820. [CrossRef]
4. Health Insurance Review and Assessment Service. National Disease Statistics of Public Interest. Available online: https://www.hira.or.kr/bbsDummy.do?brdBltNo=10980&brdScnBltNo=4&pageIndex=1&pageIndex2=1&pgmid=HIRAA020041000100 (accessed on 19 November 2024).
5. Korea Disease Control and Prevention Agency. Trends in Myocardial Infarction and Stroke Incidence and Fatality Rates; p. v. Available online: https://www.kdca.go.kr/board/board.es?act=view&bid=0015&list_no=726797&mid=a20501010000&utm (accessed on 21 November 2024).
6. Chen, L.-K.; Liu, L.-K.; Woo, J.; Assantachai, P.; Auyeung, T.-W.; Bahyah, K.S.; Chou, M.-Y.; Chen, L.-Y.; Hsu, P.-S.; Krairit, O.; et al. Sarcopenia in Asia: Consensus report of the Asian Working Group for Sarcopenia. *J. Am. Med. Dir. Assoc.* **2014**, *15*, 95–101. [CrossRef]
7. Oh, T.Y. A study on strengthening exercise for stroke patients through comparison of literature between domestic and foreign. *J. Korean Soc. Integr. Med.* **2019**, *7*, 113–124.
8. Choi, A.-Y.; Lim, J.-H.; Kim, B.-G. Effects of muscle strength exercise on muscle mass and muscle strength in patients with stroke: A systematic review and meta-analysis. *J. Exerc. Rehabil.* **2024**, *20*, 146–157. [CrossRef]
9. McNeil, C.J.; Rice, C.L. Fatigability is increased with age during velocity-dependent contractions of the dorsiflexors. *J. Gerontol. A Biol. Sci. Med. Sci.* **2007**, *62*, 624–629. [CrossRef]
10. Reuben, D.B.; Magasi, S.; McCreath, H.E.; Bohannon, R.W.; Wang, Y.-C.; Bubela, D.J.; Rymer, W.Z.; Beaumont, J.; Rine, R.M.; Lai, J.-S.; et al. Motor assessment using the NIH Toolbox. *Neurology* **2013**, *80* (Suppl. S3), S65–S75. [CrossRef]
11. Billinger, S.A.; Arena, R.; Bernhardt, J.; Eng, J.J.; Franklin, B.A.; Johnson, C.M.; MacKay-Lyons, M.; Macko, R.F.; Mead, G.E.; Roth, E.J.; et al. Physical activity and exercise recommendations for stroke survivors: A statement for healthcare professionals from the American Heart Association/American Stroke Association. *Stroke* **2014**, *45*, 2532–2553. [CrossRef]
12. Wist, S.; Clivaz, J.; Sattelmayer, M. Muscle strengthening for hemiparesis after stroke: A meta-analysis. *Ann. Phys. Rehabil. Med.* **2016**, *59*, 114–124. [CrossRef]
13. Kraemer, W.J.; Ratamess, N.A. Fundamentals of resistance training: Progression and exercise prescription. *Med. Sci. Sports Exerc.* **2004**, *36*, 674–688. [CrossRef] [PubMed]

14. Bohannon, R.W. Grip strength: An indispensable biomarker for older adults. *Clin. Interv. Aging* **2019**, *14*, 1681–1691. [CrossRef] [PubMed]
15. Liu, G.; Xue, Y.; Wang, S.; Zhang, Y.; Geng, Q. Association between hand grip strength and stroke in China: A prospective cohort study. *Aging* **2021**, *13*, 8204–8213. [CrossRef]
16. Massy-Westropp, N.; Rankin, W.; Ahern, M.; Krishnan, J.; Hearn, T.C. Measuring grip strength in normal adults: Reference ranges and a comparison of electronic and hydraulic instruments. *J Hand Surg Am.* **2004**, *29*, 514–519. [CrossRef]
17. Sunderland, A.; Tinson, D.; Bradley, L.; Hewer, R.L. Arm function after stroke. An evaluation of grip strength as a measure of recovery and a prognostic indicator. *J. Neurol. Neurosurg. Psychiatry* **1989**, *52*, 1267–1272. [CrossRef]
18. Forrest, K.Y.Z.; Williams, A.M.; Leeds, M.J.; Robare, J.F.; Bechard, T.J. Patterns and correlates of grip strength in older Americans. *Curr. Aging Sci.* **2018**, *11*, 63–70. [CrossRef]
19. Savino, E.; Sioulis, F.; Guerra, G.; Cavalieri, M.; Zuliani, G.; Guralnik, J.M.; Volpato, S. Potential prognostic value of handgrip strength in older hospitalized patients. *J. Frailty Aging* **2012**, *1*, 32–38. [CrossRef]
20. McAniff, C.M.; Bohannon, R.W. Validity of grip strength dynamometry in acute rehabilitation. *J. Phys. Ther. Sci.* **2002**, *14*, 41–46. [CrossRef]
21. Shang, X.; Meng, X.; Xiao, X.; Xie, Z.; Yuan, X. Grip training improves handgrip strength, cognition, and brain white matter in minor acute ischemic stroke patients. *Clin. Neurol. Neurosurg.* **2021**, *209*, 106886. [CrossRef]
22. Milne, J.S.; Maule, M.M. A longitudinal study of handgrip and dementia in older people. *Age Ageing* **1984**, *13*, 42–48. [CrossRef]
23. Rijk, J.M.; Roos, P.R.; Deckx, L.; van den Akker, M.; Buntinx, F. Prognostic value of handgrip strength in people aged 60 years and older: A systematic review and meta-analysis. *Geriatr. Gerontol. Int.* **2016**, *16*, 5–20. [CrossRef] [PubMed]
24. Wu, Y.; Wang, W.; Liu, T.; Zhang, D. Association of grip strength with risk of all-cause mortality, cardiovascular diseases, and cancer in community-dwelling populations: A meta-analysis of prospective cohort studies. *J. Am. Med. Dir. Assoc.* **2017**, *18*, 551.e17–551.e35. [CrossRef] [PubMed]
25. García-Hermoso, A.; Cavero-Redondo, I.; Ramírez-Vélez, R.; Ruiz, J.R.; Ortega, F.B.; Lee, D.-C.; Martínez-Vizcaíno, V. Muscular strength as a predictor of all-cause mortality in an apparently healthy population: A systematic review and meta-analysis of data from approximately 2 million men and women. *Arch. Phys. Med. Rehabil.* **2018**, *99*, 2100–2113.e5. [CrossRef] [PubMed]
26. Chen, L.-K.; Woo, J.; Assantachai, P.; Auyeung, T.-W.; Chou, M.-Y.; Iijima, K.; Jang, H.C.; Kang, L.; Kim, M.; Kim, S.; et al. Asian Working Group for Sarcopenia: 2019 consensus update on sarcopenia diagnosis and treatment. *J. Am. Med. Dir. Assoc.* **2020**, *21*, 300–307.e2. [CrossRef]
27. Wang, C.-Y.; Chen, L.-Y. Grip strength in older adults: Test-retest reliability and cutoff for subjective weakness of using the hands in heavy tasks. *Arch. Phys. Med. Rehabil.* **2010**, *91*, 1747–1751. [CrossRef]
28. Lindberg, P.G.; Roche, N.; Robertson, J.; Roby-Brami, A.; Bussel, B.; Maier, M.A. Affected and unaffected quantitative aspects of grip force control in hemiparetic patients after stroke. *Brain Res.* **2012**, *1452*, 96–107. [CrossRef]
29. Park, I.B.; Baik, S.H. Epidemiologic characteristics of diabetes mellitus in Korea: Current status of diabetic patients using Korean health insurance database. *Korean Diabetes J.* **2009**, *33*, 357–362. [CrossRef]
30. The Korea National Health and Nutrition Examination Survey. Available online: https://knhanes.kdca.go.kr/knhanes/main.do (accessed on 11 November 2024).
31. Alloubani, A.; Saleh, A.; Abdelhafiz, I. Hypertension and diabetes mellitus as a predictive risk factors for stroke. *Diabetes Metab. Syndr.* **2018**, *12*, 577–584. [CrossRef]
32. Kroshian, G.; Joseph, J.; Kinlay, S.; Peralta, A.O.; Hoffmeister, P.S.; Singh, J.P.; Yuyun, M.F. Atrial fibrillation and risk of adverse outcomes in heart failure with reduced, mildly reduced, and preserved ejection fraction: A systematic review and meta-analysis. *J. Cardiovasc. Electrophysiol.* **2024**, *35*, 715–726. [CrossRef]
33. Biggerstaff, B.J. Comparing diagnostic tests: A simple graphic using likelihood ratios. *Stat. Med.* **2000**, *19*, 649–663. [CrossRef]
34. Baik, I. Optimal cutoff points of waist circumference for the criteria of abdominal obesity: Comparison with the criteria of the International Diabetes Federation. *Circ. J.* **2009**, *73*, 2068–2075. [CrossRef] [PubMed]
35. Leong, D.P.; Teo, K.K.; Rangarajan, S.; Lopez-Jaramillo, P.; Avezum, A.; Orlandini, A.; Seron, P.; Ahmed, S.H.; Rosengren, A.; Kelishadi, R.; et al. Prognostic value of grip strength: Findings from the Prospective Urban Rural Epidemiology (PURE) study. *Lancet* **2015**, *386*, 266–273. [CrossRef] [PubMed]
36. Wu, H.; Liu, M.; Chi, V.T.Q.; Wang, J.; Zhang, Q.; Liu, L.; Meng, G.; Yao, Z.; Bao, X.; Gu, Y.; et al. Handgrip strength is inversely associated with metabolic syndrome and its separate components in middle aged and older adults: A large-scale population-based study. *Metabolism* **2019**, *93*, 61–67. [CrossRef]
37. World Health Organization. Stroke, Cerebrovascular Accident. Available online: https://www.emro.who.int/health-topics/stroke-cerebrovascular-accident/index.html (accessed on 20 January 2025).
38. Wolf, P.A. Stroke risk profiles. *Stroke* **2009**, *40* (Suppl. S1), S73–S74. [CrossRef]

39. Celis-Morales, C.A.; Welsh, P.; Lyall, D.M.; Steell, L.; Petermann, F.; Anderson, J.; Iliodromiti, S.; Sillars, A.; Graham, N.; Mackay, D.F.; et al. Associations of grip strength with cardiovascular, respiratory, and cancer outcomes and all cause mortality: Prospective cohort study of half a million UK Biobank participants. *BMJ* **2018**, *361*, k1651. [CrossRef]
40. Bohannon, R.W. Hand-grip dynamometry predicts future outcomes in aging adults. *J. Geriatr. Phys. Ther.* **2008**, *31*, 3–10. [CrossRef]
41. Rantanen, T.; Volpato, S.; Ferrucci, L.; Heikkinen, E.; Fried, L.P.; Guralnik, J.M. Handgrip strength and cause-specific and total mortality in older disabled women: Exploring the mechanism. *J. Am. Geriatr. Soc.* **2003**, *51*, 636–641. [CrossRef]
42. Silventoinen, K.; Magnusson, P.K.E.; Tynelius, P.; Batty, G.D.; Rasmussen, F. Association of body size and muscle strength with incidence of coronary heart disease and cerebrovascular diseases: A population-based cohort study of one million Swedish men. *Int. J. Epidemiol.* **2009**, *38*, 110–118. [CrossRef]
43. Strand, B.H.; Cooper, R.; Bergland, A.; Jørgensen, L.; Schirmer, H.; Skirbekk, V.; Emaus, N. The association of grip strength from midlife onwards with all-cause and cause-specific mortality over 17 years of follow-up in the Tromsø Study. *J. Epidemiol. Community Health* **2016**, *70*, 1214–1221. [CrossRef]
44. Yoon, E.S.; Park, S.H. Associations between relative handgrip strength and incidence of type 2 diabetes mellitus in middle-aged and older adults: Finding from the Korean genome and epidemiology study. *Exerc. Sci.* **2020**, *29*, 377–384. [CrossRef]
45. Kim, G.H.; Song, B.K.; Kim, J.W.; Lefferts, E.C.; Brellenthin, A.G.; Lee, D.-C.; Kim, Y.-M.; Kim, M.K.; Choi, B.Y.; Kim, Y.S. Associations between relative grip strength and type 2 diabetes mellitus: The Yangpyeong cohort of the Korean genome and epidemiology study. *PLoS ONE* **2021**, *16*, e0256550. [CrossRef]
46. Lee, J.H.; Kim, B.H. Relationship between grip strength and diagnosis of chronic diseases and mental health in people aged 60 years of older: Analysis of Korean national health and nutrition examination survey. *Korean J. Sport* **2024**, *22*, 339–362. [CrossRef]
47. Lim, H.J.; Kim, E.J. Trends of Physical Activity Among Korean Adults Using Complex Samples Analysis: Based on the 2014 KNHANES. *Korean J. Meas. Eval. Phys. Educ. Sport Sci.* **2018**, *20*, 1–14. [CrossRef]
48. Kittilsen, H.T.; Goleva-Fjellet, S.; Freberg, B.I.; Nicolaisen, I.; Støa, E.M.; Bratland-Sanda, S.; Helgerud, J.; Wang, E.; Sæbø, M.; Støren, Ø. Responses to maximal strength training in different age and gender groups. *Front. Physiol.* **2021**, *12*, 636972. [CrossRef]
49. Ransom, K.V.; Traylor, M.K.; Batman, G.B.; Mulekar, M.S.; Hill, B.D.; Nelson, A.R.; Keller, J.L. Arterial stiffness mediates the association between age and processing speed at low levels of microvascular function in humans across the adult lifespan. *Am. J. Physiol. Heart Circ. Physiol.* **2024**, *326*, H346–H356. [CrossRef]
50. Beyer, S.E.; Sanghvi, M.M.; Aung, N.; Hosking, A.; Cooper, J.A.; Paiva, J.M.; Lee, A.M.; Fung, K.; Lukaschuk, E.; Carapella, V.; et al. Prospective association between handgrip strength and cardiac structure and function in UK adults. *PLoS ONE* **2018**, *13*, e0193124. [CrossRef]
51. Farrell, S.W.; Leonard, D.; Li, Q.; Barlow, C.E.; Shuval, K.; Berry, J.D.; Pavlovic, A.; DeFina, L.F. Association between baseline levels of muscular strength and risk of stroke in later life: The Cooper Center Longitudinal Study. *J. Sport Health Sci.* **2024**, *13*, 642–649. [CrossRef]
52. Reeve, E.H.; Barnes, J.N.; Moir, M.E.; Walker, A.E. Impact of arterial stiffness on cerebrovascular function: A review of evidence from humans and preclinical models. *Am. J. Physiol. Heart Circ. Physiol.* **2024**, *326*, H689–H704. [CrossRef]
53. Perna, R.; Temple, J. Rehabilitation outcomes: Ischemic versus hemorrhagic strokes. *Behav. Neurol.* **2015**, *2015*, 891651. [CrossRef]
54. Feng, T.; Zhao, C.; Dong, J.; Xue, Z.; Cai, F.; Li, X.; Hu, Z.; Xue, X. The effect of unaffected side resistance training on upper limb function reconstruction and prevention of sarcopenia in stroke patients: A randomized controlled trial. *Sci. Rep.* **2024**, *14*, 25330. [CrossRef]
55. Kothari, R.U.; Pancioli, A.; Liu, T.; Brott, T.; Broderick, J. Cincinnati prehospital stroke scale: Reproducibility and validity. *Ann. Emerg. Med.* **1999**, *33*, 373–378. [CrossRef] [PubMed]
56. Kidwell, C.S.; Starkman, S.; Eckstein, M.; Weems, K.W.J.L.; Saver, J.L. Identifying stroke in the field. Prospective validation of the Los Angeles prehospital stroke screen (LAPSS). *Stroke* **2000**, *31*, 71–76. [CrossRef] [PubMed]
57. Malmstrom, T.K.; Morley, J.E. SARC-F: A simple questionnaire to rapidly diagnose sarcopenia. *J. Am. Med. Dir. Assoc.* **2013**, *14*, 531–532. [CrossRef] [PubMed]
58. Hong, S.-H.; Byeon, J.-Y.; Min, J.-H.; Park, D.-H.; Cho, W.-H.; Jeon, J.Y. Relationship Between Handgrip Strength and the Prevalence of Diabetes Mellitus Among Korean Adults: Korean National Health and Nutrition Examination Survey, 2014–2018. *Exerc. Sci.* **2021**, *30*, 110–121. [CrossRef]

healthcare MDPI

Protocol

A Network of Sites and Upskilled Therapists to Deliver Best-Practice Stroke Rehabilitation of the Arm: Protocol for a Knowledge Translation Study

Leeanne M. Carey [1,2,*], Liana S. Cahill [1,3], Jannette M. Blennerhassett [2,4], Michael Nilsson [5,6], Natasha A. Lannin [1,7], Vincent Thijs [2,4,8], Susan Hillier [9], Dominique A. Cadilhac [2,10], Geoffrey A. Donnan [8,11], Meg E. Morris [12,13], Leonid Churilov [8], Marion Walker [14], Shanthi Ramanathan [5,15], Michael Pollack [6,16], Esther May [17], Geoffrey C. Cloud [7,18], Sharon McGowan [19], Tissa Wijeratne [20,21], Marc Budge [10,22], Fiona McKinnon [23], John Olver [24], Toni Hogg [25], Michael Murray [4], Brendon Haslam [1,2], Irene Koukoulas [1,2], Brittni Nielsen [1,26], Yvonne Mak-Yuen [1,2,23], Megan Turville [1,2], Cheryl Neilson [1], Anna Butler [1,2], Joosup Kim [2,10] and Thomas A. Matyas [1,2]

1 Occupational Therapy, School of Allied Health Human Services and Sport, La Trobe University, Melbourne, VIC 3086, Australia; liana.cahill@acu.edu.au (L.S.C.); natasha.lannin@monash.edu (N.A.L.); b.haslam@latrobe.edu.au (B.H.); i.koukoulas@latrobe.edu.au (I.K.); b.nielsen@cgmc.org.au (B.N.); y.mak-yuen@latrobe.edu.au (Y.M.-Y.); m.turville@latrobe.edu.au (M.T.); c.neilson@latrobe.edu.au (C.N.); anna.butler@latrobe.edu.au (A.B.); t.matyas@latrobe.edu.au (T.A.M.)
2 Austin Campus, Florey Institute of Neuroscience and Mental Health, Heidelberg, VIC 3084, Australia; jannette.blennerhassett@austin.org.au (J.M.B.); vincent.thijs@florey.edu.au (V.T.); dominique.cadilhac@monash.edu (D.A.C.); joosup.kim@monash.edu (J.K.)
3 School of Allied Health (Melbourne Campus), Australian Catholic University, Fitzroy, VIC 3065, Australia
4 Austin Health, Heidelberg, VIC 3084, Australia; michael.murray@austin.org.au
5 College of Health, Medicine and Wellbeing, The University of Newcastle, Callaghan, NSW 2308, Australia; michael.nilsson@newcastle.edu.au (M.N.); shanthi.ramanathan@hmri.org.au (S.R.)
6 Centre for Rehab Innovations, The University of Newcastle, Callaghan, NSW 2308, Australia; michael.pollack@health.nsw.gov.au
7 Department of Neuroscience, Central Clinical School, Faculty of Medicine, Nursing and Health Sciences, Monash University, Melbourne, VIC 3800, Australia; g.cloud@alfred.org.au
8 Faculty of Medicine Dentistry and Health Sciences, The University of Melbourne, Melbourne, VIC 3010, Australia; geoffrey.donnan@unimelb.edu.au (G.A.D.); leonidc@unimelb.edu.au (L.C.)
9 Allied Health and Human Performance, University of South Australia, Adelaide, SA 5001, Australia; susan.hillier@unisa.edu.au
10 Clinical Sciences at Monash Health, Faculty of Medicine, Nursing and Health Sciences, Monash University, Melbourne, VIC 3800, Australia; mbudge@bendigohealth.org.au
11 Melbourne Brain Centre, Royal Melbourne Hospital, Parkville, VIC 3050, Australia
12 Academic and Research Collaborative in Health, La Trobe University, Melbourne, VIC 3086, Australia; m.morris@latrobe.edu.au
13 The Victorian Rehabilitation Centre, Healthscope Limited, Melbourne, VIC 3150, Australia
14 School of Medicine, University of Nottingham, Nottingham NG7 2UH, UK; marion.walker@nottingham.ac.uk
15 Health Economics and Impact, Hunter Medical Research Institute, New Lambton, NSW 2305, Australia
16 Hunter New England Health, New Lambton, NSW 2305, Australia
17 UniSA Health, University of South Australia, Adelaide, SA 5001, Australia; esther.may@unisa.edu.au
18 Department of Neurology, Alfred Health, Melbourne, VIC 3004, Australia
19 National Stroke Foundation, Melbourne, VIC 3000, Australia; sharon.mcgowan@ranzcp.org
20 Department of Medicine, Melbourne Medical School, The University of Melbourne, Melbourne, VIC 3010, Australia; twi@unimelb.edu.au
21 Department of Neurology and Stroke Services, Western Health, Sunshine Hospital, Footscray, VIC 3021, Australia
22 Bendigo Health, Bendigo, VIC 3550, Australia
23 St. Vincent's Hospital, Melbourne, VIC 3065, Australia; fiona.mckinnon@svha.org.au
24 Epworth Healthcare, Richmond, VIC 3121, Australia; john.olver@epworth.org.au
25 Barwon Health, Geelong, VIC 3220, Australia
26 Department of Occupational Therapy, Alfred Health, Melbourne, VIC 3004, Australia
* Correspondence: l.carey@latrobe.edu.au

Abstract: Implementation of evidence-informed rehabilitation of the upper limb is variable, and outcomes for stroke survivors are often suboptimal. We established a national partnership of clinicians, survivors of stroke, researchers, healthcare organizations, and policy makers to facilitate change. The objectives of this study are to increase access to best-evidence rehabilitation of the upper limb and improve outcomes for stroke survivors. This prospective pragmatic, knowledge translation study involves four new specialist therapy centers to deliver best-evidence upper-limb sensory rehabilitation (known as SENSe therapy) for survivors of stroke in the community. A knowledge-transfer intervention will be used to upskill therapists and guide implementation. Specialist centers will deliver SENSe therapy, an effective and recommended therapy, to stroke survivors in the community. Outcomes include number of successful deliveries of SENSe therapy by credentialled therapists; improved somatosensory function for stroke survivors; improved performance in self-selected activities, arm use, and quality of life; treatment fidelity and confidence to deliver therapy; and for future implementation, expert therapist effect and cost-effectiveness. In summary, we will determine the effect of a national partnership to increase access to evidence-based upper-limb sensory rehabilitation following stroke. If effective, this knowledge-transfer intervention could be used to optimize the delivery of other complex, evidence-based rehabilitation interventions.

Keywords: stroke; implementation science; neurological rehabilitation; stroke rehabilitation; somatosensory; healthcare services; occupational therapy; physiotherapy

1. Introduction

Implementation of evidence-based stroke rehabilitation interventions improves patient outcomes [1,2]. Evidence-based therapies for the upper limb after stroke are recommended in clinical practice guidelines [3,4] and in international best-practice guidelines [5,6]. Yet, there is inconsistent access to and delivery of quality, evidence-based stroke rehabilitation, leading to suboptimal outcomes [3,7,8]. The need for and potential benefit of implementation interventions to promote the uptake of best-evidence rehabilitation are highlighted [9–11].

There are currently very few knowledge-transfer interventions of known effectiveness to facilitate practice change for complex interventions in stroke rehabilitation, and the certainty of the evidence is very low [11]. We developed an implementation intervention to drive behavior change in clinical and community settings [12]. The intervention is guided by the Theoretical Domains Framework [13–15], with translation strategies from the Behavior Change Wheel [16]. The intervention targets the delivery of science-based rehabilitation that requires knowledge and skill of the rehabilitation therapist, an application of knowledge translation that is virtually untested in the field of stroke rehabilitation [12].

Major evidence–practice gaps in stroke rehabilitation have been identified in addressing the loss of body sensation after stroke nationally [17] and internationally [18], contributing to poor arm use and reduced ability to return to previous life activities after stroke [19–21]. Impaired sensation is experienced by one in two stroke survivors [22–25]. This loss is beyond any reduction experienced with healthy aging [22,23]. As survivors of stroke report: "It is like the hand is blind" and "…I couldn't really do daily stuff... I couldn't hold anything, things were just dropping…so I had nothing, there was nothing there" [26]. Many learn non-use of their hand, leading to secondary problems and restricting return to valued activities and work [19,20,22,27]. In addition, upper limb sensory loss is a factor contributing to inferior results in rehabilitation outcomes [19,28–30], and adequate sensation is a prerequisite for full motor recovery of the paretic upper limb [31].

Despite the high prevalence and negative impact on function, it has been highlighted that loss of body sensations is a 'neglected' area of stroke rehabilitation [32]. Rehabilitation therapists often use a compensatory, rather than restorative, approach to somatosensory loss and recovery [17,18]. Yet, use of compensation potentially reinforces learned non-use of the limb with negative long-term consequences. In our national survey, less than half of healthcare professionals reported satisfaction with the treatments they were using, or confidence in their ability to treat somatosensory impairment after stroke, indicating a readiness to change practice [17]. Barriers to implementation of best-practice sensory rehabilitation identified by therapists include low therapist confidence; lack of skills; inconsistent access to resources; and reduced quality of therapy delivery [17,33].

The purpose of this study is to increase access to best-evidence rehabilitation of the upper limb and improve outcomes for stroke survivors. Our focus is on delivery of best-evidence somatosensory rehabilitation, given the evidence–practice gap identified nationally and internationally [17,18]. Specifically, we will use a knowledge transfer intervention to upskill therapists and deliver recommended best-evidence somatosensory rehabilitation to more survivors of stroke.

A neuroscience-based approach to rehabilitation of somatosensory impairment, known as SENSe (Study of the Effectiveness of Neurorehabilitation on Sensation) [34] (http://youtu.be/G9V3I30pn68; accessed on 2 October 2023), has been systematically developed and tested, consistent with the Medical Research Council Framework for the development and evaluation of complex interventions [35]. SENSe therapy has demonstrated efficacy across a series of studies [36,37], including a double-blinded randomized controlled trial [34], with reported improvements in somatosensory capacity [34] and performance of valued occupations [26]. Survivors of stroke report the positive experience and benefits of being involved in SENSe therapy, demonstrating acceptability of this therapy for this population [26]. SENSe therapy is recommended in clinical practice guidelines for stroke [3] and in best-practice International Standards for Arm Rehabilitation Post-stroke [5].

Skill and experience of the therapist may impact implementation and delivery of evidence-based complex interventions. This is particularly evident when service delivery requires a high level of skill from therapists [11,38]. Investigation of the impact of therapist experience on therapy outcomes is therefore warranted. Further, while evidence is growing about health outcomes from implementation interventions across various settings and health professional groups [11,39], there is a paucity of data on their cost-effectiveness to inform whether the investment of resources justifies the additional benefits that might be achieved. Therefore, this study will also investigate cost-effectiveness of the intervention.

We have created a partnership of survivors of stroke, clinicians, researchers, healthcare organizations, and policy makers to (i) increase access to evidence-based SENSe therapy delivered by therapists via a network of clinical practice settings and specialist SENSe therapy centers, and (ii) improve outcomes for survivors of stroke with somatosensory impairment of the arm/hand. The partnership is supported with a National Health and Medical Research Council Partnership grant from Australia (GNT 1134495), which has allowed us to create a centralized knowledge-translation hub and four specialist therapy centers.

Two complementary studies, SENSe Implement [12] and SENSe CONNECT (ACTRN12618001389291), are being undertaken to address the identified gap and achieve our overall aims. Together, the studies will permit investigation across different modes of delivery and skill levels of therapists and will involve approximately 100 therapists and 250 stroke survivors. The first study, SENSe Implement [12] (ACTRN12615000933550), focuses on testing the effectiveness of our knowledge-transfer intervention to change clinician behavior in existing rehabilitation services. Specifically, the aim is to determine whether evidence-based knowledge-translation strategies change the practice of occupational therapists and physiotherapists in the assessment and treatment of sensory loss of the upper limb after stroke to improve patient outcomes. This study is being conducted as a pragmatic, before–after study involving eight Australian healthcare networks and existing sub-acute and community rehabilitation services (see [12] for further details).

The second study detailed here is known as SENSe CONNECT (ACTRN12618001389291). The SENSe CONNECT study is designed to increase access to evidence-based SENSe therapy via specialist SENSe therapy centers and skilled therapists. Four new specialist SENSe therapy centers, across three states in Australia, are planned to complement and extend current services. This model of service delivery differs from the current practice model being tested in the SENSe Implement study. The focus for SENSe CONNECT is on increased access for survivors of stroke living in the community. We will create a centralized hub to lead the knowledge-translation intervention and provide upskilling of therapists. A network of specialist SENSe therapy centers and community of therapists will be linked with the hub to facilitate implementation and sustainability. Web-based resources will be developed to further support therapists and help sustain practice change. Some of the broader contextual aspects of implementation [40,41] will also be investigated in the SENSe CONNECT study, including impact of therapist expertise on outcomes and cost-effectiveness. The specific aims of the current SENSe CONNECT study are to

- Increase access to evidence-based SENSe therapy delivered via a network of specialist SENSe therapy centers and skilled therapists.
- Improve outcomes for survivors of stroke with somatosensory impairment of the arm/hand (primary outcome—somatosensory function; secondary outcomes—performance of self-selected valued activities, arm use, and quality of life).
- Achieve high treatment fidelity for therapists in the delivery of upper-limb sensory rehabilitation following a tailored, evidence-informed knowledge-transfer intervention.
- Explore the association of the amount of therapist experience in SENSe delivery with outcomes for stroke survivors.
- Evaluate the cost-effectiveness of the knowledge-translation intervention in terms of the amount of improvement in SENSe therapy outcomes, i.e., somatosensory function, performance in valued activities, arm use, and quality of life.

2. Materials and Methods

2.1. Study Design

The overall knowledge translation study involves a centralized hub, 4 specialist SENSe therapy centers, and 11 healthcare networks to deliver evidence-based upper-limb sensory rehabilitation for stroke survivors. The SENSe CONNECT arm detailed here is a prospective, pragmatic knowledge-translation study, involving four specialist SENSe therapy centers and stroke survivors in the community. Inclusion criteria are broad to test broader treatment effectiveness, and therapy will be delivered using a within-participant wait list control design [42].

2.1.1. Centralized Translation Hub

A centralized hub was created to lead the knowledge translation intervention and provide upskilling of therapists. This includes a multimodal approach to upskilling therapists [12], which is supported with a therapy training manual and a suite of training videos. Therapists are credentialled and treatment fidelity is monitored and supported using document audit and fidelity observations and feedback [43]. The network of specialist services and community of therapists will facilitate implementation and sustainability. Web-based resources have been developed (https://sensetherapy.net.au/; accessed on 2 October 2023) to further support therapists and help sustain practice change via a community of practice. An overview of the network of sites and centers involved is provided in Figure 1.

2.1.2. Specialist SENSe Therapy Centers and SENSe CONNECT Protocol

Four specialist SENSe therapy centers have been set up to deliver SENSe therapy to stroke survivors across three states in Australia. The new specialist therapy centers are linked with healthcare networks and universities or research institutes. The SENSe therapy centers will permit delivery of therapy to stroke survivors living in the community. Therapy may be delivered at the center or in the client's home.

Occupational therapists and physiotherapists skilled and credentialled in SENSe therapy will deliver SENSe therapy to stroke survivors across the specialist therapy centers, using a pragmatic, within-subject wait list design [42]. The wait list design will evaluate change in outcomes over a 6-week period of usual care not associated with SENSe therapy, compared to a 6-week period of SENSe therapy delivered by credentialled therapists. During the wait list phase, participants will receive usual care, which will be monitored. Upper-limb therapy will not be restricted for participants during the control wait list phase; rather, participants will receive 'usual care' conditions [44]. Consistent with an independent review and analysis of 'usual care' usually received in health services in Australia (based on national audit and knowledge-translation study), this will usually not involve specific sensory rehabilitation, such as SENSe therapy [44]. Participants may continue to receive usual care during the SENSe therapy intervention period. Our prior controlled clinical trials provide evidence that exposure to sensory stimuli alone and/or current usual care is not usually sufficient to affect clinically significant improvement in somatosensory function [34,36,37]. All services and usual care received will be monitored.

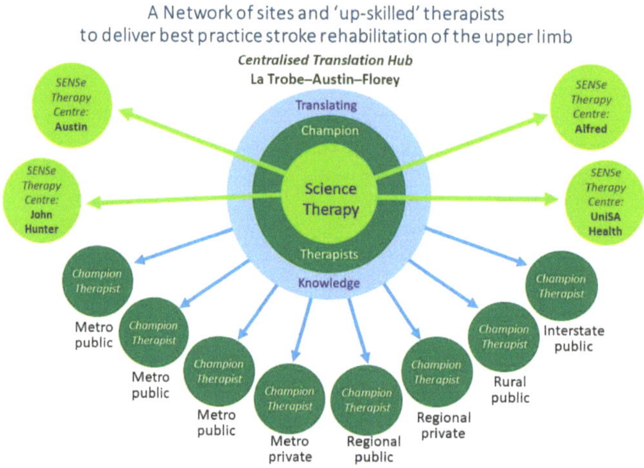

Figure 1. Diagram of the centralized translation hub and delivery sites, with champion therapists at existing health settings (SENSe Implement study) and specialist therapy centers (SENSe CONNECT study). Each interact with and are supported by the central hub.

Stroke survivors attending specialist SENSe therapy centers will be assessed on four occasions: baseline (i.e., Assessment 1, A1); after 6 weeks of usual care (i.e., A2); after 6 weeks of SENSe therapy (i.e., A3); and at follow up, 12 weeks post A3 (i.e., A4). All participants attending SENSe therapy centers will receive SENSe therapy (10 sessions) over a 6-week period. Assessors for health outcomes of stroke survivors will be blinded to study design and timing of therapy delivery. Researchers and statisticians involved in the data analysis will also be blinded to study design and timing of therapy delivery.

SENSe therapists will not be blinded due to pragmatic reasons. It is planned that each therapist will deliver SENSe therapy to up to 12 stroke survivors. A secondary analysis will permit investigation of the association between stroke survivor outcomes achieved and the therapist's amount of experience in delivering SENSe therapy. The study is approved by Austin Human Research Ethics Committee (HREC/18/Austin/153), and all experiments will be performed in accordance with the Declaration of Helsinki. Site-specific ethics approvals were also obtained. All participants will give voluntary informed consent.

Sample size: Stroke survivors—The SENSe CONNECT study design requires a within-subject, repeated measures analysis. The within-group analysis from the original SENSe randomized controlled trial (RCT) revealed a Cohen d of 0.366 for the somatosensory function outcome (repeated measures, small group $n = 22/50$; [34]). To achieve a within-group effect of d = 0.366 for a power of 0.8, a minimum sample of $n = 61$ is required. In the current study, the proposed sample size of $n = 72$ to 192 (i.e., 18 to 48 deliveries at each of the 4 centers) achieves this minimum and allows for dropout or poor recruitment.

Assuming the variability in changes found in the SENSe RCT is replicated in the delivery of SENSe therapy, a maximum sample size of n = 192 will have a high degree of precision for estimating the effect size obtained within the SENSe therapy centers. The larger sample size will also facilitate generalizability of effect estimates to the broader target population of survivors of stroke living in the community. Therapists—At each specialist SENSe therapy center, it is planned that 3 or 4 therapists will each deliver SENSe therapy to 6 to 12 stroke survivors (i.e., 18 to 48 deliveries at each site; 72 to 192 across sites). A sample of 12 to 16 therapists was chosen to maximize replication across upskilled therapists while exploring the association between the amount of experience in delivery of SENSe therapy and therapy outcomes.

2.2. Participants

Participants for the SENSe CONNECT study include both therapists and stroke survivors.

Therapists: Inclusion criteria—Qualified occupational therapist or physiotherapist; current registration to practice; and willing to participate in the upskilling in SENSe therapy, undertake evaluation, and actively participate in mentoring and treatment fidelity activities to develop competency to deliver SENSe therapy. There are no additional exclusion criteria for the participants who are therapists. Replacement therapists will be recruited as needed. As a pragmatic implementation trial, restrictions will not be imposed on therapist participants' experience or number of stroke survivors treated. However, demographic information for all therapist participants will be collected to ascertain relationships between stroke survivor outcomes and therapist characteristics.

Stroke survivors: People with stroke living in the community and presenting with new or chronic somatosensory impairment will be recruited. Stroke survivors may be referred via partner organizations, neurologists, rehabilitation physicians, general practitioners, other organizations, or self-referral. Inclusion criteria: A clinical diagnosis of stroke (including infarct or hemorrhage, people with a second stroke, no restriction on time since stroke); impaired touch sensation, limb position sense, and/or tactile object recognition of the upper limb, identified clinically and with screening tests; medically stable; able to give informed consent; able to comprehend simple instructions; willing to commit time to participate in the SENSe therapy program; and living in the community. Key exclusion criteria: Sensory impairment not due to stroke; severe unilateral spatial neglect (measured via line bisection and shape cancellation task); prior history of other central nervous system dysfunction with an unstable or progressive prognosis; severe to moderate cognitive impairment (i.e., not able to comprehend simple instructions or sustain attention needed to participate in treatment); not able to give informed consent; physical limitations that prevent participation in therapy tasks (e.g., contracture of the hand, or unhealed wounds); and unable to participate in a clinical appointment lasting 30 min. Thus, the design tests effectiveness with relatively unselected survivors of stroke in the community.

2.3. Setting

Specialist SENSe therapy centers will be based at four metropolitan sites in Australia, each having a link with a health setting and an academic or research organization. Sites are Austin Health (link with Florey Institute of Neuroscience and Mental Health and La Trobe University) and Alfred Health (link with Monash University) in Melbourne, Victoria; John Hunter Hospital (link with University of Newcastle) in Newcastle, NSW; and UniSA Health (link with University of South Australia) in Adelaide, SA.

2.4. Outcomes

Access to evidence-based sensory rehabilitation: The primary outcome is the number of complete deliveries of SENSe therapy at the SENSe therapy center by therapists credentialled in SENSe therapy. A delivery will be counted as complete if it meets the criterion of at least 7 sessions delivered with a stroke survivor.

Stroke survivors: The primary outcome is change in arm somatosensory function, pre–post SENSe therapy, across three somatosensory domains, measured using standardized, quantitative somatosensory measures and a normalized summary impairment index calibrated to normed age-matched performance [34,45]. The index will be derived from scores on the Tactile Discrimination Test [46], Wrist Position Sense Test [47], and functional Tactile Object Recognition Test [48]. Each of these quantitative measures assesses the person's ability to discriminate different somatosensations; i.e., texture discrimination, wrist joint proprioception, and haptic object recognition of the upper limb. Comparable ranges of impairment from just noticeable to extreme impairment defined for each measure enable the normalization of the three test scales for comparison in clinical and research settings [45].

The following secondary outcomes will also be assessed: client-rated performance and satisfaction of valued activities, using the Canadian Occupational Performance Measure (COPM) [49] and clinician-rated performance on the same valued activities using the Performance Quality Rating Scale for Somatosensation after Stroke [50]; arm use, using Motor Activity Log-14 [51]; and health-related quality of life, using the Assessment of Quality of Life (AQoL-6D) [52]. See Table 1 for the schedule of study outcomes.

Table 1. Study Schedule of Assessments: SENSe CONNECT.

Outcome	Measure	A1 (Baseline)	A2 (6 Weeks Post A1)	A3 (6 Weeks Post A2)	A4 (12 Weeks Post A3)
		Survivor of Stroke			
Arm somatosensory function	Tactile Discrimination Test (TDT)	X	X	X	X
	Wrist Position Sense Test (WPST)	X	X	X	X
	Functional Tactile Object Recognition Test (fTORT)	X	X	X	X
Performance of valued activities	Canadian Occupational Performance Measure (COPM)	X	X	X	X
	Performance Quality Rating Scale for Somatosensation after Stroke	X	X	X	X
Arm use	Motor Activity Log (MAL)-14 item version	X	X	X	X
Health-related quality of life	Australian Quality of Life (AQoL-6D)	X	X	X	X
Resource utilization	Resource Use and Productivity Questionnaire	X	X	X	X
Other	National Institute of Health Stroke Scale (NIHSS)	X			
	Modified Rankin Scale (mRS)	X			
	Montreal Cognitive Assessment (MoCA)	X			
	Jebsen Taylor Hand Function Test (JTHFT)	X			
		SENSe Therapist			
Treatment fidelity	Customized Documentation Audit Checklist	Post delivery of SENSe therapy to each survivor of stroke.			
Practice behavior change	Pre–Post Implementation Questionnaires	Prior to first delivery of SENSe therapy and after delivery of therapy to 12th survivor of stroke, or last scheduled delivery for that therapist.			

Therapists: Treatment fidelity is a primary outcome for therapists and will be assessed as the ability to deliver SENSe therapy with high fidelity measured with a criterion-based checklist (comprising 29 components core to the delivery of SENSe therapy; 80% fidelity) and customized documentation audit checklist [43]. Fidelity will be assessed by an independent person, using a document audit, for each therapist after delivery of each 6-week program of SENSe therapy. In addition, a sample of treatment sessions (early, middle, and late in the sequence of 10 sessions for the stroke participant) will be observed and rated by an independent person using a session-based treatment fidelity checklist. Therapist participants will also be assessed for change in practice behaviors related to SENSe therapy (secondary outcome), specifically change in knowledge, skill, and confidence levels. These outcomes will be assessed using pre–post implementation questionnaires [12] adapted for the SENSe CONNECT study. The pre-questionnaire will be completed prior to upskilling, credentialing, and first delivery of SENSe therapy. The post-implementation questionnaire will be completed after delivery of therapy to the 12th stroke survivor treated, or following the last scheduled delivery of therapy, for that therapist.

Therapist experience effect: Therapist experience will be measured according to the number of completed deliveries of the SENSe therapy program, with delivery of 7 or more sessions per stroke survivor the criterion for a completed delivery. Each therapist is anticipated to deliver SENSe therapy to 6 to 12 survivors of stroke.

Resource utilization and therapy costs: Resources used by survivors of stroke will be collected at all assessment occasions for the usual care wait list and intervention periods using a patient/carer survey. Resources will be assigned prices to convert these into costs using contemporaneous Australian reference sources. Costs will be inflated/deflated for a common reference year (e.g., 2022) using the Total Health Price Index [53], as required. Program level costs of intervention delivery: SENSe therapy costs will include the cost of upskilling therapists, equipment, and delivering the intervention according to the model of care established, as well as determining the cost of usual care. The type and quantity of each resource used will be collected in natural units, e.g., number of sessions and time taken to train therapists.

2.5. Implementation Intervention

The current knowledge-translation study and implementation intervention developed by the research team are based on the Theoretical Domains Framework [14], and guided by strategies from the Behaviour Change Wheel [16] to facilitate practice change and Normalisation Process Theory [54] to enhance sustainability. Specifically, the multi-component implementation intervention to support knowledge translation includes (i) interactive training workshops, (ii) establishing a clinical lead and site champions; (iii) provision of educational materials and structured therapy booklets; and (iv) use of treatment fidelity checklists [43] to guide feedback on therapy and to assess outcomes.

Upskilling of therapists: Occupational therapists and physiotherapists will be upskilled in delivery of SENSe therapy by a trained clinical lead researcher from the central hub using multimedia resources. Training includes a 1.5-day interactive workshop, involving theory (1 h), practical hands-on SENSe training sessions (7 h), and applied treatment planning (2 h), and is supported by 3 independent learning modules that include supervised practice tasks and case scenarios (estimated to take 1 to 2 h each); the total time is approximately 13 to 16 h. Therapists are credentialed, via observation of a simulated therapy session at the end of the upskilling process. Participant therapists will also receive supervision and mentoring during delivery of SENSe therapy. This will be primarily via the treatment fidelity observations and audit feedback. Therapists are introduced to the treatment fidelity checklist [43] during upskilling sessions and encouraged to use it for self-evaluation. The treatment fidelity criterion checklist is also used by SENSe therapy trainers to provide feedback to therapists on treatment notes and observed therapy delivery.

2.6. SENSe Therapy Intervention

SENSe (Study of the Effectiveness of Neurorehabilitation on Sensation; [34]), is a science- and evidence-based rehabilitation therapy designed to help people with stroke regain a sense of touch and use it in daily activities (http://youtu.be/G9V3I30pn68; accessed on 2 October 2023). As such, the focus is on restoration of function rather than compensation. Clinical practice protocols and therapy tools [55] have been produced to facilitate implementation and quality delivery in clinical settings. The intervention will be delivered face to face by skilled and credentialled occupational therapists and/or physiotherapists within specialist SENSe therapy centers. SENSe therapy involves modules of sensory discrimination training of texture discrimination, sensing the position of the upper limb in space (proprioception), recognizing objects through the sense of touch, and learning how to apply these skills in daily tasks identified by the person with stroke (Figure 2). Seven training principles are used during the process of somatosensory discrimination training as follows: select; attentive exploration; feedback; calibrate; anticipate; repeat and progress; and transfer (http://youtu.be/G9V3I30pn68; accessed on 2 October 2023). Specially designed training tools are used and include grids and texture training wheels of surfaces with varying surface features, graded for large, medium, and fine surface differences; box-like apparatus and protractor scales for training wrist position sense; and graded sets of objects for functional tactile object recognition that train discrimination and recognition of object weight, crushability, shape, size, temperature, texture, and functional motion. The client selects two valued activities that they believe are impacted by their sensory loss to focus on in therapy. They are guided to discover the sensory challenges in the activity and how they can use their new skills to perform the task better. Examples include using a knife or fork, finding money in a wallet, doing up buttons, and using a remote-control device. The intervention will be tailored according to the level of impairment and functional goals of the stroke participant. The dose is 10 1-hour sessions, over a period of 6 weeks. The frequency of sessions is approximately twice a week. The number, duration, and specific content of all sessions are monitored using customized training forms.

(a) (b) (c) (d)

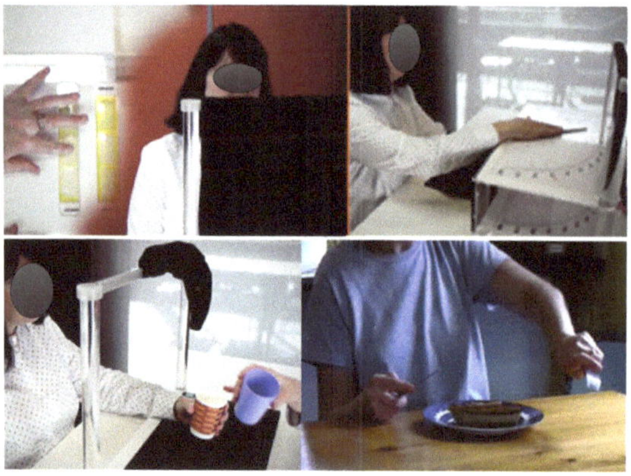

Figure 2. Images of SENSe therapy specialized equipment and activities used in training modules, including (**a**) discrimination of texture grids; (**b**) training of wrist proprioception using the box-like apparatus and protractor scales; (**c**) training of graded sets of everyday objects that vary in objects with varying diagnostic attributes such as crushability, shape, size, and weight; and (**d**) training in the context of self-chosen valued activities impacted by sensory loss.

2.7. Methods to Facilitate Sustainability

A community of practice (CoP) will be developed to support therapists in the implementation of evidence-based SENSe therapy. Initially, this community will be developed locally as part of the peer group upskilling of therapists at SENSe therapy centers. A website and online presence will be developed to enhance this CoP and provide ongoing education and peer support in the sustained implementation of evidence-based SENSe therapy. The website will connect therapists, provide support and information with case scenarios, and permit interactive feedback.

2.8. Data Analysis

Data management and data statement: Due to the personal nature of the data and original ethics approval, the data will not be made available broadly. De-identified data may be made available for related research and analyses by the research group and collaborators with additional ethics approval. Data will be entered using the REDCap electronic data capture tools [56], hosted at the Florey Institute of Neuroscience and Mental Health, by the site coordinator or trained delegate. REDCap features are in place to ensure valid data capture (e.g., data range checks), and data quality checking procedures are in place to ensure accuracy at initial entry and subsequently checked by a second independent researcher. Data will be de-identified for analyses. All data will be kept secure and confidential as per the approved ethics protocol.

Access to evidence-based sensory rehabilitation: The number of stroke survivors who receive SENSe therapy by therapists credentialled in SENSe therapy will be calculated. Successful completion of SENSe therapy for a survivor of stroke is determined as delivery of 7 or more therapy sessions. The number of attempted deliveries of SENSe therapy that did not meet the criterion for successful completion will also be counted.

Effect of SENSe therapy: We will evaluate the therapeutic gain in arm somatosensory function for stroke survivors (primary outcome) during the SENSe therapy phase compared to that of the usual care phase by estimating the mean within-person difference between the two trends and the associated 95% confidence intervals. The magnitude of change in arm somatosensory function under the two conditions will be calculated as a standardized effect size and compared to the benchmark effect size obtained in the original SENSe RCT (comparable cohort) [34]. Statistical estimates of change will be reported with 95% confidence intervals, and the extent of overlap across studies in these estimates of change will be described. Confidence intervals for the difference between mean change scores from the present and benchmarked study [34] will also be obtained. The analysis design will include the SENSe therapy center as a variable, to evaluate its potential systematic effect. Individual participant characteristics that may impact magnitude of therapeutic gain, such as age and time post-stroke, will be explored. Improvement in secondary outcomes, i.e., clinician-rated performance in valued activities, arm use, and quality of life, will also be evaluated pre–post therapy. Depending on verification of the normal distribution assumption, either a t-distribution or a bootstrapping method will be used to obtain the confidence interval. Maintenance of the intervention effect will be evaluated at the 12-week follow up (A4).

Treatment fidelity and behavior change: High fidelity delivery will be defined as a score of 80% or higher on the SENSe treatment fidelity checklists [43]. Audit data from treatment sessions will be independently summarized for each SENSe therapy treatment program delivered. The number of therapy deliveries achieving high treatment fidelity will be summarized. Pre- and post-implementation questionnaires of therapist knowledge, confidence, and ability to deliver SENSe therapy will be summarized and response tendencies will be examined using contingency tables, McNemar's test, and graphical representation.

Therapist experience effect: The availability of 6 to 12 sequential cases treated with SENSe therapy by each of the 12 to 16 therapists will allow exploration of the hypothesis that a trend towards better outcomes arises with experience of therapy delivery. Individual therapeutic gain scores will be adjusted for initial sensory impairment, consistent with our prior analysis of which individual variables affect therapeutic gain [57]. Growth curve models will be explored for the sequence of adjusted therapeutic gains from each of the therapists (n = 12–16) to evaluate the autocorrelation structure of residuals and the viability of a common model. A pooled estimate of the effect of treatment experience will then be obtained via a meta-analysis, or hierarchical linear modelling if a common trajectory form is applicable.

Economic evaluation: We will report a cost description analysis for usual care and the SENSe therapy interventions and summarize these data as part of a cost consequence analysis [58] presenting the disaggregated costs and primary and secondary outcomes for stroke participants. The incremental cost-effectiveness of SENSe therapy compared to monitored wait list usual care will also be evaluated as the cost per achievement of improved arm somatosensory function (primary outcome for stroke survivor). We will also use simulation modelling to estimate the incremental cost per Quality Adjusted Life Year gained with SENSe therapy, drawing data from the study and the published RCT for SENSe [34]. One-way sensitivity and multivariable uncertainty analyses will be performed to assess the robustness of results. The findings from the economic evaluation will be used to inform business cases for future adoption of SENSe within the Australian healthcare context and may have relevance to other countries with similar funding models for healthcare. Results will be reported according to the Consolidated Health Economic Evaluation Reporting Standards (CHEERS) [59,60].

2.9. Research Impact Evaluation

The potential translational impact of the research will be evaluated using the Framework for the Assessment of Impact and Translation (FAIT) [61]. A program logic model that defines aims, activities, outputs, stakeholders, and impact will guide this process. Impact will be evaluated in relation to the following domains: advance knowledge, e.g., publication metrics, presentations, and social media; capacity and capability building, including partnerships and networks, formal education training, upskilling of therapists, and integration with policy/practice; implementation, in relation to clinical practice change and research practice change; community benefit, including access to services and health outcomes for stroke survivors; economic benefits, such as employment-created, cost-effectiveness of SENSe therapy, commercialization, grants leveraged, potential downstream savings, and increase in potential lifetime earnings; and policy and legislation, including policy representation, policy relationships built and direct translation to policy.

2.10. Patient and Public Involvement

People who have experienced a stroke have identified the practice gap and helped drive this research from its inception. The Stroke Foundation, an Australian public advocacy group, is a partner in this program of research. Survivors of stroke and Stroke Foundation representatives are named on the successful Partnership grant and involved in group meetings. They have engaged in discussions and formulation of the research questions, design, and conduct of the study, choice of outcome measures, and recruitment to the study both at the initial project planning stage and during team meetings. They have also contributed to plans for dissemination and impact. Involvement is consistent with Stroke Foundation guidelines for involvement of people with lived experience in research.

3. Discussion

Access to best-evidence rehabilitation therapies after stroke continues to be an issue in Australia [3] and globally [7,62–64]. To address this issue, and to demonstrate a much-needed approach for stroke rehabilitation knowledge translation, we created a model based on a collaborative partnership approach, to meet the specific needs of stroke rehabilitation stakeholders, and to complement existing services. The centralized hub and specialist therapy centers created are designed to provide a vehicle to increase access to best-practice therapy through connecting all key stakeholders: stroke survivors, clinicians, healthcare organizations, research institutes, universities, policy makers, funders, and the Stroke Foundation. Thus, our approach not only addresses change at the 'micro' level of health (i.e., individual therapists) but also at the organizational or macro-system level of healthcare, with the formation of our partnership and creation of a translation hub and specialist therapy centers. It is anticipated that sustainability will be enhanced by the structure that links the central hub with local sites and skilled, credentialled therapists. Involvement of all stakeholders will help maximize meaningful and sustained policy and practice change.

We chose to focus on the evidence–practice gap of sensory rehabilitation after stroke, identified nationally [17] and internationally [18]. Consistent with recommendations for moving research evidence into practice [65], we sought to implement SENSe therapy as this therapy makes explicit the details of the intervention with therapy protocols [55], and has guidelines to assess for treatment fidelity [43]. SENSe therapy is underpinned by strong evidence including a double-blind RCT [34]. A pooled analysis of individual differences indicates adult survivors of stroke with varying age, lesion of left or right hemisphere, severity of impairment, cognition, and varying time post-stroke can benefit from SENSe therapy [57]. Despite this therapy being recommended in international best-practice guidelines for rehabilitation of the upper limb [5] and national stroke guidelines [3], adoption in clinical practice has been slow.

The knowledge-translation approach and implementation intervention outlined in this protocol may provide a foundation for creating a template for knowledge translation of evidence-based stroke rehabilitation, optimized for application to therapies that are predicated on skilled delivery by therapists, as is the case for SENSe therapy. While it is acknowledged that this implementation intervention addresses only one unmet need of stroke survivors (when many have multiple deficits and needs), the knowledge translation approach has potential for broader application in specialist upskilling and creation of networks of sites to support specialized, evidence-based therapeutic interventions.

A pragmatic approach was selected to evaluate the effectiveness of our implementation intervention in real-world clinical practice and community settings, and across a range of therapists, to maximize generalizability of the results [66]. Further, we will have the opportunity to explore a therapist experience effect on SENSe outcomes. Cost-effectiveness data may be used to improve resource allocation in different service settings. It is anticipated that the costs of services provided by such centers and services could be covered by national health and disability schemes and/or private health insurers. Dissemination will be enhanced via a knowledge translation hub, specialist therapy centers, websites (e.g., https://sensetherapy.net.au/; accessed on 2 October 2023), and a community of skilled therapists embedded in a range of healthcare settings.

Limitations: Increased access to delivery of evidence-based SENSe therapy via specialist SENSe therapy centers, the primary outcome, will likely be impacted by restrictions imposed during the COVID-19 pandemic. The ability to administer the protocol as planned and deliver SENSe therapy without interruption will also likely be impacted. Changed service demands associated with the pandemic may also influence recruitment and retention of therapists and delivery of usual care. Any protocol variations and impacts of the pandemic will be monitored and reported. As a pragmatic trial, factors such as individual characteristics of treating therapists (e.g., prior expertise, number of years of practice, number of stroke survivors treated before upskilling) and survivors of stroke (e.g., age, time since stroke, concomitant impairments) will not be controlled for. These factors will, however, be monitored and explored for their potential influence on outcomes in our planned analyses. Therapists who deliver usual care will be different from those who deliver SENSe therapy. It is recognized that this may impact outcomes. It is noted, however, that involvement of different therapists in this pragmatic design is consistent with variation in therapist experience typically experienced. Further, it is not possible for the SENSe therapists to deliver usual care following upskilling, as the specialist training may bias their usual care approach. Usual care will not be restricted, nor will it involve standard protocols. Rather, there will be monitoring and comparison to usual care as defined in our aligned SENSe Implement study, which included a phase of delivery of usual care (n = 86 patients) before therapists were upskilled in existing healthcare services, and with an independent analysis of the care usually received in health services based on a national audit [44]. To date, there are no results to present for the current prospective study.

4. Conclusions

The potential impact of this study lies in bringing together producers and users of knowledge as partners to create a network of sites and 'upskilled' therapists to deliver best-practice stroke rehabilitation. It is hoped that through linking the evidence, therapists, and stroke survivors, this interconnected network will enable increased access to evidence-based upper-limb therapy in stroke rehabilitation and better outcomes for people who experience impaired somatosensation after stroke. If successful, there is potential for this approach to be transferred to other specialized evidence-based rehabilitation interventions.

Author Contributions: L.M.C. is the lead chief investigator for the study, conceptualized and planned the study, and assembled the team. All authors contributed to aspects of the study design. M.N., N.A.L., V.T., S.H., D.A.C., G.A.D., M.E.M., L.C., M.W. and S.R. also contributed to conception as chief investigators or associate investigator (S.R.), and M.P., E.M., G.C.C., S.M., T.W., M.B., F.M., J.O., T.H. and M.M. also contributed to execution as partner investigators. L.S.C., J.M.B., B.H., I.K., B.N., Y.M.-Y., M.T., C.N., A.B. and J.K. have trial management and data collection responsibilities. T.A.M. and L.C. planned the data analysis. L.S.C. developed the implementation intervention with input from L.M.C. and N.A.L., and C.N. contributed to the sustainability design. B.N., L.M.C. and B.H. developed the treatment fidelity checklist. L.M.C. developed the SENSe intervention, with input from T.A.M., L.M.C., B.H., Y.M.-Y., L.S.C. and M.T designed, led, and conducted staff training. D.A.C., S.R., L.S.C., J.K. and L.M.C. designed the economic and impact evaluations. L.M.C. wrote the draft manuscript and revised it, with input from all authors. All authors have read and agreed to the published version of the manuscript.

Funding: This work is funded by the National Health and Medical Research Council (NHMRC) of Australia, Partnership grant (GNT1134495). We also acknowledge funding support for development of SENSe therapy from NHMRC Project grants (GNT191214, GNT307902, GNT1022694), and ongoing development from an NHMRC Ideas grant (GNT2004443) and NHMRC Centre of Research Excellence (GNT1077898). We acknowledge support for L.M.C. from NHMRC (GNT307905); for N.A.L. from Heart Foundation (GNT102055); and for L.S.C., M.T., and Y.M.-Y. from La Trobe University scholarships and Australian Government Research Training Scholarships. The funding bodies do not have any role in the design of the study; collection, analysis, and interpretation of data; nor in writing the manuscript.

Institutional Review Board Statement: The study is being conducted in accordance with the Declaration of Helsinki and has received central ethical approval by the Ethics Committee of Austin Health for studies involving humans (HREC/18/Austin/153; approved 21/08/2018) and site approvals by individual sites.

Informed Consent Statement: Informed consent is obtained from all participants involved in the study.

Data Availability Statement: The datasets generated and/or analyzed during the current study are not publicly available due to the personal nature of the data and original ethics approval, but may be available from the corresponding author on reasonable request.

Acknowledgments: We would like to acknowledge the time and interest in the study by stroke participants, and therapists involved in assessment and delivery of SENSe therapy. We acknowledge K. Bayly who contributed to the early conception of the work, assisted with development of materials to upskill therapists in SENSe therapy, and served as a lived experience advisor for the study. We also acknowledge involvement of the administering institution (La Trobe University), collaborating organizations (Florey Institute of Neuroscience and Mental Health, Monash University, The University of Newcastle, University of South Australia, University of Nottingham), partner organizations (Alfred Health, Austin Health, Bendigo Health, Barwon Health, Epworth Healthcare, Hunter New England Health, National Stroke Foundation, St. Vincent's Hospital Melbourne, UniSA Health, Western Health), and all participating sites, and thank those involved for their interest and ongoing contribution to the program of research.

Conflicts of Interest: L.M.C. is the lead originator of the SENSe approach to sensory rehabilitation. SENSe resources have been developed and are available via the not-for-profit Florey Institute of Neuroscience and Mental Health. L.M.C. has no financial interest in the sale of these resources. There is no patent or intended application for any patent associated with these resources. L.M.C. has conducted workshops on the SENSe approach and has been invited to give lectures and conference presentations on the approach. L.M.C. conceptualized the study but is not directly involved in data collection. All other authors declare that they have no competing interests. The funders had no role in the design of the study; in the collection, analyses, or interpretation of data; in the writing of the manuscript; or in the decision to publish the protocol.

References

1. Duncan, P.W.; Horner, R.D.; Reker, D.M.; Samsa, G.P.; Hoenig, H.; Hamilton, B.; LaClair, B.J.; Dudley, T.K. Adherence to postacute rehabilitation guidelines is associated with functional recovery in stroke. *Stroke* **2002**, *33*, 167–177. [CrossRef]
2. Donnellan, C.; Sweetman, S.; Shelley, E. Health professionals' adherence to stroke clinical guidelines: A review of the literature. *Health Policy* **2013**, *111*, 245–263. [CrossRef]
3. Stroke Foundation. *Clinical Guidelines for Stroke Management 2022 (Living Guidelines)*; Stroke Foundation: Melbourne, Australia, 2022; Available online: https://informme.org.au/en/Guidelines/Clinical-Guidelines-for-Stroke-Management (accessed on 21 October 2023).
4. Intercollegiate Stroke Working Party. *National Clinical Guideline for Stroke for the United Kingdom and Ireland*; Royal College of Physicians: London, UK, 2023.
5. Wolf, S.L.; Kwakkel, G.; Bayley, M.; McDonnell, M.N.; For the Upper Extremity Stroke Algorithm Working Group. Best practice for arm recovery post stroke: An international application. *Physiotherapy* **2016**, *102*, 1–4. [CrossRef] [PubMed]
6. Mead, G.E.; Sposato, L.A.; Sampaio Silva, G.; Yperzeele, L.; Wu, S.; Kutlubaev, M.; Cheyne, J.; Wahab, K.; Urrutia, V.C.; Sharma, V.K.; et al. A systematic review and synthesis of global stroke guidelines on behalf of the World Stroke Organization. *Int. J. Stroke* **2023**, *18*, 499–531. [CrossRef] [PubMed]
7. Sentinel Stroke National Audit Programme (SSNAP). *National Results Clinical Audit, UK*; Kings College: London, UK, 2023; Available online: https://www.strokeaudit.org/ (accessed on 18 August 2023).
8. World Health Organization. Rehabilitation 2030 Initiative. 2023. Available online: https://www.who.int/initiatives/rehabilitation-2030 (accessed on 18 August 2023).
9. Gagliardi, A.R.; Alhabib, S. Trends in guideline implementation: A scoping systematic review. *Implement. Sci.* **2015**, *10*, 54. [CrossRef] [PubMed]
10. Platz, T. Evidence-based guidelines and clinical pathways in stroke rehabilitation-an international perspective. *Front. Neurol.* **2019**, *10*, 200. [CrossRef] [PubMed]
11. Cahill, L.S.; Carey, L.M.; Lannin, N.A.; Turville, M.; Neilson, C.L.; Lynch, E.A.; McKinstry, C.E.; Han, J.X.; O'Connor, D. Implementation interventions to promote the uptake of evidence-based practices in stroke rehabilitation. *Cochrane Database Syst. Rev.* **2020**, *10*, 1–154. [CrossRef]
12. Cahill, L.S.; Lannin, N.A.; Mak-Yuen, Y.Y.; Turville, M.L.; Carey, L.M. Changing practice in the assessment and treatment of somatosensory loss in stroke survivors: Protocol for a knowledge translation study. *BMC Health Serv. Res.* **2018**, *18*, 34. [CrossRef]
13. Michie, S.; Johnston, M.; Abraham, C.; Lawton, R.; Parker, D.; Walker, A.; on behalf of the "Psychological Theory" group. Making psychological theory useful for implementing evidence based practice: A consensus approach. *Qual. Saf. Health Care* **2005**, *14*, 26–33. [CrossRef]
14. Cane, J.; O'Connor, D.; Michie, S. Validation of the theoretical domains framework for use in behaviour change and implementation research. *Implement. Sci.* **2012**, *7*, 37. [CrossRef]
15. Atkins, L.; Francis, J.; Islam, R.; O'Connor, D.; Patey, A.; Ivers, N.; Foy, R.; Duncan, E.M.; Colquhoun, H.; Grimshaw, J.M.; et al. A guide to using the theoretical domains framework of behaviour change to investigate implementation problems. *Implement. Sci.* **2017**, *12*, 77. [CrossRef] [PubMed]
16. Michie, S.; van Stralen, M.M.; West, R. The behavior change wheel: A new method for characterising and designing behavior change interventions. *Implement. Sci.* **2011**, *6*, 42. [CrossRef] [PubMed]
17. Pumpa, L.; Cahill, L.S.; Carey, L.M. Somatosensory assessment and treatment after stroke: An evidence-practice gap. *Aust. Occup. Ther. J.* **2015**, *62*, 93–104. [CrossRef] [PubMed]
18. Doyle, S.; Bennett, S.; Gustafsson, L. Occupational therapy for upper limb post-stroke sensory impairments: A survey. *Br. J. Occup. Ther.* **2013**, *76*, 434–442. [CrossRef]
19. Meyer, S.; Karttunen, A.H.; Thijs, V.; Feys, H.; Verheyden, G. How do somatosensory deficits in the arm and hand relate to upper limb impairment, activity and participation problems after stroke? *A systematic review. Phys. Ther.* **2014**, *94*, 14. [CrossRef]
20. Carey, L.M.; Lamp, G.; Turville, M. The state of the science of somatosensory function and its impact on daily life in adults and older adults, and following stroke: A scoping review. *OTJR Occup. Particip. Health* **2016**, *36* (Suppl. S2), 27S–41S. [CrossRef]
21. Carlsson, H.; Gard, G.; Brogårdh, C. Upper-limb sensory impairments after stroke: Self-reported experiences of daily life and rehabilitation. *J. Rehabil. Med.* **2018**, *50*, 45–51. [CrossRef]
22. Carey, L.M.; Matyas, T.A. Frequency of discriminative sensory loss in the hand after stroke. *J. Rehabil. Med.* **2011**, *43*, 257–263. [CrossRef]
23. Kim, J.S.; Choi-Kwon, S. Discriminative sensory dysfunction after unilateral stroke. *Stroke* **1996**, *27*, 677–682. [CrossRef]
24. Tyson, S.F.; Hanley, M.; Chillala, J.; Selley, A.B.; Tallis, R.C. Sensory loss in hospital-admitted people with stroke: Characteristics, associated factors, and relationship with function. *Neurorehabil. Neural Repair* **2008**, *22*, 166–172. [CrossRef]
25. Kessner, S.S.; Schlemm, E.; Cheng, B.; Bingel, U.; Fiehler, J.; Gerloff, C.; Thomalla, G. Somatosensory deficits after ischemic stroke. *Stroke* **2019**, *50*, 1116–1123. [CrossRef] [PubMed]

26. Turville, M.L.; Walker, J.; Blennerhassett, J.M.; Carey, L.M. Experiences of upper limb somatosensory retraining in persons with stroke: An interpretative phenomenological analysis. *Front. Neurosci.* **2019**, *13*, 12. [CrossRef] [PubMed]
27. Carey, L.M.; Matyas, T.; Baum, C. Effects of somatosensory impairment on participation after stroke. *Am. J. Occup. Ther.* **2018**, *72*, 7203205100p1–7203205100p10. [CrossRef] [PubMed]
28. Patel, A.T.; Duncan, P.W.; Lai, S.-M.; Studenski, S. The relation between impairments and functional outcomes poststroke. *Arch. Phys. Med. Rehabil.* **2000**, *81*, 1357–1363. [CrossRef] [PubMed]
29. Reding, M.J.; Potes, E. Rehabilitation outcome following initial unilateral hemispheric stroke: Life table analysis approach. *Stroke* **1988**, *19*, 1354–1358. [CrossRef] [PubMed]
30. Borstad, A.L.; Nichols-Larsen, D.S. Assessing and treating higher level somatosensory impairments post stroke. *Top. Stroke Rehabil.* **2014**, *21*, 290–295. [CrossRef]
31. Zandvliet, S.B.; Kwakkel, G.; Nijland, R.H.M.; van Wegen, E.E.H.; Meskers, C.G.M. Is recovery of somatosensory impairment conditional for upper-limb motor recovery early after stroke? *Neurorehabil. Neural Repair* **2020**, *34*, 403–416. [CrossRef]
32. Kalra, L. Stroke rehabilitation 2009: Old chestnuts and new insights. *Stroke* **2010**, *41*, e88–e90. [CrossRef]
33. Moncion, K.; Biasin, L.; Jagroop, D.; Bayley, M.; Danells, C.; Mansfield, A.; Tang, A. Barriers and facilitators to aerobic exercise implementation in stroke rehabilitation: A scoping review. *J. Neurol Phys. Ther.* **2020**, *44*, 179–187. [CrossRef]
34. Carey, L.; Macdonell, R.; Matyas, T.A. SENSe: Study of the Effectiveness of Neurorehabilitation on Sensation: A randomized controlled trial. *Neurorehabil. Neural Repair* **2011**, *25*, 304–313. [CrossRef]
35. Medical Research Council. *A Framework for Development and Evaluation of RCTs for Complex Interventions to Improve Health*; Medical Research Council: London, UK, 2000.
36. Carey, L.M.; Matyas, T.A.; Oke, L.E. Sensory loss in stroke patients: Effective training of tactile and proprioceptive discrimination. *Arch. Phys. Med. Rehabil.* **1993**, *74*, 602–611. [CrossRef] [PubMed]
37. Carey, L.M.; Matyas, T.A. Training of somatosensory discrimination after stroke: Facilitation of stimulus generalization. *Am. J. Phys. Med. Rehabil.* **2005**, *84*, 428–442. [CrossRef] [PubMed]
38. Juckett, L.A.; Wengerd, L.R.; Faieta, J.; Griffin, C.E. Evidence-based practice implementation in stroke rehabilitation: A scoping review of barriers and facilitators. *Am. J. Occup. Ther.* **2019**, *74*, 7401205050p1–7401205050p14. [CrossRef] [PubMed]
39. Squires, J.E.; Sullivan, K.J.; Eccles, M.P.; Worswick, J.; Grimshaw, J.M. Are multifaceted interventions more effective than single-component interventions in changing health-care professionals' behaviours? *An overview of systematic reviews. Implement. Sci.* **2014**, *9*, 152. [CrossRef] [PubMed]
40. Li, S.-A.; Jeffs, L.; Barwick, M.; Stevens, B. Organizational contextual features that influence the implementation of evidence-based practices across healthcare settings: A systematic integrative review. *Syst. Rev.* **2018**, *7*, 72. [CrossRef]
41. Nilsen, P.; Bernhardsson, S. Context matters in implementation science: A scoping review of determinant frameworks that describe contextual determinants for implementation outcomes. *BMC Health Serv. Res.* **2019**, *19*, 189. [CrossRef]
42. Hart, T.; Bagiella, E. Design and implementation of clinical trials in rehabilitation research. *Arch. Phys. Med. Rehabil.* **2012**, *93*, S117–S126. [CrossRef]
43. Nielsen, B.; Tse, T.; Haslam, B.; Carey, L.M. Development of an audit checklist to evaluate treatment fidelity of a complex rehabilitation intervention. *Disabil. Rehabil.* **2023**, *45*, 1131–1138. [CrossRef]
44. Cahill, L.S.; Lannin, N.A.; Purvis, T.; Cadilhac, D.A.; Mak-Yuen, Y.; O'Connor, D.A.; Carey, L.M. What is "usual care" in the rehabilitation of upper limb sensory loss after stroke? Results from a national audit and knowledge translation study. *Disabil. Rehabil.* **2022**, *44*, 6462–6470. [CrossRef]
45. Matyas, T.A.; Mak-Yuen, Y.Y.K.; Boelsen-Robinson, T.P.; Carey, L.M. Calibration of impairment severity to enable comparison across somatosensory domains. *Brain Sci.* **2023**, *13*, 654. [CrossRef]
46. Mak-Yuen, Y.Y.K.; Matyas, T.A.; Carey, L.M. Characterizing touch discrimination impairment from pooled stroke samples using the Tactile Discrimination Test: Updated criteria for interpretation and brief test version for use in clinical practice settings. *Brain Sci.* **2023**, *13*, 533. [CrossRef]
47. Carey, L.M.; Oke, L.E.; Matyas, T.A. Impaired limb position sense after stroke: A quantitative test for clinical use. *Arch. Phys. Med. Rehabil.* **1996**, *77*, 1271–1278. [CrossRef] [PubMed]
48. Carey, L.M.; Mak-Yuen, Y.Y.K.; Matyas, T.A. The functional Tactile Object Recognition Test: A unidimensional measure with excellent internal consistency for haptic sensing of real objects after stroke. *Front. Neurosci.* **2020**, *14*, 542590. [CrossRef] [PubMed]
49. Law, M.; Baptise, S.; Carswell, A.; McColl, M.A.; Polatajko, H.J.; Pollock, N. *Canadian Occupational Performance Measure*, 4th ed.; CAOT Publications ACE: Ottawa, ON, Cananda, 2005.
50. Wanklyn, T.; Webster, K.E.; Nielsen, B.; Mak-Yuen, Y.; Haslam, B.S.; Carey, L.M. The performance quality rating scale for somatosensation after stroke: A pilot study. *OTJR Occup. Particip. Health* **2023**, *43*, 280–287. [CrossRef] [PubMed]
51. Uswatte, G.; Taub, E.; Morris, D.; Vignolo, M.; McCulloch, K. Reliability and validity of the upper-extremity motor activity log-14 for measuring real-world arm use. *Stroke* **2005**, *36*, 2493–2496. [CrossRef] [PubMed]
52. Richardson, J.R.J.; Peacock, S.J.; Hawthorne, G.; Iezzi, A.A.; Elsworth, G.; Day, N. Construction of the descriptive system for the assessment of quality of life AQoL-6D utility instrument. *Health Qual. Life Outcomes* **2012**, *10*, 38. [CrossRef] [PubMed]
53. Australian Government, Australian Institute of Health and Wellbeing. Health Expenditure Australia 2019–2020. 2021. Available online: https://www.aihw.gov.au/reports/health-welfare-expenditure/health-expenditure (accessed on 2 July 2023).

54. May, C.; Finch, T. Implementing, embedding, and integrating practices: An outline of normalization process theory. *Sociology* **2009**, *43*, 535–554. [CrossRef]
55. Carey, L. *Sense: Helping Stroke Survivors Regain a Sense of Touch: A Manual and DVD for Therapists*; Florey Institute of Neuroscience and Mental Health: Melbourne, Australia, 2012.
56. Harris, P.A.; Taylor, R.; Thielke, R.; Payne, J.; Gonzalez, N.; Conde, J.G. Research electronic data capture (redcap)--A metadata-driven methodology and workflow process for providing translational research informatics support. *J. Biomed. Inf.* **2009**, *42*, 377–381. [CrossRef]
57. Turville, M.L.; Matyas, T.A.; Blennerhassett, J.M.; Carey, L.M. Initial severity of somatosensory impairment influences response to upper limb sensory retraining post-stroke. *NeuroRehabilitation* **2018**, *43*, 413–423. [CrossRef]
58. Szewczyk, Z.; Reeves, P.; Kingsland, M.; Doherty, E.; Elliott, E.; Wolfenden, L.; Tsang, T.W.; Dunlop, A.; Searles, A.; Wiggers, J. Cost, cost-consequence and cost-effectiveness evaluation of a practice change intervention to increase routine provision of antenatal care addressing maternal alcohol consumption. *Implement. Sci.* **2022**, *17*, 14. [CrossRef]
59. Husereau, D.; Drummond, M.; Petrou, S.; Carswell, C.; Moher, D.; Greenberg, D.; Augustovski, F.; Briggs, A.H.; Mauskopf, J.; Loder, E. Consolidated Health Economic Evaluation Reporting Standards (CHEERS) statement. *BMJ* **2013**, *346*, f1049. [CrossRef] [PubMed]
60. Husereau, D.; Drummond, M.; Augustovski, F.; de Bekker-Grob, E.; Briggs, A.H.; Carswell, C.; Caulley, L.; Chaiyakunapruk, N.; Greenberg, D.; Loder, E.; et al. Consolidated Health Economic Evaluation Reporting Standards 2022 (CHEERS 2022) statement: Updated reporting guidance for health economic evaluations. *BMC Med.* **2022**, *20*, 23. [CrossRef] [PubMed]
61. Searles, A.M.; Doran, C.; Attia, J.; Knight, D.; Wiggers, J.; Deeming, S.; Mattes, J.; Webb, B.; Hannan, S.; Ling, R.; et al. An approach to measuring and encouraging research translation and research impact. *Health Res. Policy Syst.* **2016**, *14*, 60. [CrossRef]
62. Teasell, R.; Meyer, M.J.; McClure, A.; Pan, C.; Murie-Fernandez, M.; Foley, N.; Salter, K. Stroke rehabilitation: An international perspective. *Top. Stroke Rehabil.* **2009**, *16*, 44–56. [CrossRef] [PubMed]
63. Cramer, S.C.; Wolf, S.L.; Adams, H.P.; Chen, D.; Dromerick, A.W.; Dunning, K.; Ellerbe, C.; Grande, A.; Janis, S.; Lansberg, M.G.; et al. Stroke recovery and rehabilitation research. *Stroke* **2017**, *48*, 813–819. [CrossRef]
64. World Health Organization. *The Need to Scale Up Rehabilitation*; World Health Organization: Geneva, Switzerland, 2017; Available online: https://apps.who.int/iris/handle/10665/331210 (accessed on 2 July 2023).
65. Walker, M.F.; Hoffmann, T.C.; Brady, M.C.; Dean, C.M.; Eng, J.J.; Farrin, A.J.; Felix, C.; Forster, A.; Langhorne, P.; Lynch, E.A.; et al. Improving the development, monitoring and reporting of stroke rehabilitation research: Consensus-based core recommendations from the stroke recovery and rehabilitation roundtable. *Int. J. Stroke* **2017**, *12*, 472–479. [CrossRef]
66. Ford, I.; Norrie, J. Pragmatic trials. *NEJM* **2016**, *375*, 454–463. [CrossRef]

healthcare

MDPI

Article

Improving Practice for Urinary Continence Care on Adult Acute Medical and Rehabilitation Wards: A Multi-Site, Co-Created Implementation Study

Dianne Lesley Marsden [1,2,3,*], Kerry Boyle [1,2,4], Jaclyn Birnie [5], Amanda Buzio [6], Joshua Dizon [3], Judith Dunne [7,8], Sandra Greensill [9], Kelvin Hill [10], Sandra Lever [11,12], Fiona Minett [13,14], Sally Ormond [1,15], Jodi Shipp [7,8], Jennifer Steel [16], Amanda Styles [5,17], John Wiggers [2,3,18], Dominique Ann-Michele Cadilhac [19,†] and Jed Duff [2,20,21,†] on behalf of the I-SCAMP Project Team

1 Hunter Stroke Service, Hunter New England Local Health District, New Lambton Heights, NSW 2305, Australia; kerry.boyle@health.nsw.gov.au (K.B.); sally.ormond@health.nsw.gov.au (S.O.)
2 College of Health, Medicine and Wellbeing, University of Newcastle, Callaghan, NSW 2308, Australia; john.wiggers@health.nsw.gov.au (J.W.); j2.duff@qut.edu.au (J.D.)
3 Hunter Medical Research Institute, New Lambton Heights, NSW 2305, Australia
4 Belmont Hospital, Hunter New England Local Health District, New Lambton Heights, NSW 2305, Australia
5 Armidale Hospital, Hunter New England Local Health District, Armidale, NSW 2350, Australia; jaclyn.birnie@health.nsw.gov.au (J.B.); amanda.styles@health.nsw.gov.au (A.S.)
6 Coffs Harbour Health Campus, Mid North Coast Local Health District, Coffs Harbour, NSW 2450, Australia
7 Rankin Park Centre, Hunter New England Local Health District, New Lambton Heights, NSW 2305, Australia; judith.dunne@health.nsw.gov.au (J.D.); jodi.shipp@health.nsw.gov.au (J.S.)
8 John Hunter Hospital, Hunter New England Local Health District, New Lambton Heights, NSW 2305, Australia
9 Rockhampton Hospital, Central Queensland Hospital and Health Service, Rockhampton, QLD 4700, Australia; sandra.greensill@health.qld.gov.au
10 Stroke Foundation, Melbourne, VIC 3000, Australia; khill@strokefoundation.org.au
11 Ryde Hospital, Northern Sydney Local Health District, Eastwood, NSW 2122, Australia
12 Susan Wakil School of Nursing and Midwifery, The University of Sydney, Sydney, NSW 2006, Australia
13 Manning Hospital, Hunter New England Local Health District, Taree, NSW 2430, Australia; fiona.minett@health.nsw.gov.au
14 Wingham Hospital, Hunter New England Local Health District, Wingham, NSW 2429, Australia
15 Calvary Mater Newcastle, Waratah, NSW 2298, Australia
16 Port Macquarie Hospital, Mid North Coast Local Health District, Port Macquarie, NSW 2444, Australia; jennifer.steel@health.nsw.gov.au
17 Tamworth Hospital, Hunter New England Local Health District, Tamworth, NSW 2340, Australia
18 Health Research and Translation, Hunter New England Local Health District, New Lambton Heights, NSW 2305, Australia
19 Stroke and Ageing Research, Faculty of Medicine, Nursing and Health Sciences, School of Clinical Sciences at Monash Health, Clayton, VIC 3168, Australia; dominique.cadilhac@monash.edu
20 School of Nursing and Centre for Healthcare Transformation, Queensland University of Technology, Brisbane, QLD 4001, Australia
21 Royal Brisbane and Womens Hospital, Queensland Health, Brisbane, QLD 4029, Australia
* Correspondence: di.marsden@health.nsw.gov.au; Tel.: +61-2-4922-3380
† Contributed equally as senior authors.

Abstract: Many adult inpatients experience urinary continence issues; however, we lack evidence on effective interventions for inpatient continence care. We conducted a before and after implementation study. We implemented our guideline-based intervention using strategies targeting identified barriers and evaluated the impact on urinary continence care provided by inpatient clinicians. Fifteen wards (acute = 3, rehabilitation = 7, acute and rehabilitation = 5) at 12 hospitals (metropolitan = 4, regional = 8) participated. We screened 2298 consecutive adult medical records for evidence of urinary continence symptoms over three 3-month periods: before implementation (T_0: n = 849), after the 6-month implementation period (T_1: n = 740), and after a 6-month maintenance period (T_2: n = 709). The records of symptomatic inpatients were audited for continence assessment, diagnosis, and management plans. All wards contributed data at T_0, and 11/15 wards contributed at T_1 and T_2 (dropouts due to COVID-19). Approximately 26% of stroke, 33% acute medical, and 50% of rehabilitation inpatients were symptomatic. The proportions of symptomatic patients (T_0: n = 283, T_1: n = 241, T_2: n = 256) receiving recommended care were: assessment T_0 = 38%, T_1 = 63%, T_2 = 68%; diagnosis T_0 = 30%, T_1 = 70%, T_2 = 71%; management plan T_0 = 7%, T_1 = 24%, T_2 = 24%. Overall, there were 4-fold increased odds for receiving assessments and management plans and 6-fold greater odds for diagnosis. These improvements were sustained at T_2. This intervention has improved inpatient continence care.

Keywords: urinary incontinence; lower urinary tract symptoms; inpatient; patient care planning; professional practice gaps; evidence-based practice; nursing process; hospital; implementation science; quality improvement

1. Introduction

Urinary continence issues include urinary incontinence (UI), defined as the involuntary loss of urine [1], and lower urinary tract symptoms (LUTS). LUTS is a term used to describe symptoms associated with urine storage such as urinary retention, bladder outlet obstruction, difficulty initiating a void, and frequency and urgency without incontinence [1]. These symptoms are common for the general population and for inpatients.

Despite up to 43% of adult inpatients experiencing urinary continence issues [2] and international recommendations for optimal urinary continence care [1,3–5], there is little reporting of effective interventions to systematically deliver urinary continence care to these inpatients [2,6]. Urinary continence care recommendations include that health services should have systems for assessment, diagnosis of UI/LUTS type, and management that are consistent with best evidence [1,4,5]. The recommendations emphasise shared decision making between clinicians, patients, and their carers. Providing guideline recommended UI/LUTS care is important, not only to minimise the direct effects of UI/LUTS but also to reduce often-associated complications. These include falls [7], urinary tract infections [8], breakdown of skin integrity [9,10], altered mood [11], and bladder overdistension [12]. Although UI/LUTS are often complex, with appropriate inpatient clinical care symptoms can be prevented, managed and even cured, and complications avoided.

As part of our formative research, in 2010 we developed a guideline-based intervention to assist stroke clinicians in three metropolitan inpatient rehabilitation units deliver evidence-based UI/LUTS care [13]. The team synthesised UI/LUTS guideline recommendations into the Stroke Continence Assessment and Management Plan (SCAMP) intervention. SCAMP presented clear, concise, and explicit recommendations for optimal inpatient continence care for people after stroke. The user-friendly intervention guided clinicians through conducting a urinary continence assessment, determining the type of UI/LUTS, and developing an individualised management plan for those with, or at risk of, symptoms. The plan was developed in conjunction with the patient or carer.

Although the details of the SCAMP invention were shared widely at Australian stroke conferences and forums, evidence–practice gaps in continence care for inpatients with stroke continued. Data from Australia in 2017–2018 indicated that a quarter of patients admitted with acute stroke [14] and 41% of inpatients undergoing stroke rehabilitation [15] had urinary incontinence. Of those people with symptoms, 18% in acute [14] and 52% in rehabilitation [15] had a documented urinary continence management plan. Acute stroke and rehabilitation nurses and clinician researchers recognised that the implementation, upscale, and spread of the SCAMP intervention had the potential to improve urinary continence practice not only for stroke but also for other patient populations.

The successful implementation, sustainability, and scalability of interventions is often very complex; however, they can be enhanced by using evidence-based theoretical approaches for implementation [16,17]. Different theoretical approaches can be used for different components of a study, including the design, the systematic planning and development, and the evaluation [16,18–20]. Theoretical approaches can be used to identify potential influencers on implementation and to select behaviour change strategies, such as audit and feedback, targeting these influencers [16,18–20]. Frameworks and models can assist researchers, managers, and clinicians to integrate best-practice care into practice through behaviour change [17]. To our knowledge, there are no previous studies that are informed by implementation frameworks and models that investigate the feasibility and effectiveness of a practice-change package to improve, then maintain inpatient UI/LUTS care.

The aim of this study was to determine if our practice-change package (implementation of our guideline-based SCAMP urinary continence care intervention) is effective and feasible for improving then maintaining urinary continence care in wards that admit acute and rehabilitation patients with various diagnoses in Australian metropolitan and regional hospitals.

The research questions were:

1.1. *Primary*

Does the implementation of our SCAMP urinary continence care intervention increase the proportion of inpatients with UI/LUTS who have an individually tailored UI/LUTS management plan?

1.2. *Secondary*

1. Does the implementation of our SCAMP urinary continence care intervention increase the proportion of:
    (a) Inpatients with UI/LUTS who have an assessment and diagnosis of type(s) of UI/LUTS?
    (b) Inpatients with UI/LUTS and their caregivers who are involved in the development of the management plan?
2. Does the implementation of our SCAMP urinary continence care intervention reduce rates of complications that can be associated with UI/LUTS?
3. What is the change in the above outcomes at 12 months after the implementation commenced?
4. Is the practice-change package feasible for wards to adopt, with good fidelity to the implementation strategies?

2. Materials and Methods

In this paper we report the changes in clinical practice observed at two time points following implementation of our intervention. The study protocol outlines the methods in detail [21]. The study was conducted as described in the protocol and is reported according to the Standards for Reporting Implementation Studies (StaRI) guidelines [22].

2.1. *Design*

We conducted a co-created, pragmatic, before and after implementation study on 15 wards at 12 hospitals in New South Wales and Queensland, Australia. Clinician representatives, predominantly nurses, from each ward were members of the project team from the outset. The study was conducted between December 2018 and February 2022. Inpatient clinicians were the target of the practice-change package. Data were collected via inpatient medical record audits over three 3-month periods: before and after the implementation period and after the maintenance period.

Frameworks

To enhance the success of our SCAMP intervention we used evidence-based theoretical approaches for implementation [16]. We used the:

- Knowledge to Action Framework as the process framework that guided development of the intervention ("knowledge creation" phase) and implementation ("action cycle" phase) [18].
- Theoretical Domains Framework to identify potential influencers on implementation (barriers and facilitators) and the accompanying COM-B model to identify strategies to address the key barriers [20]. The Theoretical Domains Framework is frequently used when assessing individual-level barriers and facilitators, rather than those at a systems level.
- RE-AIM Framework (reach (R), effectiveness (E), adoption (A), implementation (I), and maintenance (M)) [19] as it is a useful structure for evaluation implementation efforts. It can be used to evaluate program elements that may improve sustainable adoption and implementation.

The selection of frameworks was part of the co-design process. Clinician researcher members of the team found these highly cited frameworks relatable, as they reflected approaches previously used in ward-based quality activities. The selected frameworks were also felt to be complementary (Theoretical Domains Framework with the COM-B) [20], generalisable (because they had been used for other studies within the Australian context), and applicable to the wards participating in this study.

2.2. Sample

2.2.1. Participating Wards

This project was instigated by stroke and rehabilitation clinicians who identified UI/LUTS inpatient care needed to be improved on their ward for people after stroke and potentially for other inpatient populations. In Australia, people after stroke are cared for on wards that admit people with a range of conditions. This care may be provided in a stroke unit embedded on the ward or as part of the general ward population. Fifteen wards at 12 hospitals from four health service districts in Australia participated in this study. The 15 wards were a convenience sample of wards that admit acute and rehabilitation patients with various diagnoses in Australian metropolitan and regional hospitals. To be eligible to participate, key ward clinicians and nurse managers had to identify that UI/LUTS care was an issue for their ward and be willing to commit resources towards improving UI and LUTS care by implementing our SCAMP intervention. The characteristics of each ward are outlined in Table 1.

2.2.2. Target Population

The target population for the SCAMP practice-change package included clinicians, predominantly nurses, working in each participating ward. These clinicians were not trained continence or urology experts. There were no exclusion criteria for clinicians as the study was a service improvement initiative. Neither clinicians nor patients were consented to receive our practice-change package.

2.2.3. Included and Excluded Medical Records

The included adult inpatient populations varied between wards but included acute stroke, acute medicine, and/or rehabilitation for any condition, including stroke (Table 1). Consecutive records of inpatients aged 18 years and older who were discharged from participating wards were included. Patients screened as having no UI/LUTS symptoms or receiving end-of-life care were excluded.

Table 1. Characteristics of participating wards, and the effect of COVID-19 at each phase of the study on each ward.

Hospital/ Location	Ward Description	Included Population(s)	Before Implementation Data Collection	Implementation Period (6 Month)	After Implementation Data Collection	Maintenance Period (6 Months) and after Maintenance Data Collection
A Major city	20 bed rehab ward	Rehab	Completed	Completed	Completed	Completed while operating under COVID-19 conditions
	20 bed rehab ward	Rehab	Completed	Completed	Completed	Completed while operating under COVID-19 conditions
	28 bed rehab ward: 20 rehab, 8 neurological. 2 overflow beds	Acute stroke, acute medicine, rehab	Completed	Completed	Completed	Completed while operating under COVID-19 conditions
B Major city	12 bed ward: 8 general medicine, 4 Acute SU	Acute stroke, acute medicine	Completed	Completed	Completed: 1 of 3 months under COVID-19 conditions	Completed while operating under COVID-19 conditions
C Major city	30 bed ward: 26 general medicine, 4 comprehensive SU	Acute stroke, acute medicine	Completed	Completed	Completed: 2 of 3 months under COVID-19 conditions	Completed while operating under COVID-19 conditions
D Regional	32 bed ward: medical and rehab	Acute stroke, rehab	Completed	Completed	Completed: 2 of 3 months under COVID-19 conditions	Completed while operating under COVID-19 conditions
E Major city	32 bed rehab ward	Rehab	Completed	Completed	Study disbanded due to onset of COVID-19 with ward lockdown/closure and furloughing of staff.	
	28 bed general medical ward	Acute stroke, acute medicine	Completed	5 months completed	Study disbanded due to onset of COVID-19 with ward lockdown/closure and furloughing of staff	
F Regional	22 bed rehab ward	Rehab	Completed	Completed	Completed: 1 of 3 months under COVID-19 conditions	Completed while operating under COVID-19 conditions
G Regional	28 bed ward: 24 general medical, 4 Acute SU	Acute stroke	Completed	Completed	Completed: 2 of 3 months under COVID-19 conditions	Completed while operating under COVID-19 conditions
H Regional	16 bed rehab hospital	Rehab	Completed	Completed	Completed: 2 of 3 months under COVID-19 conditions	Completed while operating under COVID-19 conditions
I Regional	28 bed ward: 4 Acute SU, 8 MAU, 16 respiratory/cardiac	Acute stroke	Completed	Completed	Completed: 3 of 3 months under COVID-19 conditions	Completed while operating under COVID-19 conditions
J Regional	24 bed ward: 20 general rehab, 4 comprehensive SU	Acute stroke	Completed	Completed	Completed: 1 of 3 months under COVID-19 conditions	Completed while operating under COVID-19 conditions
K Regional	18 bed hospital: 8 rehab, 10 general medical	Rehab	Completed	Study disbanded due to onset of COVID-19		
L Regional	16 bed rehab ward	Rehab	Completed	Study disbanded due to onset of COVID-19		

SU = stroke unit, Rehab = rehabilitation, MAU = Medical Assessment Unit.

2.3. Data Collection

2.3.1. Medical Record Audit

The medical record audit tool used for data collection was developed for this study. It was based on questions in the Australian Stroke Foundation national audits [14,15,23] and the content of the SCAMP decision support tool. The audit tool was piloted, and all data collectors received education before its use.

Data were collected from medical records over three 3-month periods: before implementation (T_0), immediately after the 6-month implementation period (T_1), and immediately after the 6-month maintenance period (T_2). T_0 data collection for all wards occurred for patients discharged in August–October 2018. The start dates for each ward to commence implementation were staggered due to local competing interests at the time, including the NSW-wide rollout of the electronic medication chart. The first three sites commenced implementation in April 2019. Their T_1 and T_2 data collection was for patients discharged in November 2019–January 2020 and in May–July 2020, respectively. The 11th and final ward that completed all data collection undertook T_1 and T_2 data collection for patients discharged in February–April 2020 and in August–October 2020, respectively.

The medical records of inpatients were screened for the presence of UI/LUTS symptoms. To reduce selection bias, we screened consecutive records of patients discharged from each ward for each month of each 3-month data collection period. For the excluded records we extracted data for demographic characteristic information, continence status, and how this was determined.

The medical records of inpatients determined to have UI/LUTS were audited. Audits were performed for 15 records for each month or for all patients discharged during that month, whichever occurred first. Audits were conducted at each hospital by the project team members from that hospital and other local clinicians with legitimate access to the records, as per local health service requirements for patient privacy and confidentiality. An online medical record audit data dictionary was available. Information regarding assessment, diagnosis, management plans including the involvement of the patient and carer in the plan, and in-hospital complications were extracted. The in-hospital complications associated with UI/LUTS included were falls [7], urinary tract infections [8], issues with skin integrity [9,10], altered mood [11], and bladder overdistension [12]. Data were extracted into and managed using the REDCap electronic data capture tool [24] hosted on a secure server at the Hunter Medical Research Institute, NSW.

2.3.2. Feasibility and Fidelity Evaluation

To assess the feasibility and the fidelity of the implementation of the intervention on each ward a recording sheet was developed. Project team members from each ward self-reported if and how they adopted an intervention strategy.

2.4. Sample Size and Power Calculation

Our primary outcome was the change ($T_1 - T_0$) in the proportion of inpatients who had an individually tailored UI/LUTS management plan. It was determined that 15 consecutive medical record audits per ward per month (i.e., pooled sample of 675 audits anticipated per data collection period) would provide >90% power to detect a 10% absolute increase (from before intervention) in the proportion of symptomatic patients with a UI/LUTS management plan (type 1 error rate of 5%). This calculation conservatively assumed 20% of patients in acute and 50% in rehabilitation wards have a plan before intervention (based on Australian Stroke Foundation national audit results for included wards) [14,15].

2.5. Study Intervention—Practice-Change Package

Our practice-change package was the SCAMP intervention that we implemented using theoretically informed implementation strategies. The practice-change package was designed to support inpatient clinicians, predominantly nurses but including educators and managers, to deliver guideline-recommended UI/LUTS care on their ward.

2.5.1. SCAMP Intervention

In 2018 our team revised the three components of SCAMP with nursing, allied health and medical experts from stroke, continence, rehabilitation, and urology to ensure they met current best-evidenced and guideline-recommended UI/LUTS care for most adult inpatient medical and rehabilitation populations. The intervention was renamed the Structured urinary Continence Assessment and Management Plan to reflect the inclusiveness of inpatient populations beyond stroke while retaining the SCAMP acronym.

The SCAMP intervention consisted of:

a. The 4-page Structured urinary Continence Assessment and Management Plan (SCAMP) decision support tool, which can be downloaded from within each of the web-based modules below. This tool guides clinicians through conducting a urinary continence assessment, determining the type of UI/LUTS, and developing an individualised management plan for those with or at risk of symptoms in conjunction with the patient or carer.
b. The associated Clinical Practice Guideline.
c. Eight web-based education modules and a local module on how to use the SCAMP decision support tool (PowerPoint presentation with voice-over). The web-based modules cover information on normal bladder function, why continence is an issue after stroke, and six common inpatient UI and LUTS types. They are hosted on the Stroke Foundation website https://informme.org.au/modules/urinary-continence-and-stroke (accessed on 17 April 2023).

2.5.2. Implementation Strategies

The key barriers identified before implementation and strategies selected with mapping to the COM-B domains are shown in Table 2. Strategies were selected to overcome the barriers identified from three sources. Firstly, we used research of known barriers to clinicians implementing continence guideline recommendations [25]. Secondly, we used the results of our before-implementation clinician questionnaire that was informed by the Theoretical Domains Framework [20], and thirdly the ward-specific barriers that local teams identified using the Behaviour Identification and Mitigation tool [26]. For this tool, local teams asked nursing, allied health, and medical clinicians about the SCAMP decision support tool and guideline. They walked through the process to simulate real-ward circumstances and to identify the barriers to implementation. From their data, each team summarised and prioritised their barriers, then developed a local action plan focused on overcoming the barriers. The practice-change package was adapted by each ward to suit their local context. This included the mode of delivery, dose, and frequency of each local intervention strategy.

2.6. Data Analysis

The T_0, T_1, and T_2 group characteristics and demographics results are presented with descriptive statistics. Categorical data are presented as count (%) or median (interquartile range; IQR) if continuous. All results are presented as aggregated summary measures. Across-period differences in patient characteristics were examined using the Kruskal–Wallis test for continuous variables and the chi-squared test for categorical variables.

Table 2. The key identified barriers and implementation strategies mapped to the COM-B model and the proportion of the 13 wards that reached the implementation phase that adopted the strategy.

Key Barriers	COM-B Model	Strategy	Strategy Adopted by Ward [n/13 (%)]
Ward leads and champions have limited knowledge and experience in conducting implementation projects	Capability—Physical and Psychological	Identify and prepare—2 implementation workshops conducted	13 (100%)
	Motivation—Reflective and Automatic	Monthly virtual community of practice meetings, out of session phone calls, and emails with project leads	13 (100%)
- UI/LUTS usually a comorbidity, not the main reason for admission so may be overlooked - Clinicians not aware of UI/LUTS evidence–practice gap - Need to change local processes to adopt formalised UI/LUTS care	Motivation—Reflective Capability—Psychological	Audit and feedback of before-implementation results to raise awareness/highlight evidence–practice gap—via ward meetings, emails	13 (100%)
	Motivation—Reflective	Conduct BIM tool to identify local barriers and facilitators	13 (100%)
	Opportunity—Physical	Develop local action plan	12 (92%)
	Motivation—Reflective Opportunity—Social	Audit and feedback—spot check audits to determine what part of the process performed well and by who and what can be improved. Feedback via safety huddles, ward meetings, emails	13 (100%)
	Opportunity—Physical	SCAMP decision support tool embedded into routine practice	13 (100%)
	Capability—Physical	Intensive education and upskilling phase to achieve a critical mass prior to launch	13 (100%)
	Motivation—Automatic	Launch/promotional activities	12 (92%)
- Ward clinicians are not experts in continence, with no/little access to community-based continence nurses - Clinicians perceive they lack knowledge, skills, and confidence in continence care, particularly diagnosis and management plans	Capability—Psychological	Education (meetings, web-based modules) to increase knowledge UI/LUTS types, using SCAMP tool	13 (100%)
	Capability—Physical	Upskilling 1:1 with ward champion/lead	13 (100%)
	Capability—PhysicalMotivation—Reflective	Local champions identified and trained as resource people	12 (92%)
	Opportunity—Physical	Local champions available throughout implementation	4 (31%)
	Motivation—Automatic	Recognition from manager/local project lead of individual staff who did well	11 (85%)
Clinicians need to remember to use SCAMP tool	Capability—Psychological	Written reminders—including posters displayed in ward/emails/SCAMP resource folder	13 (100%)
	Opportunity—Physical	Verbal reminders—including safety huddles/1:1s/ward meetings	13 (100%)
Maintaining improvements	Capability—Psychological	SCAMP education embedded into onboarding of new nursing staff	13 (100%)
	Motivation—Reflective	Spot check audit and feedback—via safety huddles, ward meetings, emails	10/11 (91%) *

* Strategy used during maintenance phase, therefore no data for the two wards that disbanded the study after the implementation phase due to the effect of the onset of COVID-19 on the two wards (Table 1).

Groups were compared with respect to change, from T_0 to T_1 and T_2 using mixed effects logistic regression models. Demographic characteristics that were found to be significantly different across study periods (i.e., Kruskal–Wallis or chi-squared $p < 0.05$) were treated as confounders and included in the regression models as adjusting covariates. This resulted in the mixed effects logistic models having a fixed effect for study period, inpatient age, and inpatient population type, as well as a random intercept for ward. The planned regression analyses were intention-to-treat and included all available data from all wards in all time-points, regardless of participation completeness throughout the study periods. A posteriori per-protocol analyses were also performed, wherein only the included observations from the wards that had complete participation throughout the study was performed to examine the effect of the practice-change package under full uptake conditions. The a posteriori per-protocol analysis was performed using a mixed effects logistic regression with them same model specifications as above. The estimates of each mixed logistic model are presented as odds ratios (OR) with 95% confidence intervals (CI) and p-values. Process data are reported as the proportion of wards that adopted an implementation strategy.

Statistical analyses were programmed using SAS v9.4 (SAS Institute, Cary, NC, USA). A priori, $p < 0.05$ was used to indicate statistical significance.

3. Results

3.1. Ward Participation

All 15 wards completed the before-implementation audit. The onset of the COVID-19 pandemic in March 2020 affected the conduct of this study, as shown in Table 1. Four wards, including three rehabilitation wards, had to withdraw; two wards were unable to commence implementation; one ward almost completed; and one had just completed implementation before they were closed. Eleven wards contributed data to the after-implementation and maintenance audits.

3.2. Characteristics of the Inpatients Whose Medical Records Were Observed

3.2.1. Screening

The medical records of 2298 inpatients were screened for the study. The age of the inpatients screened were consistent over the three data collection periods: median years (Q1, Q3) T_0 = 78 (68, 86), T_1 = 76 (65, 84), and T_2 = 76 (65, 84). For the records screened at each data collection period, approximately 52% were female, 4% identified as Aboriginal or Torres Strait Islander, 70% were in a large city hospital, and 30% were in a regional hospital. The proportion of inpatients with UI/LUTS of those screened during each data collection period were T_0 = 33% (283/849), T_1 = 33% (241/740), and T_2 = 36% (256/709). The proportions with UI/LUTS of those screened varied by patient population: acute stroke T_0 = 30% (58/191), T_1 = 24% (44/194), and T_2 = 23% (44/190); acute medicine T_0 = 26% (92/359), T_1 = 33% (125/385), and T_2 = 33% (113/342); rehabilitation T_0 = 44% (133/299), T_1 = 43% (69/161), and T_2 = 56% (99/177). Inpatients with UI/LUTs compared with those without were 5–8 years older and more likely to be female.

For the inpatients screened as not having UI/LUTS, the method of determining their continence status changed over the three study periods. The proportion who had a documented continence assessment increased from T_0 = 8% (43/566) to T_1 = 44% (220/499) and T_2 = 40% (183/453). For the remainder of the records the auditors had to determine the continence status from the progress notes.

3.2.2. Audits

From the medical record screening, 34% of inpatients were deemed to have UI/LUTS, and their records were audited (inpatients with UI/LUTS = 780: T_0 = 283, T_1 = 241, T_2 = 256). The demographic characteristics for these inpatients, and the statistical significance of the difference in distributions of these characteristics between study periods are shown in

Table 3. Patient age at admission and inpatient population type were identified as potential confounders and were included as adjusting covariates in the regression models.

Table 3. Demographic characteristics of patients deemed to have UI/LUTS across study periods and indicating any significant difference in the distribution of the characteristic across study periods.

Demographic Characteristic		Before Implementation (n = 283)	After Implementation (n = 214)	Maintenance (n = 232)	*p*-Value
Age at admission (years)	Median (Q1, Q3)	83 (72, 88)	81 (69, 87)	78 (70, 85)	0.004 **
Age group	18–64	36 (13%)	37 (17%)	40 (17%)	0.020 **
	65–74	47 (17%)	42 (20%)	46 (20%)	
	75–84	83 (29%)	65 (30%)	86 (37%)	
	85+	117 (41%)	70 (33%)	60 (26%)	
Sex	Female	161 (57%)	119 (56%)	134 (58%)	0.631
	Male	122 (43%)	93 (44%)	97 (42%)	
	Other	0	1 (0.5%)	0	
Indigenous status *	Indigenous	3 (1.1%)	9 (4.2%)	9 (3.9%)	0.065
Location of hospital	Large city	199 (70%)	164 (77%)	163 (70%)	0.220
	Regional	84 (30%)	50 (23%)	69 (30%)	
Patient population	Acute stroke	58 (20%)	41 (19%)	38 (16%)	0.003 **
	Acute Medical	92 (33%)	104 (49%)	95 (41%)	
	Rehabilitation	133 (47%)	69 (32%)	99 (43%)	

* Indigenous status: inpatient self-identified as Aboriginal and/or Torres Strait Islander. ** $p < 0.05$.

3.3. Clinical Care Delivery Outcomes

Changes in clinical practice and the proportions of in-hospital complications associated with UI/LUTS are presented in Table 4, Figure 1, and described below. The results of the intention-to-treat and per protocol analyses were very similar and with identical conclusions; therefore, only the intention-to-treat results are presented.

Implementation of our practice-change package resulted in substantial and statistically significant improvements in continence care. The adjusted odds ratios were approximately 4-fold higher after implementation for receiving a continence assessment [OR (95% CI): 4.4 (2.7–7.0)] or management plan [OR (95% CI): 4.3 (2.3–7.9)]. Receiving a diagnosis of UI/LUTS type(s) was approximately 6-fold higher [OR (95% CI): 6.5 (4.1–10.2)]. The improvements for each of these practice components was sustained from after implementation to the maintenance period.

The proportion of inpatients who received all three components (assessment, diagnosis, and management plan) rose by 18%, from 3% (9/283) before implementation to 21% (44/214) after implementation and 21% (49/232) during the maintenance period. The documented involvement of inpatients or carers in the development of the management plan was low and unchanged across the three timeframes.

3.4. Patient Complication Outcomes

There was no statistically significant difference in the proportion of inpatients with complications associated with UI/LUTS across the three study periods (range: falls 7–8%; urinary tract infections 12–17%; issues with skin integrity 2–4%; altered mood 4–9%; and bladder overdistension 5–8%). A third of inpatients in each of the three audit periods experienced one or more complication often related to UI/LUTS (Figure 1).

Table 4. Adjusted mixed logistic regression results for aspects of care and complications: intention-to-treat analyses.

Outcome	Study Period Comparison	Intention-to-Treat Analysis *		
		OR (95% CI)	*p*-Value	N in Model
Inpatient assessed for UI/LUTS	After implementation vs. Before implementation	4.38 (2.73, 7.03)	<0.001	721
	Maintenance vs. Before implementation	4.70 (2.94, 7.52)	<0.001	
	Maintenance vs. After implementation	1.07 (0.70, 1.65)	0.745	
Inpatient received diagnosis of UI/LUTS type	After implementation vs. Before implementation	6.49 (4.13, 10.20)	<0.001	729
	Maintenance vs. Before implementation	6.01 (3.82, 9.48)	<0.001	
	Maintenance vs. After implementation	0.93 (0.60, 1.42)	0.726	
Inpatient received UI/LUTS management plan	After implementation vs. Before implementation	4.29 (2.32, 7.94)	<0.001	712
	Maintenance vs. Before implementation	4.03 (2.16, 7.50)	<0.001	
	Maintenance vs. After implementation	0.94 (0.59, 1.49)	0.788	
In-hospital complication often associated with UI/LUTS	After implementation vs. Before implementation	1.42 (0.93, 2.16)	0.106	729
	Maintenance vs. Before implementation	1.48 (0.98, 2.22)	0.061	
	Maintenance vs. After implementation	1.04 (0.69, 1.57)	0.841	
Inpatient involved in the development of UI/LUTS management plan	After implementation vs. Before implementation	0.95 (0.29, 3.08)	0.925	127
	Maintenance vs. Before implementation	0.48 (0.15, 1.57)	0.224	
	Maintenance vs. After implementation	0.51 (0.21, 1.21)	0.125	
Carer involved in the development of management plan	After implementation vs. Before implementation	1.41 (0.32, 6.22)	0.646	127
	Maintenance vs. Before implementation	1.45 (0.34, 6.22)	0.612	
	Maintenance vs. After implementation	1.03 (0.37, 2.84)	0.956	

* Adjusted for patient age and patient population (acute stroke, acute medicine, or rehabilitation).

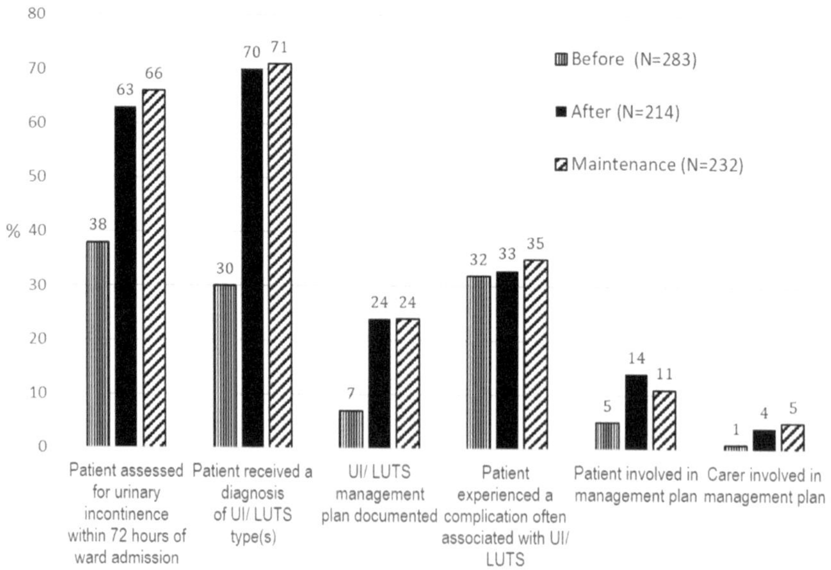

Figure 1. Proportion (%) of inpatients receiving components of UI/LUTS care and experiencing one or more complications often associated with UI/LUTS across the three study periods.

3.5. Feasibility and Fidelity Evaluation

It was feasible for all 13 wards that proceeded to implementation to adopt the practice-change package. The package appears scalable, as the wards included acute (n = 3), rehabilitation (n = 5), and acute and rehabilitation (n = 5) wards in four metropolitan and six regional hospitals. The proportion of wards that adopted each implementation strategy are shown in Table 2. Of the 18 strategies, 12 (67%) were adopted by 100% of wards and 5 (28%) were adopted by 85–92% of wards. Although 92% of the wards started with champions being trained and assigned, this dropped to 31% throughout the implementation phase. This was due to clinicians being on leave, resignations, and changes in personnel in specified roles, such as clinical nurse educators.

4. Discussion

In this study we demonstrated a reduction in the evidence–practice gap in UI/LUTS care following the implementation of our SCAMP intervention that targeted inpatient clinicians. After implementation, the proportion of inpatients with UI/LUTS receiving a UI/LUTS assessment, diagnosis of UI/LUTS type(s), and a management plan increased substantially. These improvements were maintained 6-months later, despite the onset of COVID-19 and the subsequent need for wards to make substantial changes in how they functioned. All thirteen wards that completed the implementation phase were able to adopt the SCAMP practice-change package with good fidelity.

Our findings confirm those of other studies that UI/LUTS is commonly experienced by inpatients but there is an evidence–practice gap regarding UI/LUTS care. Across our three medical record audits, 23–30% of acute stroke, 26–33% of acute medical, and 43 to 56% of patients undergoing rehabilitation were deemed to have UI/LUTS. This is in keeping with the studies reviewed by Ostaszkiewicz et al. [2]. These researchers identified that inpatient UI/LUTS prevalence ranged from 11 to 43% across a range of ward types including intensive care, surgical, medical, rehabilitation, and geriatrics. The low proportion of inpatients with UI/LUTS receiving a UI/LUTS assessment (38%), diagnosis of type (30%), and management plans (7%) observed in our before-implementation audit are similar to those found in other studies. In a study by Zurcher et al. (2011), 51% (41/78) of elderly inpatients screened positive for urinary incontinence [27]. However, of these patients with UI, only 24% (10/41) had this documented in their medical record and 5% (2/41) had a documented diagnosis of incontinence type [27]. In a study by Trad et al. (2019), their audit of 100 inpatient medical records for two surgical and two medical wards indicated that 87% of patients had a urinary continence assessment; however, only 14% had a diagnosis of type and 15% received conservative interventions that were tailored to their specific type of incontinence [28].

In the current study we were able to improve, then maintain the proportion of inpatients with UI/LUTS who received three key recommended elements of inpatient urinary continence care. The improvement from before to after implementation in receiving a UI/LUTS assessment (25%), diagnosis of type(s) (40%), and receiving a management plan (17%) are comparatively large improvements for implementation studies. Behaviour change improvements of between 4% and 12% have been reported for multifaceted interventions [29]. The improvements we saw may be due to our multifaceted intervention targeting the identified barriers and facilitators. Education programs alone regarding urinary incontinence for nurses have been shown to improve knowledge but have had mixed effects on attitudes and practice [30].

Our study is one of two studies that we have identified that addresses inpatient UI/LUTS care through theoretically informed implementation and the only one to include a maintenance period. This is despite UI/LUTS being common for inpatients, with well-recognised and considerable evidence–practice gaps in inpatient continence care. This deficit of studies for inpatient UI/LUTS care is reflected in two recent reviews investigating randomised controlled [31,32] and before–after [31] implementation studies of nursing practice. Only two studies addressing urinary continence practice were included in these reviews: one conducted in an outpatient setting [31,32] and one in a nursing home [32]. Similarly to our study, the inpatient continence care implementation study conducted by Trad et al. included a decision tool to guide assessment and management, and education was part of their intervention [28]. These strategies aimed to address their identified barrier of clinician lack of knowledge in continence care. Although the Trad et al. study showed substantial improvement from before to after implementation in assessment (87% to 99%), diagnosis (14% to 75%), and management plans (24 to 74%), there was no subsequent evaluation to determine if these improvements were maintained.

Unfortunately, the proportion of patients with documented involvement of the carer and patient in management planning was low (≤5%) and remained unchanged. This low level of engagement was similar to the study by Trad et al., where no patients received education about incontinence management before implementation and only 5% did after implementation [28]. Although the SCAMP decision tool has a prompt to include the patient and carer in the management plan and to provide them with education, our practice-change package did not include specific training for clinicians for this. The Australian National Safety and Quality Health Service Standards recommend hospitals provide education, training, and resources to equip clinicians to partner with patients in their care [33]. This may be specifically required for UI/LUTS as this can be a sensitive and often taboo topic for patients and clinicians.

The proportion of inpatients experiencing complications did not change, with approximately one third of inpatients experiencing one or more complications that are often associated with UI/LUTS. In our study, urinary tract infections and falls were the most common complications. Urinary tract infections were experienced by 12–17% of inpatients, which is much higher than the 2% who experienced a hospital-acquired urinary tract infection reported by Mitchell et al. [34]. The 8% of patients who had a fall is similar to the 10% identified in general medicine wards in five urban hospitals in Canada [35]. Reducing complications is important to reduce excess morbidity, mortality, and healthcare expenditure. Further investigation is required to determine if our practice-change package can influence complication rates.

Our practice-change package was feasible to adopt for all 13 wards that completed five or more months of the 6-month implementation phase. There was a high level of fidelity for most implementation strategies. This success is likely due to our co-creation approach. From the outset, project leads and champions (predominantly nurses) from each ward, experts in continence and implementation, clinician researchers, and academic nurse researchers were included on the team. End-user members ensured our practice-change package was not only best evidenced but clinically relevant and applicable. Project leads and champions led the practice change on their wards. The lack of a continence nurse within any of the hospitals was recognised from the outset as a barrier to supporting the practice change. This required the upskilling of ward project leads and nurse champions, not only in implementation and conducting the research but also in UI/LUTS care. The monthly virtual team meetings functioned to progress the research and formed a community of practice for the ward leads and champions. The members were able to share their successes, challenges, and locally tailored strategies, in addition to being upskilled in conducting research. Anecdotally, the ward-based project team members reported that although the research was challenging due to time and resource constraints, it was very rewarding to see it succeed and to have the opportunity for personal and professional growth. These themes are similar to those identified by Trad et al. in their inpatient continence care study [28].

4.1. Strengths and Limitations

This study has several strengths. We have reported our findings according to the Standards for Reporting Implementation Studies (StaRI) [22] to facilitate replication by other researchers. To determine if any improvements were sustained, we included a maintenance period evaluation. Our practice-change package was tested in metropolitan and regional hospitals and on acute and rehabilitation wards for three patient groups: acute stroke, acute medical, and rehabilitation. This may increase the generalisability and potential scalability of the package. SCAMP may also be applicable to other health conditions and health care settings where providing optimal UI/LUTS care is challenging. To assist other wards improve UI/LUTS care, elements of the intervention (the 4-page Structured urinary Continence Assessment and Management Plan (SCAMP) decision support tool and eight web-based education modules) are freely available on the Stroke Foundation website [https://informme.org.au/modules/urinary-continence-and-stroke (accessed on 17 April 2023)].

There are limitations to this study. We used a before and after design using retrospective medical record audits of consecutive records. A limitation of this study design is that the observed differences cannot be directly attributed to the intervention. Data were extracted by clinicians for their own ward, which has the potential for response bias. However, the use of self-reported, retrospective clinical audits is conventional practice for improvement activities. This potential bias could be mitigated in future research by using blinded assessors. This study was undertaken with only a small amount of research funding (less than AUD 90,000) and required considerable in-kind support from the staff and managers of the participating wards. With this understanding, local clinicians and managers self-selected their ward to participate and the population type to be included in the study. This may limit the generalisability due to potential selection bias. The findings may overestimate the potential effect for wards that admit a low proportion of patients who experience UI/LUTS. Although we describe the implementation strategies and self-reported fidelity, we were not resourced to investigate fully the mode of delivery, dose, and frequencies of each intervention strategy undertaken on each ward. This is a recognised challenge of implementation studies [36].

4.2. Recommendations for Further Research

Given the success of this study, further investigations are warranted through larger hybrid design implementation studies using more robust randomised controlled designs, such as step-wedge or cluster randomised controlled trials. These trials could test: the effectiveness by hospital location and type of patient population; the mode of delivery, dose, and frequencies of each intervention strategy; the effect on patient-level outcomes, including continence status, type, co-morbidities, quality of life, and severity of any complications; and scalability and spread. An analysis of the potential economic implications (cost and consequences) for hospitals implementing the SCAMP practice-change package is underway. Our practice-change package was developed from a Western medicine perspective. Further research is required to determine how urinary continence care can be addressed through a cultural lens to ensure we deliver culturally safe and appropriate care for First Nations peoples.

5. Conclusions

UI/LUTS is commonly experienced by inpatients, and there is a considerable evidence–practice gap in inpatient continence care. We designed our SCAMP practice-change package for ward clinicians, particularly nurses, who were not trained continence experts to deliver UI/LUTS-guideline-recommended care as part of their usual care. The package was adopted with good fidelity across acute and rehabilitation wards in metropolitan and regional hospitals. Although we improved assessment, diagnosis, and management by what would be considered a good outcome in an intervention study, a large proportion of inpatients still did not receive guideline-recommended care and complication rates did not improve. Further work should be conducted to reduce this evidence–practice gap.

Author Contributions: Conceptualization, D.L.M., K.B., J.W., D.A.-M.C. and J.D. (Jed Duff); Methodology, D.L.M., K.B., J.B., A.B., J.D. (Judith Dunne), S.G., K.H., S.L., F.M., S.O., J.S. (Jodi Shipp), J.S. (Jennifer Steel), A.S., D.A.-M.C. and J.D. (Jed Duff); Validation, D.A.-M.C.; Formal analysis, D.L.M., J.D. (Joshua Dizon), D.A.-M.C. and J.D. (Jed Duff); Investigation, D.L.M., K.B., J.B., A.B., J.D. (Judith Dunne), S.G., S.L., F.M., S.O., J.S. (Jodi Shipp), J.S. (Jennifer Steel) and A.S.; Resources,

D.L.M., K.B. and K.H.; Data curation, D.L.M., K.B. and J.D. (Joshua Dizon); Writing—original draft, D.L.M., D.A.-M.C. and J.D. (Jed Duff); Writing—review and editing, D.L.M., K.B., J.B., A.B., J.D. (Joshua Dizon), J.D. (Judith Dunne), S.G., S.L., F.M., S.O., J.S. (Jodi Shipp), J.S. (Jennifer Steel), A.S., J.W., D.A.-M.C. and J.D. (Jed Duff); Visualization, D.L.M., J.D. (Joshua Dizon), K.H., D.A.-M.C. and J.D. (Jed Duff); Supervision, D.L.M.; Project administration, D.L.M. and K.B.; Funding acquisition, D.L.M., D.A.-M.C. and J.D. (Jed Duff). All authors have read and agreed to the published version of the manuscript.

Funding: This research was supported by the Hunter Stroke Service (Hunter New England Local Health District). The project received small project grants from: the Hunter New England Local Health District Improvement Grant and statistical support grant, NSW Agency for Clinical Innovation Research Grant Scheme, Priority Research Centre for Stroke and Brain Injury (University of Newcastle), and NSW Nursing and Midwifery Strategy Reserve Funding. The funders had no role in the design of the study; in the collection, analyses, or interpretation of data; in the writing of the manuscript; or in the decision to publish the results.

Institutional Review Board Statement: The study was conducted in accordance with the Declaration of Helsinki and approved by the Hunter New England Human Research Ethics Committee (HNEHREC Reference No: 2019/ETH03881 29 October 2018).

Informed Consent Statement: Patient consent was waived as this study involved retrospective audits of routinely collected data.

Data Availability Statement: The data presented in this study are available on request from the corresponding author. The data are not publicly available as they were collected via medical record audit of data routinely collected in hospital. Patients whose records were audited have not consented to data sharing.

Acknowledgments: We would like to acknowledge and pay tribute to our colleague and friend Louise-Anne Jordan who sadly passed away in November 2019. Louise led the initial development of the SCAMP intervention in 2008-10 and played an integral part in the study protocol. We would like to acknowledge the non-author contributors to the I-SCAMP Project Team: *Support with conducting the project:* Annalese Johnson, Michael Pollack *Assistance with data collection, and implementation of the intervention:* Emily Saul, Michelle Coad, Jeremy Mulder, Soo Cho, Virginia Mapurazi, Helen Wheat, Helen King *Assistance with study design and for overseeing the statistical analysis:* Hunter Medical Research Institute- Christopher Oldmeadow. We would also thank for: *Assistance with data collection:* Janelle Turton, Tanya Gibson, Tracey Power, Chantelle Phee, Jiny James, Esta Luo, Minyi Luo, Samantha Hoskins, Colette Sanctuary, Joseph Cheah, Erin Saville, Kim Parrey, Abbey Klingbiel, Andrea Thatcher, Amanda Pearson, Veena Venu, Emma McCartney, Fiona Bioletti, Shae Miller, Catherine Williams. *Assistance with developing the data extraction tool in REDcap*: Hunter Stroke Service—Monique Hourn, Hunter Medical Research Institute—Alix Hall.

Conflicts of Interest: Authors D.L.M., K.B., J.B., A.B., J.D. (Judith Dunne), F.M., S.O., M.P., J.S. (Jodi Shipp), S.L., J.S. (Jennifer Steel), A.S., and J.W. are employees of NSW Health (New South Wales, Australia). S.G. is an employee of Queensland Health (Queensland Australia). K.H. is an employee of the Stroke Foundation. J.D. (Joshua Dizon) is an employee of the Hunter Medical Research Institute. J.D. (Jed Duff) is an employee of Queensland University of Technology and worked for the University of Newcastle during the study, where he now is a conjoint professor. D.A.-M.C. receives a Senior Research Fellowship from the National Health and Medical Research Council (1154273).

References

1. Abrams, P.; Cardozo, L.; Wagg, A.; Wein, A. *Incontinence*, 6th ed.; International Continence Society (ICS) & International Consultation on Urological Diseases (ICUD): Tokyo, Japan, 2017.
2. Ostaszkiewicz, J.; O'Connell, B.; Millar, L. Incontinence: Managed or mismanaged in hospital settings? *Int. J. Nurs. Pract.* **2008**, *14*, 495–502. [CrossRef] [PubMed]
3. Nambiar, A.K.; Bosch, R.; Cruz, F.; Lemack, G.E.; Thiruchelvam, N.; Tubaro, A.; Bedretdinova, D.A.; Ambuhl, D.; Farag, F.; Lombardo, R.; et al. EAU Guidelines on Assessment and Nonsurgical Management of Urinary Incontinence. *Eur. Urol.* **2018**, *73*, 596–609. [CrossRef] [PubMed]
4. Australian Commission on Safety and Quality in Health Care. *Hospital-Acquired Complications Information Kit*; ACSQHC: Sydney, Austrilia, 2018.

5. Stroke Foundation. Clinical Guidelines for Stroke Management. 2022. Available online: https://informme.org.au/en/Guidelines/Clinical-Guidelines-for-Stroke-Management (accessed on 12 December 2022).
6. Slark, J.; Stewart, L. Advances in nursing assessment and management of urinary incontinence for stroke survivors. *Br. J. Neurosci. Nurs.* **2017**, *13*, S16–S23. [CrossRef]
7. Moon, S.; Chung, H.S.; Kim, Y.J.; Kim, S.J.; Kwon, O.; Lee, Y.G.; Yu, J.M.; Cho, S.T. The impact of urinary incontinence on falls: A systematic review and meta-analysis. *PLoS ONE* **2021**, *16*, e0251711, PMCID:PMC8133449. [CrossRef] [PubMed]
8. Storme, O.; Tiran Saucedo, J.; Garcia-Mora, A.; Dehesa-Davila, M.; Naber, K.G. Risk factors and predisposing conditions for urinary tract infection. *Ther. Adv. Urol.* **2019**, *11*, 1756287218814382, PMCID:PMC6502981. [CrossRef] [PubMed]
9. Lachenbruch, C.; Ribble, D.; Emmons, K.; VanGilder, C. Pressure Ulcer Risk in the Incontinent Patient: Analysis of Incontinence and Hospital-Acquired Pressure Ulcers From the International Pressure Ulcer Prevalence Survey. *J. Wound Ostomy Cont. Nurs.* **2016**, *43*, 235–241. [CrossRef] [PubMed]
10. Barakat-Johnson, M.; Barnett, C.; Lai, M.; Wand, T.; White, K. Incontinence, Incontinence-Associated Dermatitis, and Pressure Injuries in a Health District in Australia: A Mixed-Methods Study. *J. Wound Ostomy Cont. Nurs.* **2018**, *45*, 349–355. [CrossRef] [PubMed]
11. Avery, J.C.; Stocks, N.P.; Duggan, P.; Braunack-Mayer, A.J.; Taylor, A.W.; Goldney, R.D.; MacLennan, A.H. Identifying the quality of life effects of urinary incontinence with depression in an Australian population. *BMC Urol.* **2013**, *13*, 11. [CrossRef]
12. Ersoz, M.; Tunc, H.; Akyuz, M.; Ozel, S. Bladder storage and emptying disorder frequencies in hemorrhagic and ischemic stroke patients with bladder dysfunction. *Cereb. Dis.* **2005**, *20*, 395–399. [CrossRef] [PubMed]
13. Jordan, L.-A.; Quain, D.; Marsden, D.; White, J.; Bullen, K.; Wright, S.; Galvin, R.; Dunne, J.; Baines, H. Managing urinary incontinence following stroke: Can we do better? *HNE Handover for Nurses and Midwives.* **2011**, *4*, 4–8. Available online: https://pdfs.semanticscholar.org/3987/b000f0aae5bdfbbc613ab71639b4e821f4c1.pdf?_ga=2.48050855.1878501815.591848991-288409287.571190931 (accessed on 28 March 2018).
14. Stroke Foundation. National Stroke Audit Acute Services Report 2017. 2017. Available online: https://informme.org.au/en/stroke-data/Acute-audits (accessed on 4 April 2018).
15. Stroke Foundation. National Stroke Audit Rehabiliation Services Report 2018. 2018. Available online: https://informme.org.au/stroke-data/Rehabilitation-audits (accessed on 12 March 2019).
16. Damschroder, L.J. Clarity out of chaos: Use of theory in implementation research. *Psychiatry Res.* **2019**, *283*, 112461. [CrossRef] [PubMed]
17. Hassett, L.; Wolfenden, L. Research Note: Designing implementation trials in physiotherapy. *J. Physiother.* **2022**, *68*, 210–212. [CrossRef] [PubMed]
18. Graham, I.D.; Logan, J.; Harrison, M.B.; Straus, S.E.; Tetroe, J.; Caswell, W.; Robinson, N. Lost in knowledge translation: Time for a map? *J. Contin. Educ. Health Prof.* **2006**, *26*, 13–24. [CrossRef] [PubMed]
19. Glasgow, R.E.; Vogt, T.M.; Boles, S.M. Evaluating the public health impact of health promotion interventions: The RE-AIM framework. *Am. J. Public Health* **1999**, *89*, 1322–1327, PMCID:PMC1508772. [CrossRef] [PubMed]
20. Atkins, L.; Francis, J.; Islam, R.; O'Connor, D.; Patey, A.; Ivers, N.; Foy, R.; Duncan, E.M.; Colquhoun, H.; Grimshaw, J.M.; et al. A guide to using the Theoretical Domains Framework of behaviour change to investigate implementation problems. *Implement Sci.* **2017**, *12*, 77, PMCID:5480145. [CrossRef] [PubMed]
21. Marsden, D.L.; Boyle, K.; Jordan, L.-A.; Dunne, J.; Shipp, J.; Minett, F.; Styles, A.; Birnie, J.; Ormond, S.; Parrey, K.; et al. Improving assessment, diagnosis, and management of urinary incontinence and lower urinary tract symptoms on acute and rehabilitation wards that admit adult patients: A protocol for a before-and-after implementation study. *JMIR Res. Protoc.* **2021**, *10*, e22902, PMCID:7892286. [CrossRef]
22. Pinnock, H.; Barwick, M.; Carpenter, C.R.; Eldridge, S.; Grandes, G.; Griffiths, C.J.; Rycroft-Malone, J.; Meissner, P.; Murray, E.; Patel, A.; et al. Standards for Reporting Implementation Studies (StaRI) Statement. *BMJ* **2017**, *356*, i6795, PMCID:PMC5421438. [CrossRef] [PubMed]
23. Harris, D.; Cadilhac, D.; Hankey, G.; Hillier, S.; Kilkenny, M.; Lalor, E. National stroke audit: The Australasian experience. *Clin. Audit.* **2010**, *2*, 25–31.
24. Harris, P.A.; Taylor, R.; Thielke, R.; Payne, J.; Gonzalez, N.; Conde, J.G. Research electronic data capture (REDCap)—A metadata-driven methodology and workflow process for providing translational research informatics support. *J. Biomed. Inform.* **2009**, *42*, 377–381, PMCID:2700030. [CrossRef] [PubMed]
25. Jordan, L.A.; Mackey, E.; Coughlan, K.; Wyer, M.; Allnutt, N.; Middleton, S. Continence management in acute stroke: A survey of current practices in Australia. *J. Adv. Nurs.* **2011**, *67*, 94–104, PMCID:20969615. [CrossRef] [PubMed]
26. Gurses, A.P.; Murphy, D.J.; Martinez, E.A.; Berenholtz, S.M.; Pronovost, P.J. A practical tool to identify and eliminate barriers to compliance with evidence-based guidelines. *Jt. Comm. J. Qual. Patient Saf.* **2009**, *35*, 526–532. [CrossRef] [PubMed]
27. Zurcher, S.; Saxer, S.; Schwendimann, R. Urinary incontinence in hospitalised elderly patients: Do nurses recognise and manage the problem? *Nurs. Res. Pract.* **2011**, *2011*, 671302, PMCID:PMC3169375. [CrossRef] [PubMed]
28. Trad, W.; Flowers, K.; Caldwell, J.; Sousa, M.S.; Vigh, G.; Lizarondo, L.; Gaudin, J.; Hooper, D.; Parker, D. Nursing assessment and management of incontinence among medical and surgical adult patients in a tertiary hospital: A best practice implementation project. *JBI Database Syst. Rev Implement Rep.* **2019**, *17*, 2578–2590. [CrossRef] [PubMed]

29. Grimshaw, J.M.; Eccles, M.P.; Lavis, J.N.; Hill, S.J.; Squires, J.E. Knowledge translation of research findings. *Implement Sci.* **2012**, *7*, 50, PMCID:PMC3462671. [CrossRef] [PubMed]
30. Ostaszkiewicz, J.; Tomlinson, E.; Hunter, K. The Effects of Education About Urinary Incontinence on Nurses' and Nursing Assistants' Knowledge, Attitudes, Continence Care Practices, and Patient Outcomes: A Systematic Review. *J. Wound Ostomy Cont. Nurs.* **2020**, *47*, 365–380. [CrossRef] [PubMed]
31. Spoon, D.; Rietbergen, T.; Huis, A.; Heinen, M.; van Dijk, M.; van Bodegom-Vos, L.; Ista, E. Implementation strategies used to implement nursing guidelines in daily practice: A systematic review. *Int. J. Nurs. Stud.* **2020**, *111*, 103748. [CrossRef] [PubMed]
32. Cassidy, C.E.; Harrison, M.B.; Godfrey, C.; Nincic, V.; Khan, P.A.; Oakley, P.; Ross-White, A.; Grantmyre, H.; Graham, I.D. Use and effects of implementation strategies for practice guidelines in nursing: A systematic review. *Implement. Sci.* **2021**, *16*, 1–29. [CrossRef]
33. Australian Commission on Safety and Quality in Health Care. *The National Safety and Quality Health Service (NSQHS) Standards—Partnering with Consumers Standard*; ACSQHC: Sydney, Austrilia, 2022.
34. Mitchell, B.G.; Ferguson, J.K.; Anderson, M.; Sear, J.; Barnett, A. Length of stay and mortality associated with healthcare-associated urinary tract infections: A multi-state model. *J. Hosp. Infect.* **2016**, *93*, 92–99. [CrossRef] [PubMed]
35. Forster, A.J.; Huang, A.; Lee, T.C.; Jennings, A.; Choudhri, O.; Backman, C. Study of a multisite prospective adverse event surveillance system. *BMJ Qual. Saf.* **2020**, *29*, 277–285, PMCID:PMC7146931. [CrossRef] [PubMed]
36. Akiba, C.F.; Powell, B.J.; Pence, B.W.; Muessig, K.; Golin, C.E.; Go, V. "We start where we are": A qualitative study of barriers and pragmatic solutions to the assessment and reporting of implementation strategy fidelity. *Implement Sci. Commun.* **2022**, *3*, 117, PMCID:PMC9617230. [CrossRef] [PubMed]

healthcare

MDPI

Article

Accelerating the Delivery of Psychological Therapies After Stroke: A Feasibility Stepped-Wedge Cluster Randomised Controlled Trial

C. Elizabeth Lightbody [1,*], Kulsum Patel [1], Emma-Joy Holland [2], Chris J. Sutton [3], Christopher Brown [3], Svetlana V. Tishkovskaya [3], Audrey Bowen [4], Jessica Read [5], Shirley Thomas [6], Temitayo Roberts [7] and Caroline L. Watkins [1]

1 School of Nursing and Midwifery, University of Central Lancashire, Preston PR1 2HE, UK; kpatel@uclan.ac.uk (K.P.); clwatkins@uclan.ac.uk (C.L.W.)
2 Population Health Sciences Institute, Faculty of Medical Sciences, Newcastle University, Newcastle upon Tyne NE2 4AX, UK; emma.holland@ncl.ac.uk
3 Lancashire Clinical Trials Unit, University of Central Lancashire, Preston PR1 2HE, UK; cjsutton3@uclan.ac.uk (C.J.S.); cbrown24@uclan.ac.uk (C.B.); stishkovskaya@uclan.ac.uk (S.V.T.)
4 Division of Psychology and Mental Health, School of Health Sciences, University of Manchester, Manchester M13 9PL, UK
5 East Lancashire Hospitals NHS Trust, Pendle Community Hospital, Leeds Rd., Nelson BB9 9SZ, UK; jessica.read@elht.nhs.uk
6 Centre for Rehabilitation and Ageing Research, School of Medicine, University of Nottingham, Nottingham NG7 2UH, UK; shirley.thomas@nottingham.ac.uk
7 NHS Cheshire and Merseyside Integrated Care Board, 1 Lakeside, 920 Centre Park, Warrington WA1 1QY, UK; temitayo.roberts@cheshireandmerseyside.nhs.uk
* Correspondence: celightbody@uclan.ac.uk

Abstract: Background: Psychological problems post-stroke are common and debilitating, yet insufficient evidence-based psychological support exists for stroke survivors, either in stroke or general mental health services. Many stroke survivors with significant needs remain unsupported. To address this problem, we need pathways to identify, treat and manage psychological difficulties after stroke. The Accelerating Delivery of Psychological Therapies after Stroke (ADOPTS) study aimed to explore the feasibility of collaboratively developing, implementing and evaluating intervention packages (IPs) to facilitate access to, and increase the provision of, psychological support post-stroke. **Methods:** Stakeholder groups were formed across four sites in north-west England, comprising stroke and psychological services, to collaboratively develop site-specific IPs incorporating a psychological care pathway, staff training, a staff manual for stroke-specific psychological support and supervision. A feasibility stepped-wedge cluster randomised trial recruited patients admitted with stroke during the usual care (pre-implementation of the IP) and intervention (post-implementation) periods. The feasibility of IP implementation and their potential usefulness were evaluated through assessing wellbeing and the support received, and through a process evaluation incorporating interviews with staff, patients and carers. Feasibility evaluation included the recruitment rate and attrition rate; exploratory analysis (mixed-effects linear or logistic regression models) was used to assess the 'promise' of the intervention in achieving psychological distress outcomes (mood (PHQ-9), anxiety (GAD-7)), assessed using validated measures at 6 weeks and 6 months. **Results:** IPs were collaboratively developed at each site but implementation took longer than the per-study-protocol duration of three months. Nineteen training sessions (152 attendees) were delivered for nursing, therapy, NHS Talking Therapies and voluntary staff. Nursing staff were underrepresented due to difficulties with releasing staff. Manuals were developed for each site, incorporating a mood screening and referral algorithm, but these were not finalised at one site. Stroke and NHS Talking Therapies champions were identified

https://doi.org/10.3390/healthcare13070824

in each site to facilitate cross-service staff supervision. A total of 270 patients were recruited over 14 months (133 usual care, 137 intervention), with 227 and 198 at 6 weeks and 6 months, respectively. Stroke staff found the training, manual and pathway helpful, and reported greater confidence in managing and referring psychological issues. NHS Talking Therapies staff found the training useful for adapting their therapy. However, the intervention took longer to implement in all sites, requiring an additional time period to be added to the stepped-wedge design. **Conclusions:** It is feasible to collaboratively develop and implement IPs for post-stroke psychological support. However, an alternative to the stepped-wedge design used here would be more appropriate for a future study. This study was registered in ISRCTN—the UK's Clinical Study Registry (trial registration: ISRCTN12868810, registration date: 4 February 2016).

Keywords: stroke; psychological support; mood disorders; feasibility studies; stepped-wedge design

1. Background

Stroke affects over 100,000 people in the UK each year [1]. Although more people than ever will survive, they may be left with disabilities [2], which in turn may affect their psychological wellbeing, with depression [3], anxiety [4], emotionalism [5] and post-traumatic stress disorder (PTSD) [6] being common. Psychological difficulties can significantly impact the individual and their recovery. Depression, affecting approximately one in three stroke survivors [3], is associated with poorer outcomes, including increased healthcare utilisation [7], poorer functional outcomes [8], reduced quality of life [9], higher rates of suicide [10] and mortality [11,12], in addition to higher costs [13].

Despite being highlighted by government bodies as an important issue for post-stroke care, psychological difficulties often go undetected [14] and psychological care remains largely unavailable to many stroke survivors [15]. A United Kingdom (UK) survey found that over one-fifth of stroke survivors felt that the emotional changes were difficult to deal with, with one-quarter waiting up to five months for psychological support [16]. One reason for this is the dearth of specialist psychology staff, with less than two-thirds of stroke units in the UK (n = 112, 61.2%) having access to clinical psychology [17]. These service gaps mean that stroke survivors, often with huge psychological needs, are left unsupported [16].

To address this problem, we need pathways to identify, treat and manage psychological difficulties after stroke. Stroke guidelines recommend a collaborative approach utilising a matched-care model [18,19] comprising three levels (or 'Steps') of care, in which people start at the most appropriate level of care for their needs. The model assumes that most patients will experience mild to moderate difficulties (Steps 1 and 2), and these patients can be best supported by stroke-specific staff. Specialist psychology staff, such as Clinical Psychologists/Neuropsychologists, provide higher level support (Step 3) to those with severe difficulties and supervise staff working at lower levels. Utilising a matched-care model allows for the best use of specialist staff's limited time, whilst ensuring patients receive the correct level of support. Evidence suggests that a collaborative, matched-care approach, where the intensity of psychological intervention is tailored to individual patient needs, can effectively address psychological problems [20–22].

However, access to specialist psychology services post-stroke varies greatly both geographically and within NHS Trusts, for example, between acute and rehabilitation services. Additionally, despite the fact that people from areas of greater deprivation have an increased risk of stroke and are more likely to experience more severe strokes [23], health inequalities based on socio-economic status may limit access to psychological support. Such factors require examination to identify and understand the barriers and facilitators to accessing and receiving psychological support.

The inconsistency in psychological care may be addressed through increasing collaboration between stroke services and generic psychology services, such as NHS Talking Therapies (formerly known as Improving Access to Psychological Therapists; IAPT), to increase access to psychological support and specialist psychology staff. NHS Talking Therapies services use a matched-care approach, similar to the stroke-specific model; whilst the stroke matched-care model comprises three steps, the NHS Talking Therapies model has four steps. In NHS Talking Therapies, junior psychology staff treat problems at Steps 1 and 2, with more senior and specialised staff treating more severe problems at Steps 3 and 4. NHS Talking Therapies have been effective in reducing anxiety and depression in the general population and have been encouraged to widen access to those with long-term conditions [24,25]. However, although many NHS Talking Therapies services have long-term condition champions, the number of services which have worked with patients following stroke is unknown. Stroke survivors may be perceived as challenging due to stroke-related impairments, such as cognitive or communication difficulties, which may hinder receiving traditional talk-based psychological therapies. Training NHS Talking Therapies teams in stroke-specific issues might increase confidence in, and capacity for the delivery of, Step 2 and 3 care for stroke survivors. Conversely, stroke services often focus on physical health, and staff may lack the knowledge, skills or experience in managing psychological distress [26]. Training stroke staff to deliver Step 1 psychological support, and in doing so, increasing their confidence, would facilitate the application of the matched-care model.

A complex intervention involving increasing collaborative work between services and delivering staff training needs robust evaluation. Challenges to implementing this complex intervention need to be understood. Therefore, it was decided that a feasibility study should be conducted to capture implementation issues to be considered for a larger trial. A stepped-wedge cluster randomised controlled trial (RCT) design [27] was selected in which all clusters (sites) started in the control phase, and each site received the intervention at staggered points in the study timeline. The cluster design also mitigated the potential contamination risks involved in an individual patient RCT for this type of service-level intervention.

The aim of the ADOPTS study was to develop and implement an intervention package and to explore the feasibility of utilising a collaborative approach to delivering post-stroke psychological care within existing NHS, social care and voluntary sector services.

The study design encompassed several components, conducted in three phases:

Phase 1: Describe current pathways for psychological support post-stroke and the challenges of provision and access.

Phase 2: Based on Phase 1 findings, develop an evidence-based intervention package to facilitate access to, and increase the effectiveness of, health, social care and voluntary sector services focused on stroke survivors' psychological needs.

Phase 3: Apply the intervention package and explore its feasibility, acceptability and potential effectiveness.

Objectives

A: Evaluate the feasibility of collaboratively developing and implementing the intervention package.

B: Assess whether the development of the intervention package impacts psychological service provision prior to its implementation.

C: Estimate the eligibility, recruitment and attrition rates for a larger trial.

D: Develop and test data collection systems, outcome measures and follow-up protocols.

E: Estimate the proportion of people with psychological distress, the time to first referral and the time to treatment.

F: Explore the potential benefit of the intervention package for patients, including for different stroke types and socio-economic subgroups.

G: Investigate the feasibility of the stepped-wedge design to evaluate the delivery of the intervention package.

2. Methods

2.1. Study Design and Ethics

A feasibility stepped-wedge cluster randomised trial with embedded process evaluation. This study was registered in ISRCTN—the UK's Clinical Study Registry (trial registration: ISRCTN12868810, registration date: 4 February 2016).

This study was reviewed by the NRES Committee Yorkshire and The Humber–Leeds East and received a favourable opinion (Rec reference 15/YH/0343).

2.2. Setting

Acute and community NHS Trusts based in four stroke services in the North of England.

2.3. Patient Carer and Public Involvement (PCPI)

A PCPI group was established for support throughout the study. Members included those with lived experience of stroke, or of caring for someone who had experienced a stroke. The group met regularly and were involved in the development of patient facing materials (information sheets, questionnaires) to ensure study materials were appropriately completed and accessible to stroke survivors and their carers, including those with communication difficulties.

2.4. Randomisation

The four stroke services (clusters) were randomised to one of two dates in pairs: two sites were randomised to start implementation at the first date and the remaining two sites were randomised to start implementation at the second date (3 months apart). Randomisation was performed by an independent statistician using computer-generated pseudo-random numbers. All clusters started in a usual care phase (no intervention delivered at any site, T1), then sequentially crossed over to the roll-out phase, which was intended to last 3 months, until all sites received the intervention (T4, see Figure 1).

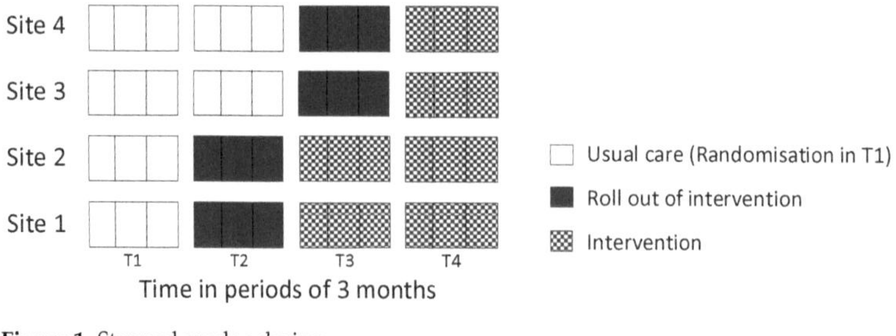

Figure 1. Stepped-wedge design.

2.5. Phase 1

Service mapping of current psychological services

To establish a picture of the psychological services across the study sites, we conducted a scoping and mapping exercise, including a patient record review, and held interviews with service users and staff. The results from the interviews will be reported in detail in future publications. To identify gaps in services and staff skills, information was sought regarding current psychological care pathways, including what psychological support was available, the mode of delivery, demands on current services and the identification of who accessed those services when they were available. This information was mapped to each site, which informed stakeholder group discussions regarding the development of intervention packages for each of the four sites during Phase 2.

Hospital Record Review

A retrospective review of patient hospital records was undertaken to explore if the process of the scoping and mapping exercise and the development of the implementation package may have had an impact on the psychological support patients received by raising staff awareness of unmet needs. Consecutive stroke patients on four acute stroke units were identified over two time points: (i) one week prior to process mapping and the development of the implementation package, and (ii) one week during the roll-out period of the implementation package. For those who consented, the hospital records were reviewed by a member of the research team who looked for instances where psychological care (e.g., psychologist, psychiatrist, mental health liaison) was recorded. Quality assurance was assessed by a second member of the research team who independently extracted data for a sample of the hospital records (4–6 for each site).

2.6. Phase 2: Feasibility Trial

Participants and setting

Consecutive stroke patients admitted to acute stroke units at each of the four sites were identified during the middle month of each 3-month period (usual care, roll-out and intervention) (see Figure 1). Eligible participants included those who had survived to day 3 post-stroke or those who were discharged prior to day 3; those living within the catchment area of an NHS Trust; and those aged $\geq$18 or over. Exclusion criteria included those who lacked capacity and had no friend/relative/carer to act as consultee. The carers of patients were also invited to participate. For participants who lacked capacity, a consultee provided assent.

Intervention

The intervention package involved providing a patient pathway for psychological support after stroke. This pathway was adopted as part of usual care; therefore, patients consented to data collection and follow-up only. While the delivery varied slightly across sites, the core aspects (referral pathway, training, manual and supervision) of the implementation strategies were consistent across all sites. The implementation package was planned to be rolled out over a 3-month period to embed the pathway in the services prior to the start of formal data collection for the intervention phase.

Data collection

Baseline data collection

Baseline data were recorded for all participants who had provided valid consent. Data were extracted from (i) patient records, including their age, sex, date of admission, stroke side and severity; (ii) face to face including communication (FAST [28]) and cognition (MoCA [29]); and (iii) from patient self-report questionnaires, including mood (PHQ-9 [30], (DISCs) [31], anxiety (GAD-7 [32]), Posttraumatic stress disorder (IES-6) [33], stroke recovery (Modified Rankin [34], Barthel (3 items) [35], Short Form Stroke Impact Scale

(SF-SIS) [36], Work and Social Adjustment Scale (WSAS) [37]) quality of life (EQ5D3L [38]) and indicators of one's social/economic context (Supplementary Table S1). Staff were also asked to complete proxy measures of patient mood (SADQ-10 [39] and Yale single item [40]) and anxiety (BOA [41]) based on their perception of how they thought the patient was feeling. All measures and questionnaires have previously been validated for use with the study population.

Outcome data collection

All participants received a postal questionnaire at 6 weeks and 6 months post-stroke. Patients were given the option of telephone or face-to-face completion. Carers who consented completed questionnaires about their observations of the patient's mood (SADQ-10 and Yale single item) and anxiety (BOA) at 6 weeks and 6 months post-stroke. Details of study measures are in Supplementary Materials Tables S1 and S2.

Statistical analysis

The analyses were conducted and reported following both the CONSORT 2010 statement extension for the reporting of stepped-wedge cluster randomised trials [42] and for reporting randomised pilot and feasibility trials [43]. As the trial aimed to assess the feasibility of intervention delivery to inform the design of a main trial, the indicative outcomes were not powered for the statistical testing of effectiveness.

Feasibility outcome measures were summarised using descriptive statistics with proportions of eligibility, recruitment, attrition rates and percentages of missing data estimated for each outcome measure at 6 weeks and 6 months.

To address the different aspects of feasibility and to inform the decision about a fully powered trial, the following participant numbers were summarised by their frequencies for each intervention group:

- Number of patients suffering from psychological distress (anxiety or depression according to the Psychological Distress Algorithm (Appendix A)) and who received psychological support at each time point;
- Number of patients with anti-depressant use at each time point;
- Number of patients when psychological treatment was first received;
- Number of patients who required a letter to be sent to their GP to notify them of a potential issue concerning psychological distress;
- Number of patients with further stroke, TIA or other major health problems which required hospital admission (electronic health records were compared to participant reported problems at each follow-up using kappa statistics);
- Number of reminders sent to encourage participants to return the questionnaires.

Baseline and demographic characteristics were summarised descriptively by the study arm using the median (interquartile range [IQR]) or proportions, as appropriate. Frequency distributions were examined for the variables describing the number of participants deemed to have anxiety or depression at baseline, at 6 weeks and at 6 months.

To explore the potential benefit of the intervention packages for different levels of deprivation, the numbers of participants suffering from psychological distress at 6 weeks and 6 months by deprivation index were examined using frequency distributions. Deprivation was measured using the Index of Multiple Deprivation (IMD) as quintiles and treated as a categorical variable.

To inform the main trial, we performed modelling of the outcome and process variables using generalised linear mixed models, with a mixed-effects logistic regression model used to model binary outcome variables (the computed psychological distress due to anxiety, psychological distress due to depression and psychological distress due to anxiety or depression) and a mixed-effects linear model for the PHQ-9 and GAD-7 scores, with site as a random effect. In addition to the intervention and cluster, the models also included time period factors and baseline outcome measures. Interaction terms between the type of stroke and the intervention group, and the IMD quintiles and the intervention group were subsequently included in the model to evaluate potential subgroup intervention effects.

The completeness of the outcome data was assessed through the response rate for the outcome questionnaires at each time point and the completion rate of the individual items. We also examined questionnaires to see if individual items were repeatedly not completed to determine participant accessibility or acceptability. Responders for psychological distress were compared to non-responders at each time point regarding their baseline characteristics and demographics, using logistic regression analysis to identify individual factors associated with non-response.

Missing data for each outcome at each time point (including baseline) was summarised overall by intervention group and by stepped-wedge design (site-by-time period). Multiple imputation was not deemed appropriate given the exploratory nature of the effectiveness analysis.

To assess the potential contamination of the usual care phase (T1) due to service mapping, the proportion of patients identified as having psychological needs, as being assessed for mood problems, as having been referred for psychological assessment/support and having started on anti-depressants before and after the service mapping were summarised and compared using logistic regression, which was adjusted for site.

For the analysis, we assumed that patients recruited during the roll-out period of the stepped-wedge design received usual care. A sensitivity analysis was conducted where participants recruited during the implementation period were assumed to have received the intervention.

Effect estimates were presented as point estimates with 95% confidence intervals. Where appropriate, the significance level was set to 5%. The descriptive analysis was performed using SPSS v.24 [44] and modelling performed using Stata v.15 [45].

2.7. Phase 3: Process Evaluation Interviews

Patient Process Evaluation Interviews

Following the roll-out of the intervention package, a sample of patients recruited to the main implementation package were interviewed to explore the acceptability of the tailored psychological service.

Participants and setting

Stroke patients and carers were purposely selected (n~12 per site) to recruit a balanced sample across sex, age (younger/older), stroke severity (mild/moderate/severe), communication abilities and time since stroke. Patients and their carers who consented were telephoned by a member of the University of Central Lancashire research team. For all of those with communication difficulties who consented to being contacted, a carer was approached, and for all of those with cognitive deficits, a consultee was contacted. Written informed consent was obtained prior to the interview commencing. Interviews were held face-to-face in the participant's home, or by telephone, depending on participant preference.

Data collection

The interviews were audio recorded. For participants with communication difficulties, interviews were video-recorded with the patient's consent. Patients and their carers (interviewed separately) were asked to describe their experiences of psychological support since their stroke, including what worked well, or which areas they felt could be improved. For participants with communication difficulties, the Supported Conversation for Adults with Aphasia (SCA™) [46] techniques were used in the design of the interview. The interviewers also used these techniques to adapt their communication methods to be tailored to individual patient needs.

Qualitative data analysis

Interviews were transcribed and analysed using thematic analysis, and interpretation was underpinned by the Theoretical Domains Framework (TDF [47]). The TDF grouped the constructs identified from theories relevant to the implementation of healthcare interventions into 14 domains. Themes were identified and key concepts developed through the interpretation of patterns and were mapped onto the domains of the TDF.

Staff Process Evaluation Interviews

Following the roll-out of the implementation package, staff were interviewed about their experiences to understand their feelings towards implementing the intervention package, including the training and supervision received, what they felt worked well and what they felt could be improved.

Participants and setting

The participants were staff working across the stroke pathway in hospitals, in the community and in generic mental health services within each of the sites, including nurses, doctors, occupational therapists, physiotherapists, allied health professionals and NHS Talking Therapies therapists, reflecting the range of staff involved in the care pathway at each site. Staff were invited by a member of the research team. Written informed consent was obtained from all staff willing to take part.

Data collection

Staff took part in a semi-structured interview based on the TDF. Interviews were held face-to-face or by telephone, or face-to-face as part of a focus group, depending on participant preference.

Qualitative data analysis

Interviews were transcribed and thematically analysed using TDF.

3. Results

3.1. Objective A: Evaluate the Feasibility of Collaboratively Developing and Implementing the Intervention Package

Stakeholder meetings were held in all four sites to inform the development and implementation of the intervention package. There were 38 attendees (Site 1 = 10, Site 2 = 11, Site 3 = 8, Site 4 = 9), and in each site they included representation from stroke services (acute, rehabilitation, community), NHS Talking Therapies, Stroke Association and patients and carers. Using information gathered from stakeholder meetings and findings from the pre-implementation interviews, an intervention package was collaboratively developed, tailored for each site. The four core components (referral pathway, training, manual and supervision) of the IP were supplemented with additional resources following suggestions by staff and patients, including an information leaflet about psychological problems post-stroke, and a card displaying useful contacts for patients. The roll-out of the intervention took longer than the intended 3 months in all sites. Therefore, an additional time period was added to the stepped-wedge design to ensure all sites experienced a full intervention period (see Figure 2). Overall, each core component was implemented to varying degrees across sites.

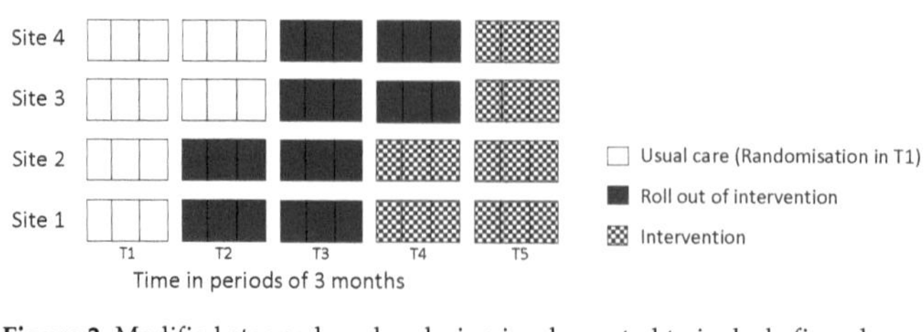

Figure 2. Modified stepped-wedge design implemented to include five phases.

3.1.1. IP Component 1: Screening and Referral Pathway

A screening and referral pathway for psychological care was developed in all four sites. In one site, the pathway was developed but not fully implemented, as it required approval and authorisation at an executive level, which was not completed during the study period. In the other three sites, the pathway was implemented and in process evaluation interviews was reported to be useful when embedded as part of practice, with staff knowing how and when to refer issues and to whom.

3.1.2. IP Component 2: Training

Training packages were developed and implemented in all sites, with training delivered separately to stroke and NHS Talking Therapies teams. Six planned training sessions were cancelled due to staff shortages; of these, three were rearranged and three did not take place because it was not possible for staff to be released. In total, nineteen training sessions were held across the four sites (Site 1: seven sessions, Site 2: two sessions, Site 3: three sessions, Site 4: two sessions; NHS Talking Therapies covering Sites 1 and 2: four sessions, NHS Talking Therapies covering Sites 3 and 4: one session). There were 152 attendees at the training sessions, including staff across various roles and levels of experience (42% therapy staff, 15% nursing staff (including HCAs), 32% NHS Talking Therapies staff and 11% Stroke Association staff). Of all staff in post across the four sites, 8% (n = 22/269) of nurses/HCAs and 59% of therapy staff (n = 64/108) attended the training sessions.

To facilitate attendance, training sessions were offered and held at different times (morning, afternoon, evening) and locations. At the suggestion of staff, training sessions were also aligned with existing team meetings. Despite this, some staff were unable to attend due to their workload, particularly nursing staff when wards were busy.

The degree of continued implementation of the training differed across sites. For example, in Site 2, training was cascaded to staff and was integrated into in-service training. In Site 4, however, the training for stroke teams was intended to be delivered by NHS Talking Therapies teams, but this was not possible during the study period due to time pressures, and so the stroke team only received written information from NHS Talking Therapies.

3.1.3. IP Component 3: Manual

A manual was developed in all four sites. In one site, the manual required authorisation at an executive level before it could be used in practice, and this authorisation was not completed within the study period. In the other three sites, the manual was implemented by stroke teams in different ways. In one site, the manual was embedded as a fundamental resource for existing and new staff; in another site, the manual was available for staff who wished to use it. Across sites, some junior staff reported being unaware that the manual existed. Staff who were aware of the manual found it a useful resource for determining when and how to screen for mood problems.

3.1.4. IP Component 4: Supervision

Supervision links were developed in all four sites, with a 'stroke champion' identified and contacts in stroke teams and NHS Talking Therapies teams named for reciprocal support. The names and contact details of these individuals were provided during training and within the manual; as such, there were differences between sites in the awareness and use of this information. Some staff reported that they had used the details of local stroke or NHS Talking Therapies champions to build links across teams. The supervision component was facilitated by stakeholder meetings and training, which allowed staff to meet and establish professional relationships and to provide assistance to each other. The contact details of stroke champions were also used in materials designed for patient use, e.g., key contact cards and information leaflets.

3.2. *Objective B: Assess Whether the Development of the Intervention Package Impacted Psychological Service Provision*

A review of patient hospital records was carried out in each site over two time points to check for potential contamination during the usual care phase due to the study set-up, service mapping and stakeholder meetings. The first hospital record review was undertaken in all sites one week prior to the study commencing, and the second held in a week during the study set-up phase. The hospital record review found no differences in how mood was routinely screened for or reported between pre-study and study set-up phases. Due to this, in the main analysis, participants recruited during the roll-out periods were assumed to have received usual care.

3.3. *Objective C: Estimate the Eligibility, Recruitment and Attrition Rates for a Larger Trial*

A total of 1066 participants were screened for eligibility across four sites. Of those screened, 674 (63%) were deemed eligible. A total of 270 (40%) patients consented to participate, with 179 (66%) in the usual care period and 91 (34%) in the intervention period (the imbalance in allocation was due to patients in the roll-out period being treated as usual care). The CONSORT diagram (Figure 3) shows the flow of participants. Following the CONSORT extension for reporting stepped-wedge cluster RCTs [42], we also included a flow chart describing a stepped-wedge design by allocated sequence, period and follow-up time (Figure 4).

The baseline and demographic characteristics of participants by study arm are shown in Table 1.

Table 1. Baseline participant characteristics, demographics and stroke and mood measures by intervention group.

	Usual Care (*N* = 179)	**Intervention (*N* = 91)**	**All (*N* = 270)**
Age, median (IQR) *n* = 269	72 (62, 81)	76 (61, 83)	73 (62, 82)
Gender ^, *n* (%)			
Female	85 (47.8)	44 (48.4)	129 (48.0)
Ethnicity ^^, *n* (%)			
White	172 (97.2)	87 (95.6)	259 (96.6)
Employment status ^^, *n* (%)			
Paid	37 (20.9)	16 (17.6)	53 (19.8)
Living situation ^^, *n* (%)			
At Home	149 (84.2)	78 (85.7)	227 (84.7)
Index of Multiple Deprivation (quintiles), *n* (%)			
1st (most deprived)	45 (25.1)	32 (35.2)	77 (28.5)
2nd	37 (20.7)	16 (17.6)	53 (19.6)
3rd	21 (11.7)	16 (17.6)	37 (13.7)
4th	38 (21.2)	13 (14.3)	51 (18.9)
5th (least deprived)	38 (21.2)	14 (15.4)	52 (19.3)
Type of stroke ^^^, *n* (%)			
Ischaemic	145 (81.9)	86 (95.6)	231 (86.5)
Intra-Cerebral Haemorrhage	32 (18.1)	4 (4.4)	36 (13.5)
Side of body affected by stroke ^^^, *n* (%)			
Left	76 (43.2)	38 (41.8)	114 (42.7)
Right	83 (47.2)	43 (47.3)	126 (47.2)
Bilateral	2 (1.1)	2 (2.2)	4 (1.5)
Neither	15 (8.5)	8 (8.8)	23 (8.6)
NIHSS score, median (IQR) *n* = 210	4 (2.5, 8.5)	5 (2, 11)	5 (2, 10)
Estimated Barthel Index, median (IQR) *n* = 265	16.3 (10, 20)	17.5 (10, 20)	17.5 (10, 20)
Modified Rankin ^^, *n* (%)			
Moderate to Severe	89 (49.7)	42 (46.2)	131 (48.9)
EQ5—VAS, median (IQR) *n* = 188	55 (40, 75)	70(50, 80)	60 (50, 80)
Sensory impairment (sight or hearing), *n* (%)	61 (34.1)	31 (34.1)	92 (34.1)
Cognitive score (MOCA), median (IQR) *, *n* = 181	23 (18, 26)	24 (19, 27)	23 (18, 26)
Cognitive impairment, n (%) *, *n* = 181	90 (73.8)	37 (62.7)	127 (70.2)
Communication score (FAST), median (IQR) *, *n* = 148	29 (26, 30)	29 (25, 30)	29 (26, 30)
Communication problems, n (%) *, *n* = 148	19 (18.6)	11 (23.9)	30 (20.3)
Current/past use of anti-depressants ^^, *n* (%)	36 (20.3)	7 (7.7)	43 (16.0)
Current/past use of psychological support ^^^, *n* (%)	31 (17.6)	10 (11.0)	41 (15.4)
Self-reported psychological difficulties, *n* (%)	80 (44.7)	39 (42.9)	119 (44.1)

* Not applicable to participants with consultee form completion. Missing data: ^ *n* = 1; ^^ *n* = 2 and ^^^ *n* = 3.

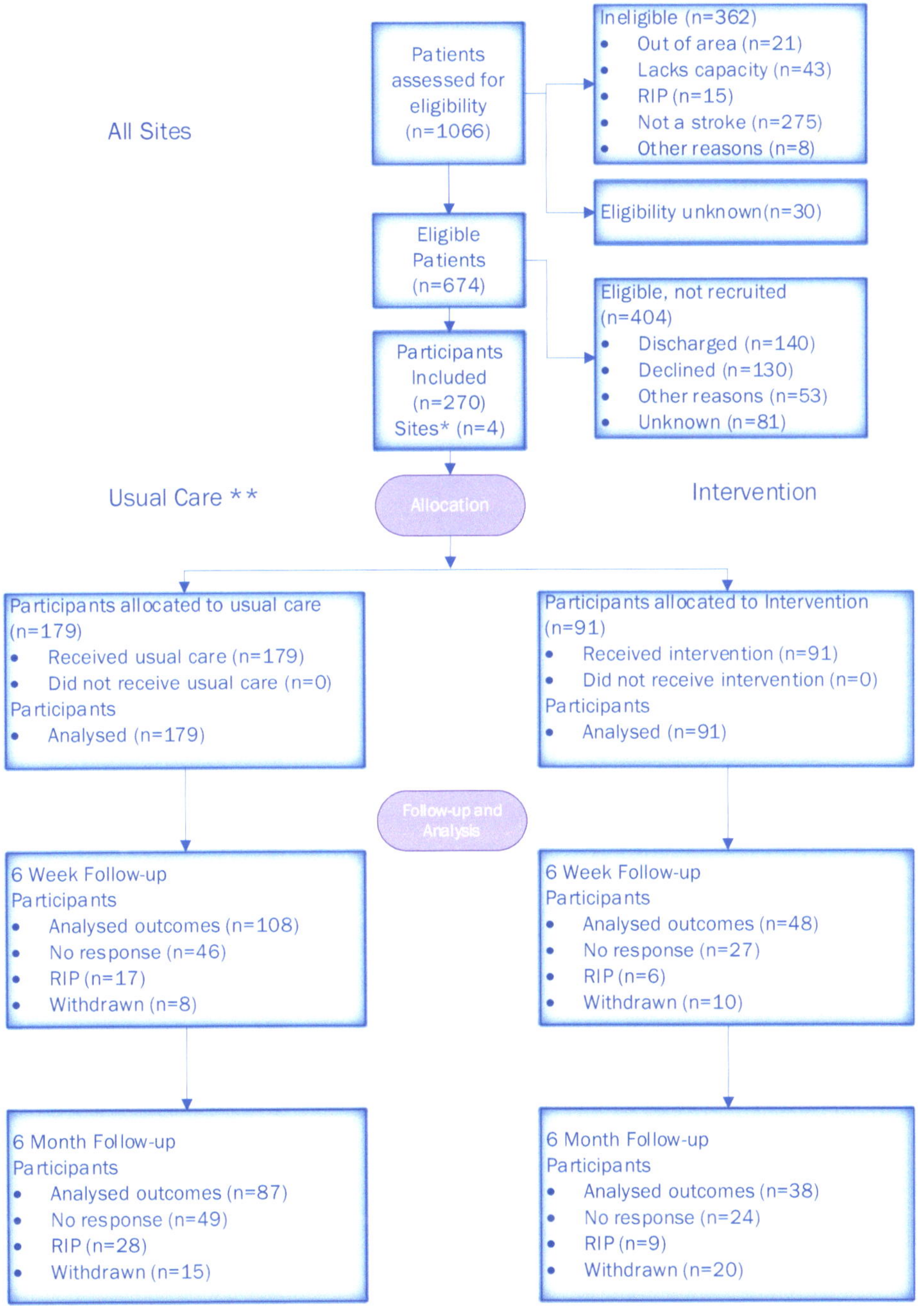

Figure 3. CONSORT diagram of participant flow through the trial. * All four sites provided data at each time point. ** Usual care included participants that were recruited during the roll-out period.

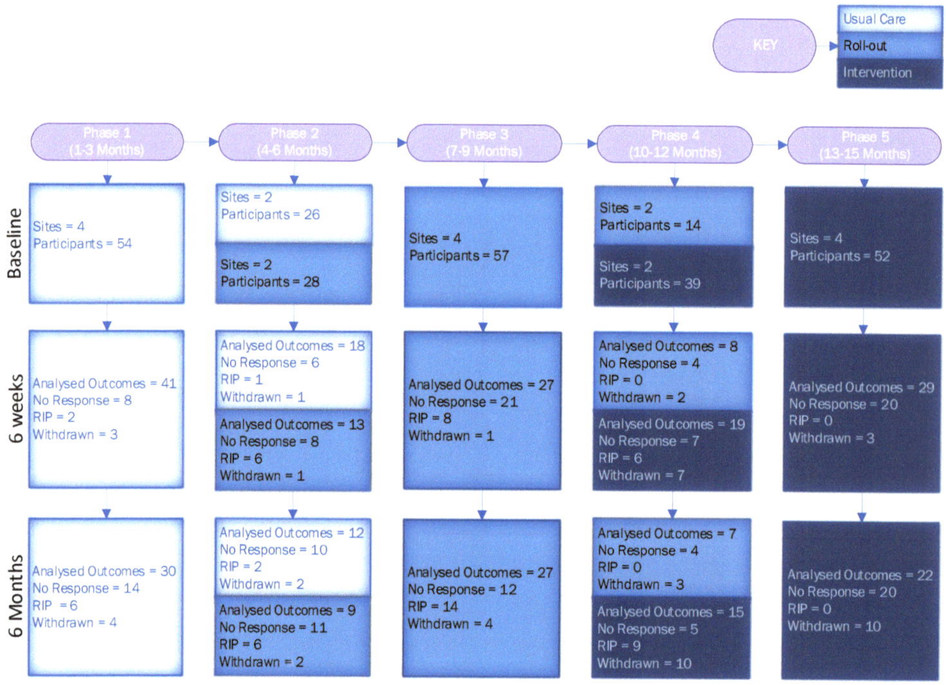

Figure 4. Flow chart of stepped-wedge design by allocated sequence, period and follow-up time.

The usual care and intervention groups were similar in terms of most characteristics. However, there were two notable differences, as shown in Table 1: (i) usual care participants were less likely to have ischaemic stroke, but more likely to have intracerebral haemorrhage; and (ii) usual care participants were more likely to use anti-depressants prior to stroke.

The attrition rate for all participants was 34% (30% usual care, 41% intervention) at 6 weeks and 40% (36% usual care, 48% intervention) at 6 months. Further details of the follow-up data are given in the CONSORT diagram (Figure 3).

3.4. Objective D: Develop and Test Data Collection Systems, Outcome Measures and Follow-Up Protocols

3.4.1. Data Collection Systems: Questionnaire Type

The number of completed questionnaires (270 at baseline, 156 (58%) at 6 weeks and 125 (46%) at 6 months) were summarised by questionnaire type at baseline, 6 weeks and 6 months, and, correspondingly, were (i) 183 (68%), 115 (74%) and 101 (81%) for the patient-reported questionnaire; (ii) 10 (3.7%), 5 (3%) and 5 (4%) for the patient-reported aphasia-friendly questionnaire; and (iii) 77 (28.5%), 36 (23%) and 19 (15%) for the consultee-reported questionnaire. The number of completed carer questionnaires at baseline, 6 weeks and 6 months were 259 (95.9%), 112 (71.8%) and 87 (69.6%), respectively.

The response rates for individual questionnaire items at baseline varied from 77% (FAST) to 100% (psychological input and self-reported psychological difficulties). Low response rates for the FAST questionnaire corresponded to more complex questions to comprehend being consistently unanswered.

3.4.2. Data Collection Systems: Outcome Measures

Table 2 gives the number of participants with anxiety or depression based on each of the measures used. Rates of psychological distress were generally higher in carer-reported measures compared to patient-reported measures. The only exception was for the Yale, where carers reported lower rates than participants. The DISCs showed the lowest proportion of participants with depression among all depression measures.

Table 2. Number of participants (%) deemed to have anxiety or depression from each questionnaire at baseline by intervention group.

Questionnaire	Problem *1	Usual Care n (%)	Intervention n (%)	All Participants n (%)
GAD-7 *2	Anxiety	26 (21.3)	11 (18.0)	37 (20.2)
BOA	Anxiety	50 (29.4)	22 (25.9)	72 (28.2)
PHQ-9 *2	Depression	29 (24.4)	10 (16.4)	39 (21.7)
SADQ-10	Depression	52 (30.1)	21 (24.4)	73 (28.5)
Yale *3	Depression	42 (33.6)	23 (35.9)	65 (34.4)
Carer Yale	Depression	52 (30.6)	20 (23.3)	72 (28.1)
DISCs	Depression	22 (17.6)	10 (15.6)	32 (16.9)

*1 Problem is determined by dichotomising the total score from each questionnaire. *2 Only applicable to returned participant-completed questionnaires. *3 Not applicable to returned consultee-completed questionnaires.

At each follow-up point, if the participants scored above a pre-determined threshold indicating that they may be experiencing psychological distress, their GP was notified (14% at 6 weeks and 17% at 6 months).

To determine the reliability of participants' self-reporting of further stroke, TIA and other major health problems, comparisons were made with hospital records at each follow-up. The agreement between self-reporting and hospital records was better at 6 weeks than 6 months; however, there were few problems reported by participants and in hospital records overall, leading to high agreement. The agreement analysis is described in Supplementary Materials Table S3.

3.4.3. Follow-Up Protocol

A total of 105/229 (46%) participants at 6 weeks and 107/198 (54%) participants at 6 months received a postal or telephone reminder to return the questionnaire. Of those who received at least one reminder, at 6 weeks, 43 (41%) returned a questionnaire; at 6 months, 42 (39%) returned a questionnaire.

The overall response rate was low at both 6 weeks and 6 months. We conducted an analysis of non-responders to identify factors associated with non-response.

At 6 weeks, the following factors were statistically significantly associated with non-response to the follow-up questionnaire: participant age (with an increase in age, the odds of non-response were lower (95% CI 0.94 to 0.99)), questionnaire type (participants who completed the consultee version of the questionnaire had a higher probability of non-responding (95% CI 1.2 to 8.2)) and cognitive problems identified at baseline (a higher probability of non-responding (95% CI 1.1 to 5.8)).

Most participants who had not responded to the 6-week follow-up did not respond at 6 months (95% CI 11.1 to 79.9). At 6 months, participants with a consultee-completed questionnaire were more likely to not respond (95% CI 1.7 to 14.4). Other factors associated with non-response were receiving psychological support at baseline (95% CI 1.5 to 19.2), and living in supported accommodation, a care/nursing home or with relatives, compared to those living in their own home (95% CI 1.6 to 21.8). Participants who were unable to work or were retired were more likely to respond compared to those in full time employment (non-response 95% CI 0.01 to 0.9, and 95% CI 0.04 to 0.4, correspondingly). Most numbers in the analysis were low, which was reflected in the wide CIs.

Tables 3 and 4 show the outcome data at 6 weeks and 6 months, respectively. The usual care and intervention groups scored similarly at both time points.

Table 3. Six-week participant measures by intervention group.

	Usual Care (n = 108)	Intervention (n = 48)	All (n = 156)
Estimated Barthel Index, median (IQR) n = 155	20 (16.3, 20)	20 (15, 20)	20 (15, 20)
Modified Rankin, n(%)			
Moderate to severe	48 (44.4)	22 (47.8)	70 (45.5)
EQ5—VAS, median (IQR) n = 119	70 (50, 87)	70 (55, 90)	70 (50, 90)
SF—SIS, median (IQR) n = 99	31 (23, 37)	30 (20, 37)	30.5 (23, 37)
WSAS, median (IQR) n = 123	12 (4, 28)	10.5 (2, 26)	12 (2, 28)
IES-6, median (IQR) n = 143	1 (0.5, 2)	1 (0.2, 2.2)	1 (0.3, 2)

Table 4. Six-month participant measures by intervention group.

	Usual Care (n = 87)	Intervention (n = 38)	All (n = 125)
Estimated Barthel Index, median (IQR) n = 122	20 (17.5, 20)	20 (15, 20)	20 (17.5, 20)
Modified Rankin, n(%)			
Moderate to severe	35 (40.2)	15 (39.5)	50 (40.0)
EQ5—VAS, median (IQR) n = 103	70 (50, 80)	70 (65, 90)	70 (50, 85)
SF—SIS, median (IQR) n = 115	32 (24, 37)	30 (21, 38)	32 (22, 37)
WSAS, median (IQR) n = 103	8 (1, 25.5)	7 (0, 28)	8 (0, 26)
IES-6, median (IQR) n = 114	0.8 (0.3, 1.7)	0.8 (0.3, 2)	0.8 (0.3, 1.8)

3.5. Objective E: Estimate the Proportion of People with Psychological Distress, Time to First Referral and Time to Treatment

3.5.1. Estimating the Proportion of People with Psychological Distress

At baseline and at each follow-up point, most participants were able to have their psychological distress status classified using an algorithm (Appendix A). The proportion of participants that were unable to be classified by the algorithm due to missing data at each time point is given in Table 5.

Table 5. Number of participants in psychological distress (%) and estimates of intervention effects by time point for anxiety, depression or either.

	Usual Care	Intervention	Total	Missing	Adjusted OR * (95% CI)
Baseline	n = 179	n = 91	n = 270		
Anxiety	52 (29.1)	22 (24.2)	74 (27.4)	5 (1.9)	N/A
Depression	84 (46.9)	36 (39.6)	120 (44.4)	2 (0.7)	N/A
Either	92 (51.4)	38 (41.8)	130 (48.2)	4 (1.5)	N/A
6 Weeks	n = 108	n = 48	n = 156		
Anxiety	27 (25.0)	10 (20.8)	37 (23.7)	4 (2.6)	0.74 (0.28, 1.93)
Depression	42 (38.9)	19 (39.6)	61 (39.1)	0 (0.0)	1.18 (0.55, 2.50)
Either	45 (41.7)	20 (41.7)	65 (41.7)	1 (0.6)	1.06 (0.50, 2.26)
6 Months **	n = 87	n = 38	n = 125		
Anxiety	16 (18.4)	7 (18.4)	23 (18.4)	4 (3.2)	1.02 (0.35, 2.98)
Depression	42 (48.3)	15 (39.5)	57 (45.6)	0 (0.0)	0.75 (0.31, 1.79)
Either	42 (48.3)	15 (39.5)	57 (45.6)	3 (2.4)	0.72 (0.30, 1.77)

* Adjusted for corresponding psychological distress status at baseline. ** Potential contamination for roll-out period included in model.

Nearly half of all participants reported some form of psychological distress at baseline. There was an imbalance in the percentage of participants experiencing psychological distress at baseline, with the usual care group having more cases of anxiety, depression or either of the two (Table 5). The intervention and control groups were similar in terms of the level of psychological distress reported at 6 weeks. At 6 weeks, almost half (42%) had some form of psychological distress.

At 6 months, the proportion of participants with anxiety was lower, but those with depression was higher compared to at baseline and at 6 weeks. At 6 months, all 23 participants with anxiety also had depression (baseline 86%; 6 weeks 89%; 6 months 100%).

3.5.2. Time to First Referral for Psychological Support/Treatment and First Treatment for Psychological Distress

Four participants were referred for psychological treatment during the study period. These participants received support 3 and 9 days after first being referred, respectively. The dates for the remaining two participants were not available.

Of those with psychological distress at baseline (n = 74), 28 (37%) had no treatment; of those with psychological distress first reported at 6 weeks and 6 months, 9/13 (69%) and 13/15 (87%) had no treatment. The percentages were similar for both the intervention and control groups.

3.6. Objective F: Explore the Potential Benefits of the Intervention Package for Patients, Including for Different Stroke and Socio-Economic Subgroups

Table 5 shows that in the usual care and the intervention group, anxiety was correspondingly 25% and 21% at 6 weeks, and at 6 months, in the usual care and the intervention group, depression was 48% and 40% and psychological distress was 48% and 40%. In the intervention group, the odds of anxiety at 6 weeks (OR = 0.74) and of depression (OR = 0.75) or either (OR = 0.72) at 6 months were lower compared to the controls (see Table 5). The trial was not powered to produce definitive results.

In addition, to explore the potential benefit of the IP for patients and assess the 'promise' of the intervention on psychological distress outcomes at 6 weeks and 6 months, the raw PHQ-9 and GAD-7 scores were analysed with a mixed-effects linear model. There was very little difference between the groups, with mean difference between the usual care and the intervention group in terms of the PHQ-9 at 6 weeks of 0.9 95%CI = (−1.1, 2.9) and at 6 months of 0.8 95%CI = (−1.3, 3.0); for GAD-7, the mean difference correspondingly at 6 weeks was 0.7 95%CI = (−1.3, 2.6) and at 6 months was −0.2 95% CI = (−2.0, 1.7), all adjusted for the baseline scores.

Potential Benefit of IPs for Patients and Subgroup Analysis of Socio-Economic Factors

The subgroup analyses of socio-economic factors (IMD) to explore the potential benefits for different socio-economic groups suggested that participants with higher deprivation (lowest quintile) were more likely to experience psychological distress post-stroke; however, the number of participants in each quintile was small. The proportion of participants with psychological distress was likely to remain at a similar level over time across all quintiles and for both the usual care and intervention groups (Figure 5).

Post-implementation process evaluation interviews with patients and carers following a stroke allowed for further exploration of the effectiveness of the IPs. Some patients described the psychological benefits of (i) staff being available and willing to initiate conversations about emotional changes following stroke and normalising the experience; (ii) being provided with information about the journey ahead to know what to expect; and (iii) access to ongoing support, including peer support and having the contact details of people who might provide support.

3.7. Objective G: Investigate the Feasibility of the Stepped-Wedge Design to Evaluate the Delivery of the Intervention Package

One significant challenge in the use of a stepped-wedge design was in implementing the IPs within the given timeframe. The study design initially comprised four time periods. However, during the 'roll-out' periods of the study, it became clear that the sites would not have enough time to agree to and complete the implementation of the IPs within the pre-specified timeframe. This included aspects of the IPs such as finalising key contact cards, patient information leaflets and setting up cross-service supervision links and staff training. It was therefore felt that an extension to the study was required, creating an additional fifth period of data collection (Figure 2) to allow extra time to ensure the IPs were agreed to and implemented, and that data collected during this fifth period would reflect a true 'intervention' period. However, despite the addition of a fifth period of data collection, the IPs were only partially implemented across the sites.

In the analysis, the measurements collected during the transition period were assigned as corresponding to the control group. We tested the sensitivity of the estimates of the intervention effect to this assumption and repeated the analysis for the dataset where participants recruited during the implementation period were assumed to have received the intervention. The sensitivity analysis results did not substantially differ from the main analysis (Supplementary Materials Table S4).

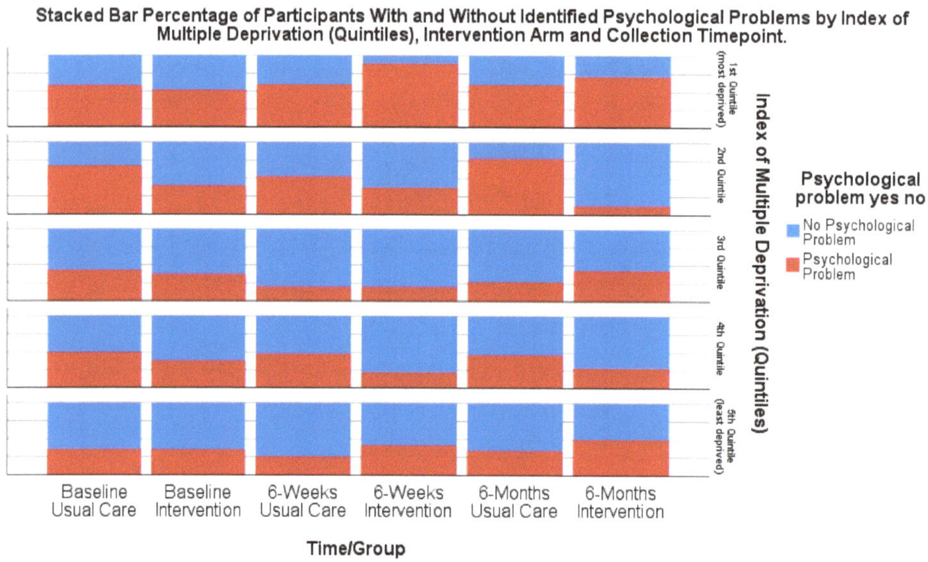

Figure 5. Bar chart of participants (%) with psychological distress at each time point by IMD quintile and intervention group.

4. Discussion

This is the first study exploring the development and implementation of an intervention package for collaborative post-stroke psychological care within the NHS, social care and voluntary sector services. Whilst it seemed feasible to develop and implement the intervention package, implementing and evaluating this within a stepped-wedge RCT was challenging. The time taken to develop this complex intervention impacted its readiness to start being implemented. The data collection procedures/systems used may be feasible for a future study with the alterations proposed. Addressing these issues is essential for optimising future implementation and evaluation.

4.1. Feasibility of Stepped-Wedge Design

A multi-site stepped-wedge RCT requires the sites to be ready for randomisation and intervention implementation at the same pre-determined time. Therefore, our sites had to achieve collaborative intervention package development (pathway, training, manual, supervision) and to implement it into practice within three months; however, this took longer than three months. Future studies should consider the following:

- A longer pre-implementation preparation period: Allocating a longer dedicated preparation phase (e.g., 6–9 months) prior to implementation may ensure readiness.
- Implementation support teams: Establishing local implementation leads or teams within each site could facilitate adaptation to service structures and improve engagement.

Achieving staff buy-in and successful implementation requires the early engagement [48,49] of a range of staff. The development of the intervention package necessitated collaboration from the start by multiple professions and lay representatives from a range of services and organisations across each site's care pathway. These services had mostly not previously collaborated, yet it was necessary here, as the intervention traversed service boundaries. However, stakeholder meetings were well attended, and staff felt the collaboration between stroke and NHS Talking Therapies services was beneficial. We did experience the known complexities of gathering stakeholders for collaborative meetings [50]; some key staff, e.g., clinical psychologists, did not attend. Furthermore, as the intervention required wide changes to implement all four components, there were delays, and all sites struggled to develop the intervention within the timeframe. Practical strategies to enhance engagement include the following:

- Incentives and recognition: Providing professional development credits or recognition for engagement in implementation efforts.
- Tailored communication strategies: Regular, targeted communication (e.g., newsletters, briefing sessions) to maintain momentum.

Previous stepped-wedge design studies of complex interventions have predominantly evaluated single component interventions, or a previously developed complex intervention, so these interventions were implementation-ready. In our study, we involved site staff in developing the intervention packages and in tailoring them to the different site service configurations. The intervention packages' pathways and manual components needed to be authorised by senior leaders pre-implementation, which one site failed to achieve. Implementation may be more successful with early leadership buy-in, which then guides service delivery staff [50]. While we largely achieved early leadership buy-in, one site's senior leader did not sign-off the intervention package. This may have impeded this site's staff engagement and ownership, as well as the package's full implementation. To address this in future studies, the following are recommended:

- Alignment strategies with service development: Aligning intervention components with existing service priorities may enhance acceptability and integration.
- Clear accountability: Defining responsibilities in implementation plans to ensure engagement.

Patient and carer involvement in intervention package development was important and led to the creation of patient-facing materials. This generated additional complexities as these materials required approval from different committees (e.g., Patient Involvement Groups) before being implemented. These groups did not meet regularly, or had a backlog of documents to review, creating further delays, and materials were not approved in all sites.

Delivering staff training took longer than the intended three months. Whilst staff were keen to receive training and it was well received, releasing staff to attend training was challenging. In stroke services, there was a greater representation of allied health professionals compared to nursing staff due to the nursing workload. In one site, training was embedded into standard service training. A future study may consider a similar approach. In one site, the inpatient psychology service agreed to deliver training to NHS Talking Therapies. However, despite frequent reminders, this was not delivered within the timeframe. We tried to be flexible in training delivery by allowing shorter sessions and using a train-the-trainer approach. Despite this, training went beyond the three-month implementation phase, with some sites training staff up to eight months later. To enhance training efficiency, future studies could consider the following:

- Flexible training delivery: Offering asynchronous online training modules with optional live question and answer sessions which may improve accessibility.
- Integrating training into service training programmes: Embedding training into existing professional development frameworks which may reduce disruption.

It was feasible to implement supervision, although it took different forms across sites. Supervision and mutual support between NHS Talking Therapies and stroke services were more successful in sites with pre-existing relations between teams. In sites without these pre-existing links, supervision was agreed, and connections developed, but these were less embedded by the study close. Mutual support and willingness to seek support may have been facilitated by established relationships. A longer implementation phase may have allowed relationships to develop between services and increased the likelihood of successful implementation. This is especially important in stroke services without access to clinical psychology, where guidance from NHS Talking Therapies would facilitate stroke staff in providing psychological support.

This pragmatic stepped-wedge cluster randomised trial is particularly well suited for heterogeneous clusters with a substantial cluster-level effect when there is evidence to support the intervention, or where sites may not wish to be randomised into the control arm [27]. However, there is the possibility that some clusters will be unable to initiate the intervention according to the pre-specified schedule, as happened in our study. As implementation exceeded the planned three-month period, we attempted to ensure that the intervention phase was truly reflected by adding a data collection period to the end of the study. Given the difficulties encountered in a four-site stepped-wedge trial, involving a greater number of sites in such a study would be challenging. A future study should consider an alternative design, e.g., a straightforward cluster randomised trial, where the implementation period is less time-bound.

4.2. Feasibility of Data Collection Procedures/Systems

Our data collection procedures were somewhat feasible but may require alterations for a future study. All sites successfully achieved recruitment and baseline data collection. Our eligibility rate was 63%, and 40% of those eligible were recruited. These figures are lower than expected based on other studies of complex interventions [51]. We widened inclusion, including those with aphasia, cognitive impairment and consultee assent. However, for some patients, consultees were not available, and overall, 37% were ineligible. Additionally, one-third of those eligible were discharged from hospital before being approached about the study.

Follow-up data collection was affected by an attrition rate of 34% at 6 weeks and 40% at 6 months; this high attrition may be in part because patients were recruited early after stroke, although this rate is lower than in another study exploring the collaborative delivery of psychological interventions [52]. The higher attrition among participants with consultees (<50% of these participants returned 6-week data, 25% at 6 months) suggests that a future study should reconsider the use of consultees given the attrition in these participants. Overall, data completion in the returned questionnaires was high. However, despite PCPI engagement to ensure the suitability of the questionnaires, completion was lower for some measures. The Work and Social Adjustment Scale (WSAS) had the highest non-completion rate. This scale was included as it is routinely collected in NHS Talking Therapies, and a stepped-wedge design is more suited to routinely collected data, as the control and intervention phases both become usual care. Within this, there was one question about work, which was not applicable for many participants. This question may not be suitable for use in post-stroke studies, and therefore its inclusion should be questioned for future studies, where an alternative design may be used, following discussion with and input from a PCPI group. Strategies to improve recruitment and retention might include the following:

- Post-discharge recruitment pathways: Allowing recruitment after hospital discharge.
- Personalised follow-up strategies: Using reminder calls, SMS messages and flexible follow-up options (e.g., visits, virtual check-ins) may improve retention.
- Simplified data collection: Streamlining questionnaires to reduce participant burden may improve response rates.

Participants' self-reporting of subsequent health problems and resource-use was fairly accurate when compared with electronic hospital records. However, with only small numbers of health problems recorded overall, interpreting the accuracy of the self-reported information was difficult. It may be feasible for a future definitive study to use electronic health records, reducing the burden on participants, whilst still obtaining relevant, accurate data for economic evaluation.

Our study-specific algorithm for classifying participants as being in psychological distress or not allowed for a high proportion (96.8–100%) of participants to be classified, depending on psychological distress type and proxy completion. However, carer-completed questionnaires were not efficient in identifying psychological distress, and could therefore be removed from a future study's algorithm.

Overall, a high number of participants had psychological distress, which reflects the wider literature [53,54]. Despite this, very few participants were referred for or received support. However, our collection of these data had limitations. Firstly, referral data were only collected from hospital records, and referrals made elsewhere (e.g., GPs) may have been missed. Secondly, follow-up questionnaires did not ask about referrals. It is possible that some participants had been referred, but were not seen by the follow-up time, as our scoping exercise showed extensive waiting list times, e.g., up to nine months for NHS Talking Therapies. Thirdly, we did not capture the informal support participants may have received, such as supportive conversations with stroke staff, which was the focus of our training. A future study should include the collection of referral data from multiple sources, informal support received and the standard of psychological care received, to determine intervention effectiveness.

Participant outcomes of psychological distress appeared to be related to socio-economic status. Although only small numbers of participants represented each deprivation index quintile, there was a trend towards participants living in higher deprivation areas being more likely to experience psychological distress. While only suggestive, this trend is reflective of evidence from the general population, highlighting the link between area deprivation and mental health [55]. Psychological support may be limited, or there may be more challenges to accessing services. Psychological services and interventions should therefore incorporate strategies to ensure equitable access. These might include the following:

- Targeted outreach: Proactive engagement in underserved areas to improve accessibility.
- Flexible service delivery models: Offering telephone or virtual psychological support to help to reduce barriers.

Whilst this study has provided valuable insights into developing and implementing a collaborative post-stroke psychological care model, this study did have some limitations. Firstly, the intervention was developed and tested within specific NHS and social care contexts, so its findings may not fully translate to other healthcare systems or resource-limited settings. Secondly, as staff were actively involved in developing the intervention, there may have been a positive bias in their perception of its feasibility and acceptability. Lastly, the study relied partly on self-reported psychological distress and service use, which may have introduced recall bias or underreporting. Despite these limitations, the study provided crucial insights into the feasibility of integrating psychological care into post-stroke services and highlighted key areas for future improvement.

5. Conclusions

In conclusion, it was feasible to collaboratively develop intervention packages and tailor all four components in all sites. Implementation was feasible for most sites but was affected by timeframes associated with the stepped-wedge design and service processes. Intervention packages, when implemented, were generally well received by staff who noticed an overall increased focus on psychological support. The stepped-wedge design meant that all sites received the intervention and, having wanted to increase post-stroke psychological provision, were all able to participate in influencing this. However, an alternative study design should be considered for a future study to facilitate the implementation of this complex intervention, with adapted data collection procedures to evaluate effectiveness. Practical recommendations include a longer implementation period, alternative trial designs, and targeted strategies for improving access and retention. Future research should explore the long-term impact of collaborative psychological interventions, assess cost-effectiveness and refine implementation strategies to optimise their scalability within routine NHS and social care settings.

Supplementary Materials: The following supporting information can be downloaded at: https://www.mdpi.com/article/10.3390/healthcare13070824/s1, Supplementary Table S1: Baseline study measures; Supplementary Table S2: The 6-week/6-month study measures; Supplementary Table S3: Hospital admissions—number (%) of participants with further stroke, TIA or other major health problems if electronic and patient-completed forms are available; Supplementary Table S4: Number of participants in psychological distress (%) and estimates of intervention effects at 6 weeks and 6 months for anxiety, depression or either, assuming those recruited in the roll-out period received the intervention.

Author Contributions: Conceptualisation: C.E.L., K.P., E.-J.H., C.J.S., A.B., S.T. and C.L.W. Methodology: C.E.L., K.P., E.-J.H., C.J.S., A.B., S.T. and C.L.W. Formal analysis: C.B. and S.V.T. Data curation: C.E.L., K.P., E.-J.H. and T.R. Writing—original draft: C.E.L., K.P. and C.B. Writing—review and editing: K.P., E.-J.H., C.J.S., C.B., S.T., A.B., S.V.T., T.R. and C.L.W. Visualisation: C.E.L., K.P., E.-J.H., C.J.S., A.B., J.R., S.T. and C.L.W. Funding acquisition: C.E.L., K.P., E.-J.H., C.J.S., A.B., J.R., S.T. and C.L.W. All authors have read and agreed to the published version of the manuscript.

Funding: This report is independent research funded by the National Institute for Health Research Applied Research Collaboration North West Coast (ARC NWC). The views expressed in this publication are those of the authors and are not necessarily those of the National Institute for Health Research or the Department of Health and Social Care.

Institutional Review Board Statement: We declare that the investigations were conducted in accordance with the principles outlined in the Declaration of Helsinki (1975, revised in 2013). Ethical approval was obtained from NRES Committee Yorkshire and The Humber–Leeds East and received a favourable opinion for study title: Accelerating Delivery Of Psychological Therapies after Stroke (ADOPTS); Rec reference 15/YH/0343: IRAS project ID167877; Date: 20 August 2015. This study was registered in ISRCTN—the UK's Clinical Study Registry (trial registration: ISRCTN12868810, registration date: 4 February 2016).

Informed Consent Statement: Informed consent was obtained from all subjects involved in this study.

Data Availability Statement: The original contributions presented in this study are included in the article/Supplementary Materials. Further inquiries can be directed to the corresponding author.

Conflicts of Interest: The authors declare no conflicts of interest.

Appendix A

Psychological Distress Algorithm

Psychological distress due to anxiety

(1) A patient will be identified as being in psychological distress for anxiety using the following algorithm:
   (i) If a patient does not have a consultee and does not have aphasia, they will be identified as being in psychological distress due to anxiety if they scored 10 or more on the GAD-7.
   (ii) If the patient has not completed the patient self-completed questionnaire and does have a consultee or carer, then the corresponding measure (GAD-7 for consultee and BOA for carer questionnaire) will be used to indicate whether a patient is in psychological distress due to anxiety. If, for either of the corresponding measures, the patient has scored above the cut-off (10 or more on the GAD-7 and 14 or more on the BOA), then the patient be identified as being in psychological distress due to anxiety.
(2) If the patient is identified as not being in psychological distress due to anxiety from either the GAD-7 or BOA, and is not identified as being in psychological distress due to anxiety from (1) above, then they will be identified as not being in psychological distress due to anxiety.
(3) If, from (1) and (2) above, the patient cannot be classed as either being in psychological distress due to anxiety or as not being in psychological distress due to anxiety, their status for psychological distress due to anxiety will be set to 'missing'.
(4) If their status for psychological distress due to anxiety is missing and the unused measure from (1) above indicated psychological distress, then they will be indicated as being in psychological distress due to anxiety.

Psychological distress due to depression

(1) A patient will be identified as being in psychological distress due to depression using the following algorithm:
   (i) If a patient completes the patient self-completed questionnaire (that is, they do not have a consultee and do not have aphasia), they will be identified as being in psychological distress due to depression if they scored 10 or more on the PHQ-9.
   (ii) If a patient does not have a consultee but does have aphasia, they will be identified as being in psychological distress due to depression if they scored 3 or more on the DISCs.
   (iii) If a patient has responded 'Yes' to the Yale question (on either the patient self-completed or aphasia-friendly patient questionnaire).
   (iv) If the patient has not completed the patient self-completed questionnaire and does have a consultee or carer, the consultee and/or carer questionnaire will be used to indicate whether a patient is in psychological distress due to depression. If a carer scored their relative/friend as 14 or more on the SADQ-10, then the patient would be identified as being in psychological distress due to depression; likewise, if the relative/friend is screened positive for mood on

the Yale question on either the consultee or carer questionnaire, the patient will be identified as being in psychological distress due to depression.

(v) A patient will also be identified as being in psychological distress due to depression if a letter has been sent to their GP.

(2) If the patient is identified as not being in psychological distress due to depression from any of the measures detailed in (1) (i)–(iv) above (PHQ-9; DISCs; patient, consultee or carer Yale question) and is not identified as being in psychological distress due to depression in (1) (v) above, then they will be identified as not being in psychological distress due to depression.

(3) If, from (1) and (2) above, the patient cannot be classed as either being in psychological distress due to depression or as not being in psychological distress due to depression, their status for psychological distress due to depression will be set to 'missing'.

(4) If their status for psychological distress due to depression is missing and an unused measure from (1) above indicated psychological distress, then they will be indicated as being in psychological distress due to depression.

Psychological distress variable

(1) A patient will be identified as being in psychological distress if they are recorded as having psychological distress due to anxiety or recorded as having psychological distress due to depression (or both).

(2) A patient will be identified as not being in psychological distress if they are recorded as not having psychological distress due to anxiety and recorded as not having psychological distress due to depression (or both).

(3) If a patient is not recorded as being in psychological distress and is recorded as 'missing' on either (or both) psychological distress due to anxiety and psychological distress due to depression, then they will be recorded as 'missing' for psychological distress.

References

1. King's College London Sentinel Stroke National Audit Programme (SSNAP) on behalf of the Intercollegiate Stroke Working Party. *State of the Nation Report 2024*; Health Quality Improvement Partnership: London, UK, 2024.
2. Feigin, V.L.; Forouzanfar, M.H.; Krishnamurthi, R.; Mensah, G.A.; Connor, M.; Bennett, D.A.; Moran, A.E.; Sacco, R.L.; Anderson, L.; Truelsen, T.; et al. Global and regional burden of stroke during 1990–2010: Findings from the Global Burden of Disease Study 2010. *Lancet* **2014**, *383*, 245–254. [PubMed]
3. Hackett, M.; Pickles, K. Part I: Frequency of depression after stroke: An updated systematic review and meta-analysis of observational studies. *Int. J. Stroke* **2014**, *9*, 1017–1025.6. [CrossRef] [PubMed]
4. Knapp, P.; Dunn-Roberts, A.; Sahib, N.; Cook, L.; Astin, F.; Kontou, E.; Thomas, S.A. Frequency of anxiety after stroke: An updated systematic review and meta-analysis of observational studies. *Int. J. Stroke* **2020**, *15*, 244–255, Erratum in *Int. J. Stroke* **2021**, *16*, NP2. [CrossRef]
5. Gillespie, D.C.; Cadden, A.P.; Lees, R.; West, R.M.; Broomfield, N.M. Prevalence of Pseudobulbar Affect following Stroke: A Systematic Review and Meta-Analysis. *J. Stroke Cerebrovasc. Dis.* **2016**, *25*, 688–694. [CrossRef] [PubMed]
6. Janssen, E.P.J.; Spauwen, P.J.J.; Bus, B.A.A.; Rijnen, S.J.M.; Ponds, R.W.H.M. Prevalence of posttraumatic stress disorder after stroke: A systematic literature review. *J. Psychosom. Res.* **2024**, *187*, 111914. [CrossRef]
7. Ghose, S.S.; Williams, L.S.; Swindle, R.W. Depression and other mental health diagnoses after stroke increase inpatient and outpatient medical utilization three years poststroke. *Med. Care* **2005**, *43*, 1259–1264. [CrossRef] [PubMed]
8. Pohjasvaara, T.; Vataja, R.; Lepparuor, A.; Kaste, M.; Erkinjuntti, T. Depression is an independent predictor of poor long-term functional outcome post-stroke. *Eur. J. Neurol.* **2001**, *8*, 315–319. [CrossRef]
9. De Wit, L.; Theuns, P.; Dejaeger, E.; Devos, S.; Gantenbein, A.R.; Kerckhofs, E.; Schuback, B.; Schupp, W.; Putman, K. Long-term impact of stroke on patients' health-related quality of life. *Disabil. Rehabil.* **2017**, *39*, 1435–1440. [CrossRef] [PubMed]
10. Pompili, M.; Venturini, P.; Lamis, D.A.; Giordano, G.; Serafini, G.; Murri, M.B.; Amore, M.; Girardi, P. Suicide in Stroke Survivors: Epidemiology and Prevention. *Drugs Aging* **2015**, *32*, 21–29. [CrossRef]
11. House, A.O.; Anderson, A.; Hackett, M. Effects of antidepressants and psychological therapies for reducing the emotional impact of stroke. *J. R. Coll. Surg. Edinb.* **2001**, *31*, 50–60.

12. Kowalska, K.; Krzywoszański, Ł.; Droś, J.; Pasińska, P.; Wilk, A.; Klimkowicz-Mrowiec, A. Early Depression Independently of Other Neuropsychiatric Conditions, Influences Disability and Mortality after Stroke (Research Study-Part of PROPOLIS Study). *Biomedicines* **2020**, *8*, 509. [CrossRef] [PubMed]
13. Husaini, B.; Levine, R.; Sharp, L.; Cain, V.; Novotny, M.; Hull, P.; Orum, G.; Samad, Z.; Sampson, U.; Moonis, M. Depression Increases Stroke Hospitalization Cost: An Analysis of 17,010 Stroke Patients in 2008 by Race and Gender. *Stroke Res. Treat.* **2013**, *2013*, 846732. [CrossRef] [PubMed] [PubMed Central]
14. Hackett, M.L.; Yapa, C.; Parag, V.; Anderson, C.S. Frequency of Depression After Stroke. *Stroke* **2005**, *36*, 1330–1340. [CrossRef] [PubMed]
15. King's College London Sentinel Stroke National Audit Programme (SSNAP) on behalf of the Intercollegiate Stroke Working Party. *Acute Organisational Audit 2021*; Health Quality Improvement Partnership: London, UK, 2022.
16. Royal College of Physicians Sentinel Stroke National Audit Programme (SSNAP). National Report 2015—Phase 2 - Post-acute stroke service provider audit. Prepared by Royal College of Physicians, Clinical Effectiveness and Evaluation Unit on behalf of the Intercollegiate Stroke Working Party. Available online: https://strokeaudit.org/Results2/PostAcute/National.aspx (accessed on 25 February 2025).
17. Gittins, M.; Vail, A.; Bowen, A.; Lugo-Palacios, D.; Paley, L.; Bray, B.; Gannon, B.; Tyson, S. Factors influencing the amount of therapy received during inpatient stroke care: An analysis of data from the UK Sentinel Stroke National Audit Programme. *Clin. Rehabil.* **2020**, *34*, 981–991. [CrossRef]
18. National Clinical Guideline for Stroke for the UK and Ireland. London: Intercollegiate Stroke Working Party. Available online: www.strokeguideline.org (accessed on 4 May 2023).
19. The British Psychological Society. Recommendations for Integrated Community Stroke Services 2023. Available online: https://www.bps.org.uk/guideline/recommendations-integrated-community-stroke-services (accessed on 25 February 2025).
20. Harriman, E.; Poh, J.; Steverson, T. A clinical psychology service in stroke rehabilitation: A review of five years of referrals and an evaluation of a matched care model. *Neuropsychol.* **2021**, *11*, 38–46. [CrossRef]
21. Wagenaar, B.H.; Petersen, I.; Rao, D.; Chwastiak, L. 7—Collaborative care models: A global perspective. In *Global Mental Health in Practice, Global Mental Health and Psychotherapy*; Stein, D.J., Bass, J.K., Hofmann, S.G., Eds.; Academic Press: Cambridge, MA, USA, 2019; pp. 153–170. ISBN 9780128149324. [CrossRef]
22. Rugkåsa, J.; Tveit, O.G.; Berteig, J.; Hussain, A.; Ruud, T. Collaborative care for mental health: A qualitative study of the experiences of patients and health professionals. *BMC Health Serv. Res.* **2020**, *20*, 844. [CrossRef] [PubMed]
23. Marshall, I.J.; Wang, Y.; Crichton, S.; McKevitt, C.; Rudd, A.G.; Wolfe, C.D.A. The effects of socioeconomic status on stroke risk and outcomes. *Lancet Neurol.* **2015**, *14*, 1206–1218. [CrossRef]
24. Fellow-Smith, E.; Moss-Morris, R.; Tylee, A.; Fossey, M.; Cohen, A.; Nixon, T. Investing in Emotional and Psychological Wellbeing for Patients with Long-Term Conditions. Available online: https://www.choiceforum.org/docs/iep.pdf (accessed on 25 February 2025).
25. Department of Health and Social Care. Long-Term Conditions Positive Practice Guide. London: Department of Health and Social Care. 2008. Available online: http://www.uea.ac.uk/documents/246046/11991919/longterm-conditions-positive-practice-guide.pdf/f9e2b540-2061-4950-a428-b2c9c3ddb35d (accessed on 25 February 2025).
26. Harrison, M.; Ryan, T.; Gardiner, C.; Jones, A. Psychological and emotional needs, assessment, and support post-stroke: A multi-perspective qualitative study. *Top. Stroke Rehabil.* **2017**, *24*, 119–125. [CrossRef]
27. Hemming, K.; Haines, T.P.; Chilton, P.J.; Girling, A.J.; Lilford, R.J. The stepped wedge cluster randomised trial: Rationale, design, analysis, and reporting. *BMJ* **2015**, *350*, 391. [CrossRef]
28. Enderby, P.M.; Wood, V.A.; Wade, D.T.; Hewer, R.L. The Frenchay Aphasia Screening Test: A short, simple test for aphasia appropriate for non-specialists. *Int. Rehabil. Med.* **1986**, *8*, 166–170. [CrossRef]
29. Nasreddine, Z.S.; Phillips, N.A.; Bedirian, V.; Charbonneau, S.; Whitehead, V.; Collin, I.; Cummings, J.L.; Chertkow, H. The Montreal Cognitive Assessment, MoCA: A brief screening tool for mild cognitive impairment. *J. Am. Geriatr. Soc.* **2005**, *53*, 695–699. [CrossRef] [PubMed]
30. Kroenke, K.; Spitzer, R.; Williams, W. The PHQ-9: Validity of a brief depression severity measure. *J. Gen. Intern. Med.* **2001**, *16*, 606–616. [CrossRef]
31. Turner-Stokes, L.; Kalmus, M.; Hirani, D.; Clegg, F. The Depression Intensity Scale Circles (DISCs): A first evaluation of a simple assessment tool for depression in the context of brain injury. *J. Neurol Neurosurg. Psychiatry* **2005**, *76*, 1273–1278. [CrossRef] [PubMed] [PubMed Central]
32. Spitzer, R.L.; Kroenke, K.; Williams, J.B.W.; Lowe, B. A brief measure for assessing generalized anxiety disorder. *Arch. Intern. Med.* **2006**, *166*, 1092–1097. [CrossRef]
33. Hosey, M.M.; Leoutsakos, J.S.; Li, X.; Dinglas, V.D.; Bienvenu, O.J.; Parker, A.M.; Hopkins, R.O.; Needham, D.M.; Neufeld, K.J. Screening for posttraumatic stress disorder in ARDS survivors: Validation of the Impact of Event Scale-6 (IES-6). *Crit Care* **2019**, *23*, 276, Erratum in *Crit Care* **2020**, *24*, 37. https://doi.org/10.1186/s13054-020-2759-0. [CrossRef] [PubMed] [PubMed Central]

34. van Swieten, J.C.; Koudstaal, P.J.; Visser, M.C.; Schouten, H.J.; van Gijn, J. Interobserver agreement for the assessment of handicap in stroke patients. *Stroke* **1988**, *19*, 604–607. [CrossRef]
35. Ellul, J.; Watkins, C.; Barer, D. Estimating total Barthel scores from just three items: The European Stroke Database 'minimum dataset' for assessing functional status at discharge from hospital. *Age Ageing* **1998**, *27*, 115–122. [CrossRef]
36. Jenkinson, C.; Fitzpatrick, R.; Crocker, H.; Peters, M. The Stroke Impact Scale: Validation in a UK setting and development of a SIS short form and SIS index. *Stroke* **2013**, *44*, 2532–2535. [CrossRef] [PubMed]
37. Mundt, J.C.; Marks, I.M.; Shear, M.K.; Greist, J.H. The Work and Social Adjustment Scale: A simple measure of impairment in functioning. *Br. J. Psychiatry* **2002**, *180*, 461–464. [CrossRef] [PubMed]
38. The EuroQol Group. EuroQol—A new facility for the measurement of health-related quality of life. *Health Policy* **1990**, *16*, 199–208. [CrossRef]
39. Sutcliffe, L.; Lincoln, N. The assessment of depression in aphasic stroke patients: The development of the stroke aphasic depression questionnaire. *Clin. Rehabil.* **1998**, *12*, 506–513. [CrossRef]
40. Mahoney, J.; Drinka, T.J.K.; Abler, R.; Gunter-Hunt, G.; Matthews, C.; Gravenstein, S.; Carnes, M. Screening for depression: Single question versus GDS. *J. Am. Geriatr. Soc.* **1994**, *9*, 1006–1008. [CrossRef]
41. Linley-Adams, B.; Morris, R.; Kneebone, I. The Behavioural Outcomes of Anxiety scale (BOA): A preliminary validation in stroke survivors. *Br. J. Clin. Psychol.* **2014**, *53*, 451–467. [CrossRef] [PubMed]
42. Hemming, K.; Taljaard, M.; McKenzie, J.E.; Hooper, R.; Copas, A.; Thompson, J.A.; Dixon-Woods, M.; Aldcroft, A.; Doussau, A.; Grayling, M.; et al. Reporting of stepped wedge cluster randomised trials: Extension of the CONSORT 2010 statement with explanation and elaboration. *BMJ* **2018**, *363*, k1614. [CrossRef]
43. Eldridge, S.M.; Chan, C.L.; Campbell, M.J.; Bond, C.M.; Hopewell, S.; Thabane, L.; Lancaster, G.A. CONSORT 2010 statement: Extension to randomised pilot and feasibility trials. *BMJ* **2016**, *355*, i5239. [CrossRef]
44. IBM Corp. *IBM SPSS Statistics for Windows, Version 24.0*; IBM Corp: Armonk, NY, USA, 2016.
45. StataCorp. *Stata Statistical Software*; Release 15; StataCorp LLC.: College Station, TX, USA, 2017.
46. Kagan, A. Supported Conversation for Adults with Aphasia (SCA). In *The SAGE Encyclopedia of Human Communication Sciences and Disorders*; Damico, J.S., Ball, M.J., Eds.; SAGE Publishing: Los Angeles, CA, USA, 2019.
47. Michie, S.; Johnston, M.; Abraham, C.; Lawton, R.; Parker, D.; Walker, A. on behalf of the 'Psychological Theory' Group: Making psychological theory useful for implementing evidence based practice: A consensus approach. *Qual. Saf. Health Care* **2005**, *14*, 26–33. [PubMed]
48. Green, A.; Aarons, G.A. A comparison of policy and direct practice stakeholder perceptions of factors affecting evidence-based practice implementation using concept mapping. *Implement Sci.* **2011**, *7*, 104. [CrossRef]
49. Palinkas, L.A.; Aarons, G.A.; Chorpita, B.F.; Hoagwood, K.; Landsverk, J.; Weisz, J.R. Cultural exchange and the implementation of evidence-based practices. *Res. Soc. Work. Pract.* **2009**, *19*, 602–612. [CrossRef]
50. Pepin, R.; Hoyt, J.; Seifert, B.; Bartels, S.J. A multi-stakeholder process to transform a community-based screening and referral program to implement evidence-based depression care. *J. Evid. Inf. Soc. Work* **2016**, *13*, 362–372. [CrossRef]
51. Bragstad, L.K.; Bronken, B.A.; Sveen, U.; Hjelle, E.G.; Kitzmuller, G.; Martinsen, R.; Kvigne, K.J.; Mangset, M.; Kirkevold, M. Implementation fidelity in a complex intervention promoting psychosocial well-being following stroke: An explanatory sequential mixed methods study. *BMC Med. Res. Methodol.* **2019**, *19*, 59. [CrossRef]
52. Coventry, P.; Lovell, K.; Dickens, C.; Bower, P.; Chew-Graham, C.; McElvenny, D.; Hann, M.; Cherrington, A.; Garrett, C.; Gibbons, C.J.; et al. Integrated primary care for patients with mental and physical multimorbidity: Cluster randomised controlled trial of collaborative care for patients with depression comorbid with diabetes or cardiovascular disease. *BMJ* **2015**, *350*, h638. [CrossRef] [PubMed]
53. Liu, L.; Xu, M.; Marshall, I.J.; Wolfe, C.D.; Wang, Y.; O'Connell, M.D. Prevalence and natural history of depression after stroke: A systematic review and meta-analysis of observational studies. *PLoS Med.* **2023**, *28*, e1004200. [CrossRef] [PubMed] [PubMed Central]
54. Tjokrowijoto, P.; Stolwyk, R.J.; Ung, D.; Kneebone, I.; Kilkenny, M.F.; Kim, J.; Olaiya, M.T.; Dalli, L.L.; Cadilhac, D.A.; Nelson, M.R.; et al. Receipt of Mental Health Treatment in People Living With Stroke: Associated Factors and Long-Term Outcomes. *Stroke* **2023**, *54*, 1519–1527, Erratum in *Stroke* **2023**, *54*, e230. [CrossRef] [PubMed]
55. Office for National Statistics (ONS), Released 6 December 2022, ONS Website, Article, Cost of Living and Depression in Adults, Great Britain: 29 September to 23 October 2022. Available online: https://www.ons.gov.uk/peoplepopulationandcommunity/healthandsocialcare/mentalhealth/articles/costoflivinganddepressioninadultsgreatbritain/29septemberto23october2022 (accessed on 25 February 2025).

healthcare

MDPI

Article

Aphasia Depression and Psychological Therapy (ADaPT): Perspectives of People with Post-Stroke Aphasia on Participating in a Modified Cognitive Behavioral Therapy

Caroline Baker [1,2,*], Sonia Thomas [3], Priscilla Tjokrowijoto [2,4,5], Brooke Ryan [2,6,7], Ian Kneebone [2,7] and Renerus Stolwyk [2,4,5]

1 Speech Pathology Department, Monash Health, Melbourne, VIC 3192, Australia
2 Centre of Research Excellence in Aphasia Recovery and Rehabilitation, Melbourne, VIC 3086, Australia; priscilla.tjokrowijoto@mh.org.au (P.T.); brooke.ryan@curtin.edu.au (B.R.); ian.kneebone@uts.edu.au (I.K.); rene.stolwyk@monash.edu (R.S.)
3 Thinking Matters, Melbourne, VIC 3184, Australia; thinkingmattersonline@gmail.com
4 Turner Institute for Brain and Mental Health, School of Psychological Sciences, Monash University, Melbourne, VIC 3800, Australia
5 Stroke and Telehealth Research, Monash-Epworth Rehabilitation Research Centre, Melbourne, VIC 3121, Australia
6 Speech Pathology, Curtin School of Allied Health, Curtin University, Perth, WA 6845, Australia
7 Graduate School of Health, University of Technology Sydney, Sydney, NSW 2007, Australia
* Correspondence: caroline.baker@monashhealth.org; Tel.: +61-3-92651000

Abstract: Aphasia, a communication disability commonly caused by stroke, can profoundly affect a person's mood and identity. We explored the experiences of stroke survivors with aphasia and depression who received a modified cognitive behavioral therapy (CBT)-based psychological intervention. The therapy is manualized with a flexible treatment protocol, including 10 individually based therapy sessions (+2 booster sessions) either via telehealth or in person. Six participants with chronic aphasia (60% of the total sample) participated in in-depth interviews that were analyzed using reflexive thematic analysis. Two core themes were derived from the data: the first theme, helpful elements of therapy—doing enjoyable activities, new ways of thinking, problem solving, working with the experienced therapist, and using telehealth; and the second theme, making progress—mood, communication, acceptance of the 'new me', and improving relationships. All participants found the therapy to be helpful in managing mood problems with various elements being beneficial depending on the individual, highlighting the importance of tailoring the intervention. Therefore, delivering modified CBT to individuals with aphasia is likely to be acceptable both in person and through telehealth. Further evaluation of the intervention and its impact on mood would be beneficial.

Keywords: stroke; aphasia; modified cognitive behavioral therapy; psychological therapy; stroke rehabilitation

1. Introduction

Acquired communication disabilities after stroke are common and can include aphasia (difficulties with verbal and written expressions, understanding, and reading); apraxia of speech/dysarthria (motor speech problems); and/or cognitive communication impairments (difficulties with conversational discourse and social skills) [1,2]. Approximately, a third of people who have a stroke experience aphasia [3]. Aphasia after stroke can have negative impacts on a person's identity and relationships, which can lead to fewer friendships and less participation in social activities [4,5]. Depression and anxiety are common mood concerns after post-stroke aphasia [6,7], reported at higher rates compared to those without aphasia [6–9]. Despite some research efforts, there is still a need for psychotherapeutic interventions that are both acceptable and effective for the mental health and wellbeing of individuals with aphasia [10,11].

Cognitive behavioral therapy (CBT) is a psychotherapy treatment that helps a person to manage their emotions, optimize their everyday activities and functioning while maintaining realistic, yet optimistic thinking [12]. One primary aim of CBT is reducing symptoms of depression, such as apathy, hopelessness, and low mood across a range of clinical populations [12]. CBT can effectively treat depression in the general, neurotypical population with comparable effects to pharmacotherapy treatment [13]. Furthermore, it has emerging support for positive effects in reducing overall symptoms and maintaining improvement in those with stroke [14,15]. However, there is currently limited evidence for the use of a CBT intervention adapted to support the specific communication and psychological needs of stroke survivors with aphasia. Despite the known high prevalence rates of mood problems in people with aphasia, stroke audits and research evidence consistently report a lack of mood assessments and appropriate psychological care and follow-up treatment with mental health specialists [16,17]. The access and provision of psychological treatments after stroke is a high priority in the research and clinical care [17]. To address this significant gap in clinical care, Aphasia Depression and Psychological Therapy (ADaPT) was developed to test feasibility and preliminary efficacy for the treatment of depression after post-stroke aphasia using a single-case-design evaluation study [18]. ADaPT is a protocolized, tailored treatment program delivered by a clinical neuropsychologist. It focuses on approaches to support communication skills and access (e.g., supported conversations and photo diaries); behavioral skills (e.g., scheduling enjoyable activities and relaxation techniques); and cognitive skills (e.g., modifying negative thoughts and problem solving) [16]. The establishment of acceptability within ADaPT is essential.

The AdaPT treatment outcome study found that the intervention was largely feasible and could be implemented with most of the participants (n = 10) via telehealth with varying degrees of aphasia severity and time post-stroke [18]. The primary outcome measure was self-reported depression. Three of the participants reported an improvement in mood during the intervention phase, which was sustained for two of these participants during follow-up sessions. An additional four participants demonstrated a delayed treatment response during the follow-up period. Three participants did not appear to benefit during the study period, one of which did not complete all of the intervention sessions [18].

This current study considered the retrospective (experienced) acceptability of ADaPT by examining patient perspectives as the participants of the intervention [19] as an additional qualitative analysis approach to the quantitative results report of the single-case series evaluation [18]. When patients find a therapy acceptable and tailored to their needs, they are more likely to engage fully, attend all sessions, and apply the strategies they learn, which is vital for achieving positive outcomes [19]. Therefore, this qualitative study followed the completion of delivery of CBT within the ADaPT single-case series study [18]. Qualitative methodology was an appropriate approach to explore the experiences of people with aphasia who participated in this modified CBT as part of an evaluation of its feasibility. It can provide an in-depth understanding of the person's experience (e.g., self-perceived helpful or unhelpful aspects of treatment), which can complement the findings gained from quantitative measures.

Specifically, the aims of the study were to: (1) explore the experiences of people with aphasia when participating in modified CBT; (2) identify their needs and preferences; and (3) provide recommendations to improve the therapy.

2. Materials and Methods

2.1. Design

Reflexive thematic analysis was chosen for the methods and data analysis as an appropriate approach to this qualitative study due to the purpose of exploring participants' experiences and perspectives of therapy. This is a common approach used in health science research as it values the researcher's subjective experience as the primary way to discern knowledge from the data. The purpose is to derive meaning and sense of the data from using the researcher's experiences and values, rather than aiming to search for objectivity and remove bias [20,21]. The approach has been used in previous research on aphasiology, for example, in exploring prognostication in post-stroke aphasia, and also in treatment studies, for example, in exploring experiences of interventions in healthcare [22,23]. Individual interviews were chosen to enable participants to have their experiences conveyed in a supportive communication environment with the researcher (CB) [24]. The research followed the Consolidated criteria for Reporting Qualitative research (COREQ) [25] (see Supplementary File Table S1).

2.2. Participant Recruitment and Eligibility

All 10 participants who completed all therapy sessions of ADaPT were considered for inclusion and invited to take part in an in-depth interview within 6 weeks of completion of the modified CBT intervention [18]. Six were interviewed; three participants declined (two due to a decline in their medical condition) and one was considered to decline as they failed to respond to 3 invitations. To be eligible to participate in the ADaPT study [18], participants had to be adults aged 18 years or older; had a diagnosis of ischemic/hemorrhagic stroke confirmed by a health practitioner; a clinical diagnosis of aphasia (Western Aphasia Battery-Revised (WAB-R) < 93.7) [26]; a self-reported low mood ($\geq$2 on the Depression Intensity Scale Circles (DISCs)) [27]; no previous history or concurrent major neurological/psychiatric diagnosis; capacity to consent (with supported communication); capacity and availability to engage; and not concurrently receiving any other psychological interventions and on stable dose of mood medications, if any. Participants were identified through the community, stroke, and aphasia organizations (e.g., social media and mail-out flyers via the Stroke Foundation and professional mailing lists) [18]. Those consenting to an interview were allocated a unique code to protect anonymity, identified throughout this manuscript using their code (P1–P6). Four participants were male and two were female, aged 58 to 71 years. All except one participant lived with a family member. Participants 1, 2, and 3 were interviewed with their spouse/carer present who provided communication support during the interview (Table 1). The mean duration of the interviews was 56 min (range: 45–75 min).

Table 1. Participant characteristics.

Variables	Participant					
	P1	P2	P3	P4	P5	P6
Age (y)	58	70	59	71	69	64
Sex	Male	Male	Male	Female	Female	Male
Education (y)	15	17	12	17	15	9
Type of stroke	L ICA dissection	L MCA ischemic	L ischemic	Subdural hematoma	L hemorrhagic	L ICA occlusion
Tpo (y)	3	1	2	1	5	0.4
Aphasia quotient (WAB-R)	40.6 (severe)	78.2 (mild)	86 (mild)	71.1 (moderate)	89.48 (mild)	93.5 (mild)
Aphasia type	Wernicke's	Anomic	Anomic	Conduction	Anomic	Anomic
Living with family?	Yes	Yes	No	Yes	Yes	Yes
Telehealth sessions (n)/10	10	10	9	10	10	9
Location	WA	NSW	Vic	NSW	NSW	Vic

Abbreviations: y = years, n = number, Tpo = time post-onset stroke, L = left, ICA= internal carotid artery, MCA = middle cerebral artery, WAB-R = Western Aphasia Battery-Revised total score and aphasia severity; WA = Western Australia, NSW = New South Wales, Vic = Victoria.

2.3. ADaPT Intervention Sessions

A full description of the intervention is provided [18]. In summary, ADaPT was tailored to the goals and needs of each participant using approaches of communication and cognitive support, behavioral activation, identity renegotiation, and cognitive therapy (challenging and modifying unhelpful thinking patterns/thoughts) [18]. The therapy sessions were conducted via a mix of in-person and telehealth sessions subject to COVID-19 pandemic restrictions and client preference.

2.4. Data Collection

The perspectives of participants with aphasia were gathered through semi-structured interviews. The topic guide was developed by the first author (CB) with revisions and suggestions offered by all co-authors (see Supplemental File Table S2 [28,29]). The topic guide included open-ended questions and prompts to support a semi-structured interview about the person's experiences, needs, preferences, and recommendations regarding the ADaPT intervention. How they experienced study procedures was also a topic of the interview, but not reported in this current study. To facilitate the interviews, total communication strategies were used (e.g., using short and simple phrases, using written key words/pictures as needed, verifying and confirming the participant's message, asking for clarification, repeating questions as needed, and engaging the support person as a communication partner) [30]. All interviews were conducted via Zoom at the participant's home, except for one person who was interviewed in person in a clinic setting. All participants consented to video recording and the interviews were transcribed verbatim. The interviewer had previously met participants for their baseline WAB-R aphasia tests prior to commencing CBT. Otherwise, the interviewer remained independent of the participants' involvement in the ADaPT study [18].

2.5. Data Analysis

The interview data were analyzed inductively using reflexive thematic analysis [20,21] with coding and derivation of themes from across the dataset (see Supplemental File Table S3 for an example of the reflexive thematic data analysis process). The analysis followed the following steps: familiarization of video/audio recordings and transcripts with repeated readings and note-taking to generate initial reflections (CB); open coding of all transcripts (CB); peer review of transcripts and codes of a third of the transcripts (ST); peer debriefing of codes (ST and CB); generation of themes within each transcript (CB); derivation of themes across transcripts (CB); peer debriefing of themes derived across the sample with all co-authors; refining, defining, and naming themes (CB); derivation of final core themes and subthemes (all authors); and producing the report (all authors) with exemplar quotes from participants with aphasia. All quotes were transcribed verbatim from the participant with aphasia, which may or may not have included language errors. The study complied with the research rigor described in Lyons and McAllister [31] (details in Supplementary File Table S1).

2.6. Ethical Statement

The Monash University Human Research Ethics Committee approved this study (HREC ID 7888). All participants provided verbal and/or written informed consent. Information and consent processes were provided in a communicatively accessible manner by the researcher (PT), consistent with stroke research inclusion recommendations for people with aphasia [32].

3. Results

The qualitative data show a complex and varied experience of participation in the ADaPT intervention, where, overall, the therapy was valued by participants and perceived as a helpful part of their aphasia and stroke rehabilitation and recovery. All participants reported that the therapy helped to manage mood problems in different ways (e.g., through doing enjoyable activities and/or modifying unhelpful thoughts). All participants perceived the benefits of managing their mood and other aspects of life (e.g., relationships).

Two core themes were derived from the qualitative data with perceptions around: (1) helpful elements of therapy and (2) making progress.

3.1. Core Theme 1: Helpful Elements of Therapy

Participants perceived the therapy sessions as personalized and adapted for their specific goals and needs at the time, rather than tasks set by the therapist to perform, regardless of their current mood and wellbeing needs. A participant particularly valued the 'flexible' 'very person-centered' approach to the ADaPT therapy. This approach led to personalized therapy goals and activities, such as writing to their grandchildren living at a distance from the participant:

> 'She [therapist] was very person-centred. . .she sent me the picture [of participant's holiday location] and so I was talking about the idea to connect to my grandchildren, and I'd thought of writing them a letter every two weeks. And so I've started doing that. . .' (P5, female).

In terms of what the participants found particularly helpful, five subthemes were derived from the data: (a) doing enjoyable activities; (b) new ways of thinking; (c) problem solving; (d) working with the experienced therapist; and (e) using telehealth.

3.1.1. Doing Enjoyable Activities

The majority of participants described how therapy helped them to consider and identify enjoyable activities, as a participant described it as:

> 'the things that gave me joy' (P5, female).

Sessions provided an opportunity to plan and schedule doing these activities, share how things went in the following session, and how this impacted on their mood. For example, a participant described how her valued activities were:

> 'simple things. . .like nice smells [putting on the oil vaporizer]. . .heat and warmth. . . listening to music and dancing.' (P5, female)

She described that the therapist helped her to focus on how far she had come and what she was able to do rather than unable to do. Another participant described going outdoors:

> 'to see the birds, as well as the dogs.' (P6, male)

He looked forward to the opportunity most days:

> 'I'll come across a couple of magpies, a mother and a baby. . .I get a bit of bread. . .I'll talk to her and feed her. . .they take food out of my hand. So things like that are really good. That makes me happy.' (P6, male)

When the person themselves or the therapist noted success in participating in such activities, it boosted their confidence and positive emotions. In contrast, for the same participant (P6, male), if activities were complex (e.g., boat improvements), there were mixed emotions due to only the partial completion of the activity:

> 'I've got new carpet in the boat. . .I'm happy with that. . .[now] it's just a matter of putting the seats back in and I just can't be bothered.' (P6, male)

Participants reported that the therapist helped them to manage physical and communication difficulties in order to participate in enjoyable activities. For example, knowledge and skill building with the therapist to prepare for planned activities for the week (P2, male discussing with his therapist going to a café with his spouse and a small group of friends). The therapist also facilitated connecting participants with other health professionals in the community, such as an occupational therapist and physiotherapist (P6, male). Some participants were restricted in their ability to participate in activities due to COVID-19. A participant reported not being able to do the things he would have liked to, which resulted in him feeling 'a little bit worse' in mood during this time:

> '. . .I was unable to get out. . .less freedom. . .It was bad. I feel myself lock in jail.' (P3, male)

3.1.2. New Ways of Thinking

Participants valued the explicit information provided by the therapist about negative thinking and how this way of thinking can be changed. All participants perceived value in the component of therapy that involved challenging and modifying their negative thoughts or unrealistic expectations of recovery. An example of how participants' valued this aspect of ADaPT was shown in the following interaction with a participant with severe aphasia:

> Interviewer: did anything surprise you in the therapy? Surprise.
>
> Spouse: which one? [From choice on worksheets]. Oh what's the evidence? [What is the evidence] I have to support my thoughts?
>
> P6, male: [pointing to 'What's the evidence?' worksheet]. 'Yeah'.
>
> Interviewer: that surprised you to think about that?
>
> P6, male: 'Yeah. Thank God, yeah, yeah.'

The participant's spouse strongly endorsed the combined techniques of doing enjoyable activities and working through challenging-thoughts worksheets. She reported that the CBT was well-organized and well-explained; she was enabled to support the completion of home-practice tasks. She observed an improved mood, engagement, and confidence in her husband, particularly with him being more involved with family and friends in social situations. In contrast, two other participants found the 'What is the evidence?' concept and worksheet the least helpful part of their therapy. They were introduced to the concept, but preferred to focus on identifying and performing enjoyable activities that were supported by the therapist.

Another participant reported how the therapist had encouraged a different way of thinking, to achieve a more positive outlook:

> '[Therapist] asked me to help whichever I think, I am thinking about the good side, about positive side. . .rather than, I just thinking about the worst.' (P3, male)

Modifying negative thoughts was considered the most helpful aspect of therapy for this participant. He reported perceived benefits in his life overall since completing ADaPT, indicating a positive impact (on a scale of 1–10, scoring 9) and with sustained improvements in mood and wellbeing:

> 'I feel less worried. . .I feel more better.' (P3, male)

Participants reported feeling enabled to incorporate this strategy into everyday routines or when needed. For example, a participant reported on their progress:

> 'So, my cup was always half empty, always. I was never in a good mood. . .I'm still like that but I can understand things a bit better. . .[the therapist] helped me look at things differently, much differently' (P6, male).

This participant was able to put strategies into place and noted improvements in working through problems and getting along with others as a:

> 'big positive impact [after intervention] because I didn't know how much I could change my thought for a better way, sees towards other people...' (P6, male).

3.1.3. Problem Solving

Participants reported facing different problems associated with a range of changes in functioning after stroke (e.g., physical, communication, and cognitive changes). They reported that the therapist helped them navigate these problems through counseling skills (e.g., active listening) and in practical ways, such as providing information resources, linking participants to community supports, and supporting their skills and confidence to use their problem-solving action plan (e.g., discussing the scenario in advance, such as a difficult conversation with their spouse). They often felt different and more vulnerable to others, particularly due to the 'invisibility' of the communication difficulties and the lack of awareness of others about stroke and communication difficulties. This was evident through descriptions provided by a participant preparing to return to driving:

> 'At the time, with those people [Road Traffic Authority workers] were not very helpful and they did not understand aphasia very much at all.' (P4, female)

This participant also experienced anxiety in what was required to return to driving her car after having a stroke. She perceived that the therapist enabled her to 'get a positive thing' from her interactions during this testing process as she felt supported with various strategies (e.g., break large task into small actions and relaxation techniques). These strategies were useful during and following the ADaPT intervention:

> 'You know when you're calm and she had different ways that I could go to do that, little things that I could do that. . .they helped me immediately with that and even now.' (P4, female)

The feeling that the therapist understood participants' problems and feelings was perceived to make a difference. Participants felt supported to take steps to work through current problems they faced rather than feeling alone.

Within ADaPT, some participants reported that home practice was difficult to complete. However, they felt supported by the therapist to complete tasks with support either from a family member or from therapy sessions with the therapist. For example, two participants were assisted by a close other (spouse/formal carer) to work through the tasks. Due to communication difficulties (talking, reading, and writing), a participant felt home practice was the least useful part of the intervention and rather completed parts of this within sessions with the therapist.

All participants perceived that the time commitment to CBT was significant but worthwhile, and that they would recommend the CBT treatment to others with aphasia. Some participants felt 'busy' with and challenged by other commitments (e.g., medical appointments and holidays), but were able to discuss and agree upon alternative therapy scheduling with the therapist. Strategies to overcome scheduling problems included offering telehealth from locations other than home (e.g., local library room), appointment reminders on the fridge, or via text message.

Some improvements to therapy were suggested by participants, which included: providing a clear understanding of the purpose of CBT to manage any potential expectations of language-based psychotherapy; simplifying some of the handouts around concepts of grief and loss/acceptance of changes in functioning post-stroke; and minimizing disruptions in the use of technology for telehealth.

3.1.4. Working with the Experienced Therapist

The working relationship with the therapist was perceived to be an important element in the experience of participants. All the participants reported a highly positive experience working with the therapist, including over video conference, and noted her ability to understand aphasia and support conversations and emotions by allowing extra time and being open and approachable:

> 'I think the relationship of a client to the therapist is an important factor. . .she listened. She took on board everything I said.' (P5, female)

This participant also described the therapist as 'flexible'. A participant noted that the therapist was the most useful part of the therapy:

> 'I think it's excellent [working with the therapist]. . .I have been really happy and very, really happy with [therapist]. . .she has helping me a lot with everything. . .she

knew how to understand with depression and anxiety mainly. . .I think she understand as a psychologist, as a person who can really relate to what is happening there.' (P4, female)

Another participant with a background in counseling prior to the stroke valued the ethics of CBT and thought it would be helpful prior to commencing the study.

Most participants appreciated the way that the therapist involved their support person in therapy, also noting her ability to explain concepts, such as modifying thoughts and using the worksheets, and 'trouble shoot' occasional technical breakdowns as needed with them.

Participants reported on the therapist's ability to help them manage stress and anxiety through the use of a range of relaxation strategies. For example, they valued using technology, such as smartphones or iPads, to listen to audio recordings of relaxation exercises by the therapist. A participant reported:

'There've been, for example for anxiety, there were different things that she's [the therapist] done at home as well as recording to calm down. . .I'll use those things and even get some apps as well. . .she's [the therapist] given me a, how can I say? It's a box. . .there of a whole lot of things that she's helping me. . .' (P4, female).

3.1.5. Using Telehealth

All participants found it acceptable to use telehealth for participation in ADaPT, with most reporting progress in their familiarity and learning of how to use it across the course of the therapy. The Zoom platform was used by all participants, with only occasional difficulties with elements of the technology. A participant living interstate from the therapist valued being able to participate in the study via Zoom. He was supported by his spouse to use Zoom and participate in ADaPT due to severe aphasia:

Interviewer: Let's talk about Zoom. What was it like to use Zoom? [offering rating scale].

P1, male: 'Okay' [pointing to the positive end of the rating scale].

The main reason described by participants that contributed to a positive view of telehealth was the convenience of not needing to travel and still being able to access the service despite living remote to the therapist. There were technical difficulties experienced by three participants, which led to some frustration and anxiety (e.g., difficulty working out how to access the Zoom link (P1, male) and the screen 'freezing' due to internet disconnection (P4, female). Despite this, most participants described being able to learn and grow in confidence in using Zoom. Three participants had a support person assist with the setup of Zoom (e.g., adjusting volume and accessing the meeting via the link). The therapist, using features such as screen sharing to support communication, was described as useful. A participant used an iPad and reported that a larger screen, such as a computer, would have been more helpful for seeing the therapist and the therapy worksheets (P3, male). All participants rated their interactions and working relationships with the therapist over Zoom as a positive experience.

3.2. Core Theme 2: Making Progress

Participants described the impact of their therapy as feeling 'positive', 'more better', 'less worried', 'different to what I am or what I was', and 'better from before to now'. They also felt better equipped with strategies to manage not only mood problems, but other life challenges associated with communication difficulties (e.g., avoiding social gatherings), 'to have the tools to try and do that [think positively]'. Subthemes included perceptions around (a) mood; (b) communication; (c) an acceptance of the 'new me'; and (d) improving relationships.

3.2.1. Mood

ADaPT was perceived to be important in helping to manage negative thoughts, which could lead to mood problems. Many participants acknowledged that managing their mood and wellbeing was a 'work in progress' and they had learned ways to avoid mood decline:

> 'it's not spiralling down [in negative thoughts]. . .I think that I have to do work on that.' (P4, female).

The therapy was also perceived to help in lifting a participant's mood through its promotion of participation in valued activities and connecting with others (e.g., talking to friends, writing to family, being present at family occasions, and attending the stroke/aphasia group). Others noted that the intervention assisted in alleviating anxiousness and stress by training strategies and techniques, such as 'changing a view or outlook on a situation towards the positive side' (P6, male); 'building self-awareness of mood symptoms' (P5, female); 'using calm breathing' (P4, female); and 'keeping a thought record journal' (P5, female).

A participant described a history of depression and being 'more reclusive' prior to the stroke and participation in ADaPT. A highly valued part of ADaPT was being supported by the therapist to build self-awareness of mood 'warning signs' and develop a depression relapse prevention plan:

> 'Largely I think my mood has improved a lot [since completing the intervention]. . .a very positive impact, but I'm aware that I'm a bit up and down in my moods and so having a strategy in case something goes wrong. . .I love that.' (P5, female)

3.2.2. Communication

Participants reported that, while the ADaPT intervention had not improved or changed their communication functioning, they described ways they had come to accept communication changes due to aphasia. A common theme was that participants described having more confidence to communicate in different situations during and following CBT, such as talking over a meal with family, attending to stroke support group, or wishing a friend a happy birthday over the phone. They also described the impact of this on their social connection, mood, and wellbeing:

> 'What a joy it was meeting the others from the stroke group. . .I've enjoyed that. . .I've been there three times so I feel I know them a bit better.' (P5, female)

3.2.3. Acceptance of the 'New Me'

A common thread across the data was the participants' perception that the therapist had helped them to accept changes in functioning post-stroke (communication, psychological, and physical abilities). In addition, they described ways that the therapist assisted participants to navigate new changes and identity with themselves and others, for example, through stroke and aphasia information provision:

> 'Everybody else around me, you know, they don't understand [stroke and aphasia]. [Therapist] she would understand those things because she knows what the problem is [aphasia]... she was actually explaining [what happened] in the brain as well. . .and then I was able to say to other people "No look this is the thing, and this is what happened.' (P4, female)

A participant described how the therapist offered her a way to think and re-name herself post-stroke—by name and as 'the new [participant's first name]' (P5, female). This participant reported this as one of the very positive things: an acceptance of her new identity. She was particularly appreciative of when the therapist took the time to speak with her and her husband about the grief following stroke and aphasia, and the reality of not returning to previous levels of functioning in terms of communication:

> 'I think what was particularly helpful was addressing ongoing grief. . .I'm not the same as I was.' (P5, female)

3.2.4. Improving relationships

The majority of the participants reported the positive impact the ADaPT intervention had on managing relationships and social interactions. Three participants described the openness of the therapist to assist them in developing strategies (e.g., modifying thoughts, behaviour change) to manage pre-existing difficult relationships such as interactions with partners/spouses:

> "I had to look at it differently [communication breakdowns with partner], different ways were written down [by therapist], which I brought home to try and go through that particular way of looking at it. . .I used to take myself out of the bad situation and look at other ways to talk to her." (P6, male)

Participants also reported feeling more socially connected to others, less isolated and more confident as the therapist supported them to increase social participation and activities (e.g., attending aphasia or stroke groups, meeting friends). A participant (P2, male) described usually feeling 'isolated' but reported the therapist assisted him to join in more with meeting a 'few people' with his wife, an activity he would usually avoid prior to commencing the intervention.

Participants valued the therapist checking on their progress in social situations in between therapy sessions. They were able to share and express their feelings on how interactions occurred, feelings varied from those of frustration to satisfaction to feelings of pride, for example, initiating a phone call to a friend or joining the local library.

4. Discussion

Understanding the experiences and needs of stroke survivors with aphasia when participating in psychotherapeutic interventions is critical to establishing feasibility, acceptability, and identifying opportunities for improvement. To date, no other studies have explored the feasibility or perceived acceptability and experiences of people with aphasia participating in CBT facilitated by a psychologist and adapted for communication disabilities. Therefore, this current study focused on the experiences and needs of people with aphasia who were enrolled in the ADaPT single-case series study (60% of total sample) [18]. Overall, this sample strongly endorsed the intervention as acceptable and a positive experience. The modified CBT intervention was an acceptable therapy approach to all participants, including the participants with moderate to severe aphasia. All participants also considered appropriate and adequate communication support systems were provided. The intervention was tailored to participants' goals and needs. Some participants preferred focusing on doing enjoyable activities, others on challenging their thinking patterns or in combination. Levels of independence in home-practice tasks varied: two participants were independent while the remaining participants required support of the therapist or spouse/carer. Five key areas were identified as helpful elements of therapy: doing enjoyable tasks; new ways of thinking; problem solving; working with the experienced therapist; and using telehealth. The participants described key areas for perceived gains in progress regarding mood, communication, accepting their new identity, and improving relationships. There was variation in experiences within each key area of therapy and within the theme of 'making progress'; however, all participants were highly satisfied with and valued the therapy indicating that ADaPT was acceptable to them.

Participant perceptions around the 'helpful elements of therapy' support concepts of 'active ingredients' or 'mediators' for change in mood symptoms or outcomes within the psychological intervention [33,34]. Participants valued identifying and doing enjoyable activities, which aligns with previous research that concluded that behavioral activation is feasible and may reduce depressive symptoms after stroke and aphasia [35,36]. Focusing on increasing goal-directed and meaningful activities may lead to improved participation and feelings of 'happiness', 'joy', and 'more confidence', as described by participants in the current study. People with severe cognitive and/or communication difficulties may be challenged with cognitive aspects of CBT, hence the behavioral elements may be more engaging for them [36]. Another key element, 'new ways of thinking', was often a new concept to participants and helpful in changing from negative to more positive thinking patterns or accepting more realistic expectations of themselves post-stroke. This matches the previous research, which reported on two case studies (one with dysarthria and one with aphasia after stroke). Both participants had a reduction in anxiety symptoms immediately post-therapy and at follow up (3 months) [37]. These findings challenge the assumption that those with aphasia cannot engage with cognitive elements of CBT. A notable finding of this study is that participants with moderate to severe communication impairments (expressive and/or receptive skills) also felt ADaPT was a valuable therapy for them to participate in. This complements the preliminary evidence in the broader ADaPT study [18] that psychological therapy, such as CBT, though complex from some perspectives, can be modified to be accessible to people with aphasia, even those with moderate to severe impairments.

The variety of experiences and preferences within ADaPT also support the need for individually tailored interventions based on the person's communication and psychological care needs, in addition to their therapy goals. This is consistent with the need for clinicians to ensure that people with aphasia are included in therapy goal setting and provided with communication support to make choices, negotiate, and agree upon goals and therapy activities [38]. This finding is consistent with solution-focused brief therapy, which views participants as the experts in their lives and enables them to achieve their goals and outcomes by drawing on their strengths, skills, and resources [39]. Furthermore, in the current study, the working relationship with the experienced therapist was highly valued and important to participants. Previous research confirms that speech pathologists report that verbal and non-verbal communication support are a vital factor to fostering a therapeutic alliance [40]. Of note, mental health practitioners report insufficient knowledge and training concerning aphasia, with a need for collaboration and interdisciplinary practice with speech-language pathologists [41]. It will be important for future research to understand the training, support, and supervision needs of ADaPT therapists to deliver therapy using modifications and approaches to support communication.

The changes participants perceived in accepting a new identity due to a disruption post-stroke are consistent with previous aphasia and identity research [4]. The findings of exploring identity as a helpful part of ADaPT aligns with the results from a subset of participants who experienced a renegotiation of post-stroke identity following solution-focused brief therapy [39]. This was possible through increasing self-respect, noticing personal strengths, and enabling the person to connect with their sense of who they are [39]. The experiences of 'self under threat' or discrepancy in identity following acquired brain injury are also central to the 'Y-shaped' model of rehabilitation [42]. The theories underpinning the model support the use of multiple approaches to address identity discrepancy, including a therapeutic focus on building social relationships and a self-awareness of thoughts, feelings, and abilities [42].

An additional notable finding of the current study is the perceived progress, in terms of communication confidence, improved mood, and knowledge of how to manage mood problems in the future (e.g., depression relapse prevention plan). These steps in progress enhanced the person's ability to move forward, in-between and beyond therapy sessions in various ways, for example, involving themselves more in social interactions, which in turn assisted in reducing feelings of isolation. With the support of the therapist, most were able to build a level of self-awareness of their capabilities to make changes and intentionally seek ways to enhance their mood and wellbeing. This in-depth exploration of self-perceived progress and beneficial changes in mood should complement our understanding of CBT, which may be a helpful therapy post-stroke, despite the inconclusive nature of RCTs and meta-analysis in stroke research [14,43].

4.1. Clinical Implications

This study reports that people with aphasia highly value and accept ADaPT delivered by an experienced therapist. While a modification of the therapy may have been key, it is important to note that participants described the therapist's understanding of aphasia and post-stroke mood problems as being important as well. In addition, experience that resulted in the therapist knowing how to personalize therapy in a flexible way to address current goals and everyday life problems was identified as critical. This indicates that simply providing the manual to therapists may not be enough to support the outcomes. Training would need to cover aphasia and stroke for those without this background, alongside the development of skills in supportive communication. The ADaPT therapist, a clinical neuropsychologist, has extensive clinical experience and skills working with people with neurological conditions, including stroke and aphasia. Professional clinical supervision by the experienced therapist will be a critical element to ensure the clinical integrity of ADaPT in future studies.

Participant suggestions for improvement in future included: enabling participants to have a clear understanding of the purpose of CBT to manage any potential expectations of language-based therapy; simplifying some handouts around concepts of grief and loss; and considerations to enhance connection and participation on telehealth.

4.2. Strengths, Limitations, and Future Directions

The study provides preliminary support for the broad applicability of ADaPT for people with aphasia; however, a future study with a larger sample of participants is required to confirm this. The ADaPT therapy was conducted during COVID-19, and so telehealth was used, which was also acceptable to participants as a mode of delivery. Despite the small sample size, there was a variation in time post-stroke onset and types/severities of aphasia of those participating in the ADaPT study, confirmed by comprehensive aphasia testing. The interviewer was independent of the therapy and single-case series study, with a background in speech pathology and communication support and access to people with aphasia. Thus, the interviewer was able to support communication to facilitate a rich and in-depth account of each participant's experience. Using a reflexive thematic analysis enabled all interdisciplinary co-researchers to contribute their expertise in working with people after stroke, aphasia, and other acquired brain injuries (all from psychology and speech pathology disciplines). A limitation of the study was not including in-depth perceptions of close others (e.g., spouse/carer) who supported the person with aphasia throughout ADaPT and the limited diversity within the sample. Those who were unable to be interviewed or declined (n = 4) may have provided different views on their experiences, which may have influenced the findings in a different way. There was also a possible recruitment bias in the broader ADaPT study [18]. This study suggests that CBT within the ADaPT study is an acceptable approach, potentially warranting further investigation in a larger trial design. Developing appropriate training in the modified therapy will be a challenge for a major trial. Future qualitative research could include experts in aphasia, including those with lived experiences in co-producing aspects of the research, for example, topic guides for interviews. It could also include prospective interviews (prior to therapy) to understand the participant's expectations of and hopes for therapy, with a possible comparison of perspectives post-therapy.

5. Conclusions

Modified CBT can be adapted for people with aphasia, including via telehealth, and it is acceptable to them. Participants identified key areas that were helpful to them and noted making progress in their mood, wellbeing, and communication confidence. The most useful parts of therapy included performing more enjoyable activities, modifying thoughts to be more helpful, and working with an experienced therapist knowledgeable in aphasia and stroke.

Supplementary Materials: The following supporting information can be downloaded at: https://www.mdpi.com/article/10.3390/healthcare12070771/s1, Table S1: Consolidated criteria for Reporting Qualitative studies (COREQ): 32-item checklist [25]; Table S2: interview topic guide; and Table S3: example of reflexive thematic data analysis process.

Author Contributions: Conceptualization, all authors; methodology, all authors; formal analysis, C.B., S.T. and B.R.; investigation, all authors; writing—original draft preparation, C.B.; writing—reviewing and editing, all authors; supervision, R.S., S.T., I.K. and B.R.; project administration, P.T., C.B., R.S. and S.T.; funding acquisition, R.S. and I.K. All authors have read and agreed to the published version of the manuscript.

Funding: This project was funded by the Centre for Research Excellence in Aphasia Recovery and Rehabilitation: National Health and Medical Research Council Australia (NHMRC APP1153236).

Institutional Review Board Statement: The study was conducted in accordance with the Declaration of Helsinki and approved by the Monash University Human Research Ethics Committee (Project ID 7888; v12_Protocol ADAPT depression and aphasia; date of approval: 24 March 2021).

Informed Consent Statement: Informed consent was obtained from all participants involved in the study. Written informed consent was obtained to present the results in peer-reviewed publications.

Data Availability Statement: This was a qualitative study exploring the experiences of participants when participating in therapy. Participant characteristic data, examples of data analysis, themes/subthemes derived from the data, and exemplar quotes from interview transcripts are provided in the manuscript and Supplementary Files.

Acknowledgments: We acknowledge the people with aphasia and their supporters who participated in the study. We also acknowledge the clinicians and researchers who shared expressions of interest with others during the participant enrolment phase for the study.

Conflicts of Interest: The authors declare no conflicts of interest.

References

1. O'Halloran, R.; Worrall, L.; Hickson, L. The number of patients with communication related impairments in acute hospital stroke units. *Int. J. Speech Lang. Pathol.* **2009**, *11*, 438–449. [CrossRef] [PubMed]
2. Baker, C.; Foster, A.M.; D'Souza, S.; Godecke, E.; Shiggins, C.; Lamborn, E.; Lanyon, L.; Kneebone, I.; Rose, M.L. Management of communication disability in the first 90 days after stroke: A scoping review. *Disabil. Rehabil.* **2022**, *44*, 8524–8538. [CrossRef] [PubMed]
3. Flowers, H.L.; Skoretz, S.A.; Silver, F.L.; Rochon, E.; Fang, J.; Flamand-Roze, C.; Martino, R. Poststroke Aphasia Frequency, Recovery, and Outcomes: A Systematic Review and Meta-Analysis. *Arch. Phys. Med. Rehabil.* **2016**, *97*, 2188–2201.e8. [CrossRef]
4. Shadden, B. Aphasia as identity theft: Theory and practice. *Aphasiology* **2005**, *19*, 211–223. [CrossRef]
5. Northcott, S.; Moss, B.; Harrison, K.; Hilari, K. A systematic review of the impact of stroke on social support and social networks: Associated factors and patterns of change. *Clin. Rehabil.* **2016**, *30*, 811–831. [CrossRef] [PubMed]
6. Kauhanen, M.L.; Korpelainen, J.T.; Hiltunen, P.; Määttä, R.; Mononen, H.; Brusin, E.; Sotaniemi, K.A.; Myllylä, V.V. Aphasia, Depression, and Non-Verbal Cognitive Impairment in Ischaemic Stroke. *Cerebrovasc. Dis.* **2000**, *10*, 455–461. [CrossRef] [PubMed]
7. Morris, R.; Eccles, A.; Ryan, B.; Kneebone, I. Prevalence of anxiety in people with aphasia after stroke. *Aphasiology* **2017**, *31*, 1410–1415. [CrossRef]
8. Hilari, K. The impact of stroke: Are people with aphasia different to those without? *Disabil. Rehabil.* **2011**, *33*, 211–218. [CrossRef]
9. Zanella, C.; Laures-Gore, J.; Dotson, V.; Belagaje, S. Incidence of post-stroke depression symptoms and potential risk factors in adults with aphasia in a comprehensive stroke center. *Top. Stroke Rehabil.* **2023**, *30*, 448–458. [CrossRef]
10. Baker, C.; Worrall, L.; Rose, M.L.; Hudson, K.; Ryan, B.; O'Byrne, L. A systematic review of rehabilitation interventions to prevent and treat depression in post-stroke aphasia. *Disabil. Rehabil.* **2018**, *40*, 1870–1892. [CrossRef]
11. Ryan, B.J.; Clunne, S.M.; Baker, C.J.; Shiggins, C.; Rose, M.L.; Kneebone, I.I. A systematic review of non-drug interventions to prevent and treat anxiety in people with aphasia after stroke. *Disabil. Rehabil.* **2022**, *44*, 4997–5006. [CrossRef] [PubMed]
12. Broomfield, N.M.; Laidlaw, K.; Hickabottom, E.; Murray, M.F.; Pendrey, R.; Whittick, J.E.; Gillespie, D.C. Post-stroke depression: The case for augmented, individually tailored cognitive behavioural therapy. *Clin. Psychol. Psychother.* **2011**, *18*, 202–217. [CrossRef] [PubMed]
13. DeRubeis, R.J.; Hollon, S.D.; Amsterdam, J.D.; Shelton, R.C.; Young, P.R.; Salomon, R.M.; O'Reardon, J.P.; Lovett, M.L.; Gladis, M.M.; Brown, L.L.; et al. Cognitive Therapy vs Medications in the Treatment of Moderate to Severe Depression. *Arch. Gen. Psychiatry* **2005**, *62*, 409–416. [CrossRef] [PubMed]
14. Wang, S.B.; Wang, Y.Y.; Zhang, Q.E.; Wu, S.L.; Ng, C.H.; Ungvari, G.S.; Chen, L.; Wang, C.X.; Jia, F.J.; Xiang, Y.T. Cognitive behavioral therapy for post-stroke depression: A meta-analysis. *J. Affect. Disord.* **2018**, *235*, 589–596. [CrossRef] [PubMed]

15. Ahrens, J.; Shao, R.; Blackport, D.; Macaluso, S.; Viana, R.; Teasell, R.; Mehta, S. Cognitive-behavioral therapy for managing depressive and anxiety symptoms after stroke: A systematic review and meta-analysis. *Top. Stroke Rehabil.* **2022**, *30*, 368–383. [CrossRef] [PubMed]
16. Stroke Foundation. *National Stroke Audit Rehabilitation Services 2020*; Stroke Foundation: Melbourne, Australia, 2020. Available online: https://informme.org.au/stroke-data/rehabilitation-audits (accessed on 20 March 2024).
17. *James Lind Alliance Priority Setting Partnership for Stroke*; Stroke Association: London, UK, 2021. Available online: https://www.stroke.org.uk/research/priority-setting-partnership (accessed on 20 March 2024).
18. Tjokrowijoto, P.; Thomas, S.; Kneebone, I.; Ryan, B.; Stolwyk, R.J. Aphasia, Depression, and Psychological Therapy (ADaPT): A single case design evaluation of a modified cognitive behavioural therapy to treat depressive symptoms in stroke survivors with aphasia. *Neuropsychol. Rehabil.* 2024; *in press*.
19. Sekhon, M.; Cartwright, M.; Francis, J.J. Acceptability of healthcare interventions: An overview of reviews and development of a theoretical framework. *BMC Health Serv. Res.* **2017**, *17*, 88. [CrossRef] [PubMed]
20. Braun, V.; Clarke, V. *Thematic Analysis: A Practical Guide*; Sage Publications: Thousand Oaks, CA, USA, 2022.
21. Braun, V.; Clarke, V. Conceptual and design thinking for thematic analysis. *Qual. Psychol.* **2022**, *9*, 3–26. [CrossRef]
22. Cheng, B.B.Y.; Ryan, B.J.; Copland, D.A.; Wallace, S.J. Prognostication in Poststroke Aphasia: Perspectives of Significant Others of People With Aphasia on Receiving Information about Recovery. *Am. J. Speech Lang. Pathol.* **2022**, *31*, 896–911. [CrossRef]
23. Gibson, B.; Umeh, K.; Davies, I.; Newson, L. The best possible self-intervention as a viable public health tool for the prevention of type 2 diabetes: A reflexive thematic analysis of public experience and engagement. *Health Expect.* **2021**, *24*, 1713–1724. [CrossRef]
24. Luck, A.; Rose, M. Interviewing people with aphasia: Insights into method adjustments from a pilot study. *Aphasiology* **2007**, *21*, 208–224. [CrossRef]
25. Tong, A.; Sainsbury, P.; Craig, J. Consolidated criteria for reporting qualitative research (COREQ): A 32-item checklist for interviews and focus groups. *Int. J. Qual. Health Care* **2007**, *19*, 349–357. [CrossRef]
26. Kertesz, A.; Raven, J.C. *The Western Aphasia Battery Revised, revised ed.*; PsychCorp: San Antonio, TX, USA, 2007.
27. Turner-Stokes, L.; Kalmus, M.; Hirani, D.; Clegg, F. The Depression Intensity Scale Circles (DISCs): A first evaluation of a simple assessment tool for depression in the context of brain injury. *J. Neurol. Neurosurg. Psychiatry* **2005**, *76*, 1273–1278. [CrossRef] [PubMed]
28. Ryan, B.; Kneebone, I.I.; Rose, M.L.; Togher, L.; Power, E.; Hoffman, T.; Khan, A.; Simmons-Mackie, N.; Carragher, M.; Worrall, L. Preventing depression in aphasia: A cluster randomised control trial of the Aphasia Action Success Knowledge (ASK) program. *Int. J. Stroke* **2023**, *18*, 996–1004. [CrossRef]
29. Worrall, L.; Ryan, B.; Hudson, K.; Kneebone, I.I.; Simmons-Mackie, N.; Khan, A.; Hoffman, T.; Power, E.; Togher, L.; Rose, M. Reducing the psychosocial impact of aphasia on mood and quality of life in people with aphasia and the impact of caregiving in family members through the Aphasia Action Success Knowledge (Aphasia ASK) program: Study protocol for a randomized controlled trial. *Trials* **2016**, *17*, 153. [CrossRef] [PubMed]
30. Wilson, C.; Kim, E. Qualitative data collection: Considerations for people with Aphasia. *Aphasiology* **2021**, *35*, 314–333. [CrossRef]
31. Lyons, R.; McAllister, L. (Eds.) *Qualitative Research in Communication Disorders: An Introduction for Students and Clinicians*; J & R Press Ltd: Havant, UK, 2019.
32. Shiggins, C.; Ryan, B.; O'Halloran, R.; Power, E.; Bernhardt, J.; Lindley, R.I.; McGurk, G.; Hankey, G.J.; Rose, M.L. Towards the Consistent Inclusion of People With Aphasia in Stroke Research Irrespective of Discipline. *Arch. Phys. Med. Rehabil.* **2022**, *103*, 2256–2263. [CrossRef]
33. Lemmens, L.H.J.M.; Müller, V.N.L.S.; Arntz, A.; Huibers, M.J.H. Mechanisms of change in psychotherapy for depression: An empirical update and evaluation of research aimed at identifying psychological mediators. *Clin. Psychol. Rev.* **2016**, *50*, 95–107. [CrossRef]
34. Lorenzo-Luaces, L. Identifying active ingredients in cognitive-behavioral therapies: What if we didn't? *Behav. Res. Ther.* **2023**, *168*, 104365. [CrossRef]
35. Thomas, S.A.; Walker, M.F.; Macniven, J.A.; Haworth, H.; Lincoln, N.B. Communication and Low Mood (CALM): A randomized controlled trial of behavioural therapy for stroke patients with aphasia. *Clin. Rehabil.* **2013**, *27*, 398–408. [CrossRef]
36. Thomas, S.A.; Drummond, A.E.; Lincoln, N.B.; Palmer, R.L.; das Nair, R.; Latimer, N.R.; Hackney, G.L.; Mandefield, L.; Walters, S.J.; Hatton, R.D.; et al. Behavioural activation therapy for post-stroke depression: The BEADS feasibility RCT. *Health Technol. Assess.* **2019**, *23*, 1–176. [CrossRef] [PubMed]
37. Kneebone, I.I.; Jeffries, F.W. Treating anxiety after stroke using cognitive-behaviour therapy: Two cases. *Neuropsychol. Rehabil.* **2013**, *23*, 798–810. [CrossRef] [PubMed]
38. Worrall, L.; Sherratt, S.; Rogers, P.; Howe, T.; Hersh, D.; Ferguson, A.; Davidson, B. What people with aphasia want: Their goals according to the ICF. *Aphasiology* **2011**, *25*, 309–322. [CrossRef]
39. Northcott, S.; Simpson, A.; Thomas, S.; Barnard, R.; Burns, K.; Hirani, S.P.; Hilari, K. "Now I Am Myself": Exploring How People With Poststroke Aphasia Experienced Solution-Focused Brief Therapy Within the SOFIA Trial. *Qual. Health Res.* **2021**, *31*, 2041–2055. [CrossRef] [PubMed]
40. Lawton, M.; Sage, K.; Haddock, G.; Conroy, P.; Serrant, L. Speech and language therapists' perspectives of therapeutic alliance construction and maintenance in aphasia rehabilitation post-stroke. *Int. J. Lang. Commun. Disord.* **2018**, *53*, 550–563. [CrossRef] [PubMed]

41. Strong, K.A.; Randolph, J. How Do You Do Talk Therapy With Someone Who Can't Talk? Perspectives From Mental Health Providers on Delivering Services to Individuals With Aphasia. *Am. J. Speech-Lang. Pathol.* **2021**, *30*, 2681–2692. [CrossRef] [PubMed]
42. Gracey, F.; Evans, J.J.; Malley, D. Capturing process and outcome in complex rehabilitation interventions: A "Y-shaped" model. *Neuropsychol. Rehabil.* **2009**, *19*, 867–890. [CrossRef]
43. Lincoln, N.B.; Flannaghan, T. Cognitive behavioral psychotherapy for depression following stroke: A randomized controlled trial. *Stroke* **2003**, *34*, 111–115. [CrossRef]

healthcare

MDPI

Article

Evaluating Feasibility of a Secondary Stroke Prevention Program

Stephanie Hunter [1], Kimberley Vogel [1], Shane O'Leary [1,2] and Jannette Maree Blennerhassett [1,3,*]

[1] Austin Health, Health Independence Program, Community Rehabilitation Service, Melbourne, VIC 3084, Australia
[2] Austin Health, Spinal Community Integration Service, Melbourne, VIC 3101, Australia
[3] Austin Health, Physiotherapy Department, Melbourne, VIC 3084, Australia
* Correspondence: jannette.blennerhassett@austin.org.au; Tel.: +61-3-94962211

Abstract: Healthy lifestyles including exercise and diet can reduce stroke risk, but stroke survivors often lack guidance to modify their lifestyles after hospital discharge. We evaluated the implementation of a new, secondary stroke prevention program involving supervised exercise, multidisciplinary education and coaching to address modifiable risk factors. The group-based program involved face-to-face and telehealth sessions. The primary outcomes were feasibility, examined via service information (referrals, uptake, participant demographics and costs), and participant acceptability (satisfaction and attendance). Secondary outcomes examined self-reported changes in lifestyle factors and pre–post scores on standardized clinical tests (e.g., waist circumference and 6-Minute Walk (6MWT)). We ran seven programs in 12 months, and 37 people participated. Attendance for education sessions was 79%, and 30/37 participants completed the full program. No adverse events occurred. Participant satisfaction was high for 'relevance' (100%), 'felt safe to exercise' (96%) and 'intend to continue' (96%). Most participants (88%) changed (on average) 2.5 lifestyle factors (diet, exercise, smoking and alcohol). Changes in clinical outcomes seemed promising, with some being statistically significant, e.g., 6MWT (MD 59 m, 95% CI 38 m to 80,159 m, $p < 0.001$) and waist circumference (MD −2.1 cm, 95%CI −3.9 cm to −1.4 cm, $p < 0.001$). The program was feasible to deliver, acceptable to participants and seemed beneficial for health. Access to similar programs may assist in secondary stroke prevention.

Keywords: secondary stroke prevention; exercise; exercise therapy; model of care; risk factors; health education; physical education and training; telerehabilitation; health risk behaviour; stroke

1. Introduction

Stroke is an episodic condition and a leading cause of disability and death worldwide [1–4]. In Australia, more than 445,087 people are living with the effects of stroke, often altering independence and quality of life, which impacts families, communities, healthcare and support services [1]. In Australia in 2020, 27,428 people had a stroke for the first time, with 24% of those people being under 55 years of age, and around 70,000 people were admitted to hospital for stroke [1]. The estimated economic impact of stroke in Australia in 2020 was AUD 6.2 billion for direct financial costs with an additional AUD 46 billion for mortality and loss of wellbeing [1]. These data also involve people who have recurrent stroke, which has an accumulative effect that increases the level of disability and demands on healthcare and further degrades quality of life [5].

The long-term risk and rate of recurrent stroke has been described as unacceptably high [6,7], especially given estimates that 80% of strokes can be prevented [2,8]. For example, a large longitudinal study in Canada found that people with stroke or transient ischaemic attack (TIA) who were clinically stable 90 days post-event had an 8-fold increase in hazard for recurrent stroke relative to matched controls at one year (HR 8.2, 95% CI 4.8

to 5.5) [6]. In Germany, a large population study found that the rate of recurrent stroke was 7.4% after 1 year and 19.4% after 5 years [9]. Therefore, there is an imperative to reduce rates of recurrent stroke [7]. Given that behavioural factors, such as exercise, diet and smoking, are estimated to account for 47% (41.3 to 54.4) of the burden of stroke [3], addressing those modifiable risk factors [7,10–12] has the potential to complement established medical and pharmacological management to reduce recurrent stroke [4,13,14]. For instance, a large population study found that people who were physically active had a 68% lower chance of stroke or death than people who were sedentary [15]. People with mild stroke or TIA have a 6-fold risk reduction for recurrent stroke if they undertake cardiovascular exercise, which is independent of receiving the recommended pharmacological management [16]. However, despite the health benefits of exercise, community-dwelling individuals with stroke are sedentary, spending the majority of their day sitting [17], a known risk factor for cardiovascular disease and stroke, including recurrent stroke [18].

Models of community care may support secondary stroke prevention [4,6], with guidelines recommending physical activity and cardiovascular exercise and referrals to support behaviour change to address modifiable risk factors [10–12,18,19]. Models of care, shown to be beneficial for health and fitness outcomes, include modified versions of cardiac rehabilitation programs [20]. The use of emerging technologies, such as telehealth and wearable devices, also has merit to support training, education, goal setting and monitoring to facilitate self-management programs [21]. Moreover, the use of telehealth has been feasible and may improve access to stroke care [22]. Factors that support people with stroke to be physically active and address lifestyle risk factors include guidance by health professionals who understand stroke, peer support and approaches that incorporate goal-directed and behavioural change [23,24]. These factors are consistent with the wishes of stroke survivors, who want more information on how to prevent stroke, including guidance on lifestyle and exercise [25,26], but these resources may not be provided routinely when people leave the hospital. When examining our local care in consecutive people with TIA, we observed that half of those people may get a brochure about the benefits of exercise, but few people were referred to health professionals to support behaviour changes for lifestyle factors (unpublished data), as recommended by current evidence-based guidelines to reduce the risk of a further stroke event [12,14,19]. These observations may be similar to other people with mild stroke who go directly home after a short hospital stay with medical and pharmacological management [27]. Given that current opinion and evidence cautions that the provision of simple advice or information about exercise may be ineffective [18], and that people with stroke or TIA may be unclear about safe and suitable exercise following a stroke event [18,23,25], we thought that providing access for community-dwelling people with stroke or TIA to modify lifestyle factors could support secondary stroke prevention. For the purpose of this study, secondary stroke prevention refers to interventions and strategies that aim to lower the risk of stroke recurrence for people who have had a stroke event, including TIA [10,12]. The program, outlined below, was designed to complement medical–surgical–pharmacological management.

Our primary aim was to evaluate the implementation of a secondary stroke prevention program provided within a Community Rehabilitation Service to see if it was feasible to deliver and acceptable for participants. The secondary aim was to evaluate if participation contributed to clinical outcomes that may help mitigate the risk of stroke. During the design and evaluation phase, we sought stakeholder, consumer and participant guidance to help ensure that the program met the needs of the participants. We hypothesised that we could design, deliver and implement a group-based program involving multidisciplinary education, supervised exercise and coaching to support people with mild stroke or TIA to modify lifestyle factors known to increase risk of further stroke. In addition, we hypothesized the program would be acceptable for participants.

2. Materials and Methods

2.1. Design and Setting

The study was an observational study that evaluated the implementation of a newly designed secondary stroke prevention program (during a 12-month period of intake, October 2021 to October 2022). The program was delivered within a community multidisciplinary rehabilitation setting, from the Health Independence Program at Austin Health, in Melbourne, Australia. Austin Health is a large metropolitan tertiary public health organization affiliated with universities for research and the teaching of medical, nursing and allied health. Austin Health admits around 500 people with a stroke event per year. Our stroke care includes an emergency department, an acute stroke unit, subacute inpatient and community rehabilitation and outpatient medical clinics. The project had ethical approval granted by the Austin Health Office for Research (reference number 20210118).

2.2. Participant Recruitment and Eligibility

People with mild stroke or TIA were invited to participate with the support of written participant information, discussion and opt-in consent. To be eligible, people needed to be community dwelling, over 18 years of age, within 4 months post stroke event, able to walk independently with or without an assistive device and living within the geographical area. Participants needed to be medically stable and have modifiable lifestyle risk factors for stroke. There were no additional exclusion criteria. People were referred to the program by allied health professionals, stroke liaison nurses or medical staff working in stroke care at Austin Health. This included acute wards, outpatient clinics (TIA and stroke prevention and rehabilitation physicians) and community rehabilitation. Eligibility and informed consent were confirmed via a triage process involving telephone contact with each person referred.

2.3. Program Format

The program was based on current guidelines [12,14,19] and comprised supervised exercise and multidisciplinary education to modify lifestyle risk factors for stroke. The program was delivered over a 12-week period and involved two phases: (1) supervised exercise and education and (2) coaching via telehealth to support self-management and behaviour change. Participants were assessed before starting to establish personal goals and preferences. Assessments were repeated midway (6 weeks) and at discharge (12 weeks) to provide feedback on progress, update the plan and support motivation. See Figure 1 and Table 1 below. The program was funded publicly at no cost to the participant. Participants were not provided with stipends.

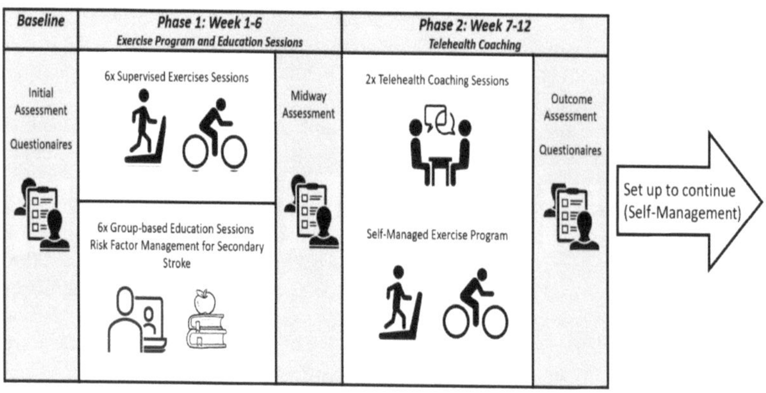

Figure 1. Infographic of secondary stroke prevention program showing assessment time points, phases and intent for continued self-management.

Phase 1 (weeks 1 to 6, Figure 1): Participants had one 60 min session of supervised, group-based, onsite exercise per week for six weeks. (Group numbers were set by the COVID-19 mitigation strategies at the time. For the first intake, exercise was supervised via telehealth). The exercise program was designed and supervised by an Exercise Physiologist to ensure that exercise was safe, suitable and tailored to the individual's ability, fitness and preferences. The key focus for exercise was moderate-intensity aerobic exercise, with coaching and guidance to support participants to learn how to feel safe and self-monitor their performance and intensity during exercise. The sessions also included discussion about behaviour change to problem solve strategies to overcome barriers for physical activity.

Table 1. Education topics.

Week	Topic	Presenter [1]
1	Welcome and overview of the program. Why should I exercise? How can I get started?	Exercise Physiologist
2	Overview of stroke and managing risk factors. Introduction to Stroke Foundation resources.	Stroke Liaison Nurse
3	Diet and Cholesterol.	Dietitian
4	Living Well after Stroke.	Occupational Therapy
5	How much exercise should I do?	Exercise Physiologist
6	Where to from here?	Exercise Physiologist

[1] Senior staff from the Community Rehabilitation Service or Stroke Service.

Phase 1 also included weekly education sessions (1 h duration) delivered in a group telehealth format (synchronous video using the Microsoft 365 Teams platform) by the multidisciplinary team from Austin Health's Community Rehabilitation Service or Stroke Service (Table 1). All presenters were experienced in working with people with stroke. The series of education sessions was designed by relevant members of the multidisciplinary team with input from consumers, was adapted to support people with mild cognitive or communication difficulties and used existing trusted online resources [2]. Each session built upon and reinforced early components of the education. The educational model was interactive to enable peer discussion and support and promoted principles of behaviour change. All presenters received a detailed handover of the participants (medical, social and stroke-related impairments and goals) to promote relevance of each topic.

Phase 2 (week 7 to 12, Figure 1): Fortnightly telehealth coaching sessions (30 min to 1 h duration, synchronous video using the Microsoft 365 Teams platform) were undertaken and conducted by an Exercise Physiologist. These aimed to taper off the professional support, while encouraging the participants to self-manage their exercise/physical activity and lifestyle risk factors [18,21]. The coaching reinforced the person's goals, checked in on their progress, and explored barriers and enablers to increase self-efficacy.

2.4. Outcome Measures

Our primary outcomes examined the feasibility and acceptability of delivering the secondary stroke prevention program. Feasibility considered the practicality of the new approach and was evaluated by collating a range of service delivery information, such as referrals (numbers and uptake), participant demographics and costs (staff time and wages). Participant acceptability was measured by participant uptake, attendance (number of sessions and proportion who completed the program) and satisfaction with the program. To determine satisfaction, we custom designed an online survey to enable participants to provide anonymous feedback about the program (using Microsoft 365 Forms). The survey focused on relevance, format (e.g., time and presentation), perceived safety and support and whether the program supported the ability to address lifestyle risk factors, as outlined by behaviour-change principles [28]. Survey responses included 5-point Likert scales and open text.

Our secondary outcomes involved clinical tests and patient-reported outcomes measured before commencing the program and at 12 weeks (discharge). The series of standardized clinical tests and validated questionnaires used are listed below. All clinical outcomes and questionnaires (with the exception of the Stroke Exercise Preference Inventory) were completed at initial assessment (before commencing program), midway (week 6) and discharge (week 12). Participants also provided self-reported information about changes in their lifestyle risk factors for stroke via the online, anonymous survey at the completion of the program (via Microsoft 365 Forms). The tests and questionnaires used are as follows:

- Blood pressure: measured using an automated machine (OMRON HEM-7203) with an inflatable cuff around the upper arm. For those with a stroke or TIA, blood pressures lower than 130/80 mmHg are recommended to reduce risk of recurrent stroke [29].
- Waist circumference (centimetres): measured at the level of the umbilicus with a tape measure being loose enough to fit one finger between the tape and participant. The Australian Heart Foundation recommends waist circumference less than 94 cm for males and less than 80 cm for females [30].
- Six-Minute Walk Test (6MWT): a widely used measure of functional walking endurance with high test–retest reliability, validity and established normative data for age and sex [31,32]. The test was conducted in a 30-metre corridor and included monitoring of cardiovascular parameters.
- Thirty-Second Sit to Stand Test: a practical test of functional leg strength and endurance with excellent test and retest reliability and validity. Scores reflect the number of times a person can complete sit to stand in 30 s from a 43 cm chair. Normative values in community-dwelling healthy adults aged 60–64 range from 12 to 17 for women and 14 to 19 for men [33].
- International Physical Activity Questionnaire (IPAQ) [34]: we used the short-form, 7-item IPAQ, which is a self-report of physical activity and sitting time over the past 7 days. The IPAQ has established test–retest reliability and validity, enabling estimates of total physical activity including vigorous intensity, moderate intensity and walking (in minutes per week) and time spent sitting (hours per week) [34].
- The Stroke Self-Efficacy Questionnaire (SSEQ) [35]: a self-reported questionnaire about level of confidence reported on a 0 to 10 scale (0 = not confident, 10 = very confident) when completing 13 activities of daily life following stroke. The SSEQ has good internal consistency and criterion validity. The overall score is the sum of all items.
- Fatigue Severity Scale (FSS) [36]: a valid and reliable scale to measure fatigue post stroke that involves rating agreement for 9 items on a 7-point Likert scale (1 = disagree, 7 = agree). Overall scores are averaged, reporting fatigue on a scale of 1 to 7, with higher scores reflecting higher levels of fatigue. The normal range is 2.3/7 or lower [37]. Scores higher than 4/7 reflect problematic fatigue in healthy adults [36].
- Stroke Exercise Preference Inventory (SEPI) [38]: a standardised questionnaire designed to explore preferences and barriers to exercise after stroke. Participants rate their level of agreement, where 0% represents 'Don't agree at all' and 100% represents 'Totally agree'. The SEPI was undertaken only at commencement to help establish participants' preferences and understand perceived barriers to physical activity.

2.5. Data Analyses

Service information (referrals, referral uptake, participant demographics, staff costs to deliver the program and program details) were collated to examine if the program was feasible to deliver. Participant acceptability was summarized by collating information such as participant uptake, attendance and satisfaction. Clinical outcomes for group data were summarized (pre and post) and then analysed statistically using paired comparisons. We used a paired-sample *t*-test for interval data that were normally distributed and the Wilcoxon signed-rank test for non-parametric data or interval data that were not normally distributed. Statistical significance was set at 0.05. Paired comparisons were also reported as mean difference and 95% confidence intervals. Self-reported changes in lifestyle factors (provided in the online survey) were summarized descriptively outlining the proportion of participants who made lifestyle changes and the number of risk factors addressed. Data from the IPAQ (physical activity in minutes and time spent sitting per week in hours) were also collated. Statistical analyses were performed using R Statistical Software (version 4.2.2; R Core Team 2022). Online surveys and descriptive data were analysed using Microsoft 365 Forms and Excel. We did not undertake an intention-to-treat analysis, nor perform a priori sample size calculations.

3. Results

3.1. Feasibility

Over the evaluation period (intake October 2021 to October 2022), 90 referrals were received for the program. At triage, 37 people consented to participate, 10 were wait listed and 43 did not proceed with the program. The reasons for not participating were as follows: offered an alternative service such as 1:1 Exercise Physiology (28); medical (4); could not access telehealth (2); program was not indicated (3) and person's choice (6). The 37 referrals that proceeded came from the acute ward (19), community rehabilitation (13), Better at Home (an inpatient bed substitution provided at home (3)), the Stroke Prevention Outpatient Clinic (1) and the external subacute rehabilitation setting (1).

Of the 37 participants, 73% were male, and the average age was 62 years. Most participants had an ischaemic stroke event (86%) and were a first presentation for a stroke event (86%). At triage, the average time since stroke event was 56 days. One-quarter of participants only received the secondary stroke prevention program, while the remainder also had Community Rehabilitation Services. For more demographic and medical information, see Table 2.

Table 2. Demographic and medical information about the 37 participants. Stroke event includes stroke or transient ischaemic attack.

Characteristics	Detail	Data
Age (years)	Average (SD) Range	62 (12) years 38 to 83 years
Gender (n)	Male Female	27 10
Type of stroke event (n)	Ischemic Haemorrhagic TIA	32 2 3
First vs. recurrent stroke event (n)	First stroke event Recurrent stroke event	32 5
Time since stroke event, at time of triage (days)	Average (SD) Range, days	55.9 (35.6) days 12 to 168 days [1]
Relevant medical condition linked to stroke event (n)	Hypertension Carotid artery stenosis/occlusion Carotid artery dissection Intracranial radiotherapy Patent foramen ovale Thoracic aortic atherosclerosis Diabetic Atrial fibrillation Arteriovenous malformation Aneurysm No other relevant medical conditions	9 4 2 1 4 1 5 6 1 1 3
Mobility, (n)	Independent without gait aid	37
Required carer help to attend program (n)	No Yes	36 1
Community Rehabilitation Services provided (n)	SSPP only Community Rehabilitation Service and SSPP	9 28

Abbreviations: n = number, SD = standard deviation, TIA = transient ischaemic attack, SSPP = secondary stroke prevention program. [1] One person was referred 168 days post stroke, with the remainder meeting the 4-month selection criteria. This participant did not complete the program so their data are not included in pairwise comparisons.

During the evaluation period, we delivered seven intakes of the program. Given that each intake had the capacity for eight participants, the overall uptake of the program during the evaluation period was 66%, while the later intakes ran at full capacity. No adverse events occurred. Seven participants did not complete the full program (defined by attending the final assessment session) for the following reasons: medically unwell unrelated to stroke (three); moved overseas (one); exacerbation of back pain (one); contracted COVID-19 (one) and returned to work (one).

We calculated that 122 staff hours were needed to deliver the 12-week program for eight participants to receive 24 occasions of service. These hours involved approximately 105 h of Exercise Physiology (for triage, assessment, education, coaching and general administration), with the remainder being for multidisciplinary education and administration. Based on 2023 award rates (including on-costs), the cost of the 12-week program was AUD 7760, and the cost per participant was AUD 970.

3.2. *Acceptability*

At triage, 83% of referrals wanted to participate in the 12-week program or an alternative service, and only 7% of people referred declined a service. Participants attended 79% of the telehealth education sessions and 83% of the supervised exercise sessions. The majority of the planned telehealth coaching sessions were completed. As mentioned previously, 81% of the participants completed the full program.

Twenty-four participants completed the online survey (65% response rate). The findings support that satisfaction was high (strongly agree and agree) for 'relevance' (100%), 'would recommend to others' (96%), 'felt safe to exercise' (96%) and 'intend to continue' (96%). See Table 3 for more details.

Table 3. Participant survey responses (n = 24 responses from 37 invited).

Survey Theme and Question	Percentage Overall Agreement [1]	Breakdown of Responses (Percentage)				
		Strongly Agree	Agree	Neutral	Disagree	Strongly Disagree
General format of program						
The stroke prevention program was relevant to me.	100	79.2	20.8	0	0	0
I would recommend this overall program to other stroke survivors.	95.8	75	10.8	4.2	0	0
The time of the telehealth sessions suited me.	95.8	50	45.8	4.2	0	0
The format of the telehealth sessions suited me.	91.7	54.2	37.5	8.3	0	0
Relevance of each education session [2]						
Exercise Physiology: Introduction to program. Benefits of exercise and how to get started.	100	62.5	37.5	0	0	0
Stroke Liaison Nurse: Overview of stroke and medical-pharmacological management.	95.8	54.2	41.7	0	4.2	0
Dietitian: Cholesterol and diet.	91.7	58.8	33.3	4.2	0	4.2
Occupational Therapy: Tips to resume life and activities.	91.7	62.7	29.2	4.2	4.2	0
Exercise Physiology: Tips to keep exercising.	100	79.2	20.8	0	0	0
Support to exercise						
I felt safe exercising at home.	95.8	66.7	29.2	4.2	0	0
There was enough follow up to help me check in on my progress.	95.8	75.0	20.8	4.2	0	0
Lifestyle and behavioural changes [3]						
Since the program started, I have changed some lifestyle factors (e.g., diet, alcohol consumption, smoking, exercise).	87.5	62.5	25.0	12.5	0	0
I understand how much exercise I need to do to minimise my risk of secondary stroke. [3]	100	66.7	33.3	0	0	0
I have the skills and resources to continue my exercise program long-term. [2]	91.7	50	41.7	8.3	0	0
I am committed to continue my exercise to meet the secondary stroke guidelines and keep me healthy. [3]	95.8	58.3	37.5	4.2	0	0

[1] Data are summarized as overall agreement (responded strongly agree or agree). [2] Respondents were not asked to explain their rating of relevance. [3] Survey structured using COM-B model of behaviour change wheel: Capability (knowledge); Opportunity; and Motivation [28].

3.3. Clinical Outcomes and Stroke Risk Mitigation

The secondary outcomes involved clinical tests and questionnaires. Paired comparisons for the group show improvements after participation that were statistically significant for waist circumference, walking endurance, functional lower limb strength and levels of physical activity and fatigue. The changes observed for self-efficacy and blood pressure showed a diverse range and were not statistically significant (see Table 4).

Table 4. Observed mean and standard deviation for group data at commencement and discharge. Change scores recorded showing mean difference with 95% confidence intervals for the group.

Outcome Measure	Initial Assessment (n = 37)	Discharge Assessment (n = 30)	Paired-Comparisons Mean Difference, [95% CI] (n = 30) [1]	*p*
Blood pressure (systolic) mmHg	125 (15)	124 (11.5)	−2.6, 95% CI [−8.4 to 3.2]	0.42
Blood pressure (diastolic) mmHg	79 (9.6)	79 (9.5)	−0.3, 95% CI [−3.7 to 3.0]	0.32
Waist circumference (cm)	100 (10.6)	98 (10.4)	−2.1, 95% CI [−2.8 to −1.4]	<0.001
6-Minute Walk Test (metres)	473 (83.6)	529 (88.6)	59, 95% CI [37.9 to 80.2]	<0.001
30 s Sit to Stand Test (repetitions)	13 (3.4)	15 (3.8)	2.4, 95% CI [0.9 to 4.0]	0.003
IPAQ total physical activity, (minutes per week)	350 (384)	582 (413)	276, 95% CI [−80 to 471]	0.008
IPAQ sitting time (hours per week)	6.2 (3.0)	4.5 (2.0)	−1.6, 95% CI [−3.1 to −0.7]	0.04
SSEQ (/130)	119 (9.6)	119 (10.1)	2.6, 95% CI [−2.5 to 7.7]	0.29
FSS (/7)	3.9 (1.5)	2.7 (1.2)	−0.9, 95% CI [−1.6 to 0]	0.08

Abbreviations: n = number, CI = confidence intervals, *p* = *p*-value, IPAQ = International Physical Activity Questionnaire, SSEQ = Stroke Self-Efficacy Questionnaire, FSS = Fatigue Severity Scale. [1] Data from the participant who was 168 days post stroke was not included in pairwise comparisons, as they did not complete the program for medical reasons unrelated to stroke.

Most participants (89%) reported that they had changed a lifestyle risk factor for stroke since attending the program (see Table 3). On average, each of those participants reported to have changed 2.5 lifestyle risk factors (diet, exercise, smoking and alcohol). Self-reports for physical activity (as reported by the IPAQ) indicated that participants increased physical activity time and reduced sedentary sitting time, and these changes were found to be statistically significant (see Table 4).

4. Discussion

The secondary stroke prevention program incorporating supervised exercise, multidisciplinary education and coaching was found to be feasible, safe and low cost to deliver. Participants found the program acceptable in terms of uptake, satisfaction and attendance. The clinical outcomes observed after participation also suggest possible benefits for addressing modifiable lifestyle factors associated with risk of recurrent stroke [3,4,10,14,18]. Our evaluation supports that this model of community care may be implemented within established multidisciplinary community teams with experience in stroke and links to acute stroke units to support people with mild stroke or transient ischaemic attack to address modifiable risk factors after leaving the hospital.

Elements of our program that may have assisted in making the model feasible to deliver and acceptable to participants require mention. The education, support and coaching were guided by evidence and principles of behaviour change [18,28]. The program employed skills and experience from a multidisciplinary team experienced in adapting programs for people with stroke [23,24]. Participants gave input to the program in terms of design, content and scheduling. During implementation, we also took on feedback from participants, staff and referrers to refine the service, making minor changes to streamline implementation (e.g., referral processes, patient information, etc.) and participant experience (e.g., provision of written handouts, emphasis for the education sessions and support to set up telehealth). This iterative process enabled us to document our model of care, permitting the possibility to share our procedures with other health services or to support research evaluation. Referral to the program was via trusted health professionals and followed up by a comprehensive triage discussion. Each person's program was individualized for relevant risk factors, preferences for physical activity, physical capacity and goals. Feedback on progress was supported by the use of standardized tests, which included patient-reported outcomes. Participants also valued the interactive and supportive culture within the group-based education and supervised exercise sessions, as they provided opportunity for peer support and sharing of lived experiences. Having an initial phase of 6 weeks for telehealth and attendance also seemed palatable and practical, irrespective of the participant's work, driving and social situation. The use of telehealth options also has scope to improve access, thus reducing impacts on carers and work schedules and overcoming barriers such as distance or transport [21,22]. It is, however, worth noting that some people required support from carers or staff to set up telehealth, leading us to recommend that future programs include options for onsite education. The inclusion of the second phase, with tapered coaching to enable the participant and clinician to communicate via telehealth, seemed helpful in reinforcing the importance of self-management for health promotion [14,18,21,26,28], while providing each patient with the opportunity and support to gain confidence to continue their chosen program.

In terms of feasibility, our program aimed to support people with mild stroke or TIA, as many of these people are not linked to health professionals for guidance to modify lifestyle risk factors for stroke, such as diet and exercise. Our referral data indicate that we captured 18% of the 500 people admitted annually to our health setting for stroke events. However, the low referral numbers for people with TIA or from the Stroke Prevention Outpatient Clinic highlights areas to target for referrals and service promotion. While our observation that few people (7%) declined a service for secondary stroke prevention may reflect a referral or selection bias, it seems that people want to improve their health outcomes and would benefit from the opportunity for support. Further, while the program ran at 66% capacity, it took time to promote a new service within our health setting and to establish clear referral pathways. At the end of the 12-month evaluation period, demand increased, and we now have a waiting list and continue to deliver the program as part of routine care.

Given that low levels of physical activity [2,3,12,17,18] and cardiovascular fitness [15,16,19] are risk factors for stroke, the observed gains for physical activity, walking endurance and lower limb function and the reduction in sitting time seemed promising. At discharge, the performance scores generally were within the normative range for the 6-Minute Walk Test [31,32] and the 30 s Sit to Stand Test [33]. On average, the group reported 4.6 h/day more physical activity and 1.6 h/day less sitting time. It was also promising that being more active did not seem to have a negative impact on fatigue. For instance, at commencement, the average level of fatigue reported approached that of being problematic [36] and improved towards normative values for healthy adults [37]. In terms of our other secondary outcomes, waist circumference scores showed improvements, but those changes were small and may not be clinically significant. No direct benefit for blood pressure was observed, but this was not surprising given that the participants were all medically stable, within the recommended range [29] and receiving pharmacological management.

The potential cost benefits of our program to reduce healthcare costs seem promising. Our 12-week program for eight people was estimated to cost AUD 7760 and may have contributed to reducing the risk of recurrent stroke given the observed increase in physical activity, walking endurance and changes in lifestyle. In comparison, the Australian weighted-average inpatient separation for stroke in 2020 costed AUD 10,209 [1], which suggests one hospital admission could fund 1.3 intakes of the secondary stroke prevention program. On approximate terms, four intakes of the program delivered to 32 people would have similar costs as three inpatient separations. The evidence supports that physical activity and exercise can reduce the risk of stroke (68% relative risk reduction [15] or reduced odds ratio of 0.4 (confidence intervals 0.2 to 0.6) [16]). Extrapolating from those data suggests that treating between two and five people (with exercise) may be needed to reduce one person from having a stroke. Given that recurrent stroke also has other economic and human costs [1,3,4,6,26], our program, which has been shown to be feasible to deliver and acceptable to participants, appears to offer good value for the money.

Several limitations of this study need consideration when interpreting and attempting to generalize from our findings. The study involved a small convenience sample of people from one healthcare setting with an established stroke unit and was from a high-income country. The participants had a range of medical conditions but were clinically stable and living independently in the community. Given the clinical nature of the program, the rate of attrition in attendance due to unrelated illness, relocation and return to work was not surprising, and seemed unrelated to the program. The study was also undertaken in the context of a program evaluation and was not designed to investigate the effectiveness of the intervention. The study was not controlled was under powered, and outcome measures were not undertaken by independent assessors. Moreover, the participants were aware of the program evaluation, and their positive views about the program were a source of potential bias. Further, while our approach did aim to change behaviour, we do not follow up participants to see if the observed changes were sustained. Given these limitations, the gains observed in the secondary outcomes should be interpreted with caution. Future controlled research is needed to determine if the program is effective, leads to sustained changes in lifestyle and reduces risk of recurrent stroke.

5. Conclusions

Our group-based program that combined supervised exercise, education and coaching to manage modifiable risk factors for stroke was feasible and low cost to deliver, acceptable to participants and may have supported beneficial clinical and health outcomes. This type of model of care has the scope to support people to address modifiable risk factors for stroke, and thus may assist in improving patient outcomes and optimizing the use of healthcare services. Further investigation of the program is needed to examine if it is effective and if changes in lifestyle are sustained.

Author Contributions: Conceptualization, J.M.B., S.H. and K.V.; methodology, J.M.B., S.H. and K.V.; formal analysis, J.M.B., S.H., S.O. and K.V.; investigation, J.M.B., S.H., S.O. and K.V.; writing—original draft preparation, J.M.B., S.H., S.O. and K.V.; writing—review and editing, J.M.B., S.H., S.O. and K.V.; supervision, J.M.B.; project administration, S.H., S.O. and K.V. All authors have read and agreed to the published version of the manuscript.

Funding: This research received no external funding.

Institutional Review Board Statement: This study was conducted in accordance with the Declaration of Helsinki and approved by the Office for Research of Austin Health (reference number 20210118, date: 9 September 2021) as a Quality Improvement activity.

Informed Consent Statement: Opt-in informed consent, supported by a written participant information sheet, was obtained from all participants involved in the study.

Data Availability Statement: This was an observational study evaluating a program of care. The project did not require registration. The minimal datasets for this project are provided in the manuscript. Further data may be shared via correspondence with the authors.

Acknowledgments: We acknowledge the contribution of the multidisciplinary team at Austin Health who were delivered the education program. We also acknowledge the support provided by the Health Independent Program to commence and deliver this program, and to Timothy J. Albiston for conducting the statistical analyses.

Conflicts of Interest: The authors declare no conflict of interest.

References

1. Deloitte Access Economics. No Postcode Untouched, Stroke in Australia 2020. Available online: https://www2.deloitte.com/au/en/pages/economics/articles/economic-impact-stroke-australia.html (accessed on 11 August 2021).
2. Stroke Foundation. Prevent Stroke. Available online: www.strokefoundation.org.au/about-stroke/prevent-stroke (accessed on 1 December 2020).
3. World Stroke Organization. "WSO Global Stroke Fact Sheet 2022". Available online: www.world-stroke.org/news-and-blog/news/wso-global-stroke-fact-sheet-2022 (accessed on 19 September 2023).
4. GBD 2019 Stroke Collaborators. Global, regional, and national burden of stroke and its risk factors, 1990–2019: A systematic analysis for the Global Burden of Disease Study 2019. *Lancet Neurol.* **2021**, *20*, 795–820. [CrossRef] [PubMed]
5. Hankey, G.J. Preventable stroke and stroke prevention. *J. Thromb. Haemost. JTH* **2005**, *3*, 1638–1645. [CrossRef] [PubMed]
6. Edwards, J.D.; Kapral, M.K.; Fang, J.; Swartz, R.H. Long-term morbidity and mortality in patients without early complications after stroke or transient ischemic attack. *CMAJ* **2017**, *189*, E954–E961. [CrossRef] [PubMed]
7. Hill, M.D. Long-term stroke prevention: We can do better. *CMAJ* **2017**, *189*, E952–E953. [CrossRef] [PubMed]
8. Hackam, D.G.; Spence, J.D. Combining multiple approaches for the secondary prevention of vascular events after stroke: A quantitative modeling study. *Stroke* **2007**, *38*, 1881–1885. [CrossRef] [PubMed]
9. Stahmeyer, J.T.; Stubenrauch, S.; Geyer, S.; Weissenborn, K.; Eberhard, S. The frequency and timing of recurrent stroke: An analysis of routine health insurance data. *Dtsch. Arztebl. Int.* **2019**, *116*, 711–777. [PubMed]
10. Kleindorfer, D.O.; Towfighi, A.; Chaturvedi, S.; Cockroft, K.M.; Gutierrez, J.; Lombardi-Hill, D.; Kamel, H.; Kernan, W.N.; Kittner, S.J.; Leira, E.C.; et al. 2021 Guideline for the prevention of stroke in patients with stroke and transient ischemic attack: A guideline from the American Heart Association/American Stroke Association. *Stroke* **2021**, *52*, e364–e467. [CrossRef] [PubMed]
11. O'Donnell, M.J.; Chin, S.L.; Rangarajan, S.; Xavier, D.; Liu, L.; Zhang, H.; Rao-Melacini, P.; Zhang, X.; Pais, P.; Agapay, S.; et al. Global and regional effects of potentially modifiable risk factors associated with acute stroke in 32 countries (INTERSTROKE): A case-control study. *Lancet* **2016**, *388*, 761–775. [CrossRef]
12. Wein, T.; Lindsay, M.P.; Cote, R.; Foley, N.; Berlingieri, J.; Bhogal, S.; Bourgoin, A.; Buck, B.H.; Cox, J.; Davidson, D.; et al. Canadian stroke best practice recommendations: Secondary prevention of stroke, sixth edition practice guidelines, update 2017. *Int. J. Stroke* **2018**, *13*, 420–443. [CrossRef]
13. Kirk, H.; Kersten, P.; Crawford, P.; Keens, A.; Ashburn, A.; Conway, J. The cardiac model of rehabilitation for reducing cardiovascular risk factors post transient ischaemic attack and stroke: A randomized controlled trial. *Clin. Rehabil.* **2014**, *28*, 339–349. [CrossRef]
14. Mead, G.E.; Sposato, L.A.; Sampaio Silva, G.; Yperzeele, L.; Wu, S.; Kutlubaev, M.; Cheyne, J.; Wahab, K.; Urrutia, V.C.; Sharma, V.K.; et al. A systematic review and synthesis of global stroke guidelines on behalf of the World Stroke Organization. *Int. J. Stroke* **2023**, *18*, 499–531. [CrossRef] [PubMed]
15. Mittleman, M.A.; Mostofsky, E. Physical, psychological and chemical triggers of acute cardiovascular events: Preventive strategies. *Circulation* **2011**, *124*, 346–354. [CrossRef] [PubMed]
16. Turan, T.N.; Nizam, A.; Lynn, M.J.; Egan, B.M.; Le, N.A.; Lopes-Virella, M.F.; Hermayer, K.L.; Harrell, J.; Derdeyn, C.P.; Fiorella, D.; et al. Relationship between risk factor control and vascular events in the SAMMPRIS trial. *Neurology* **2017**, *88*, 379–385. [CrossRef] [PubMed]
17. English, C.; Healy, G.N.; Coates, A.; Lewis, L.; Olds, T.; Bernhardt, J. Sitting and activity time in people with stroke. *Phys. Ther.* **2016**, *96*, 193–201. [CrossRef] [PubMed]
18. Prior, P.L.; Suskin, N. Exercise for stroke prevention. *Stroke Vasc. Neurol.* **2018**, *3*, 59–68. [CrossRef] [PubMed]
19. Billinger, S.A.; Arena, R.; Bernhardt, J.; Eng, J.J.; Franklin, B.A.; Johnson, C.M.; MacKay-Lyons, M.; Macko, R.F.; Mead, G.E.; Roth, E.J.; et al. Physical activity and exercise recommendations for stroke survivors: A statement for healthcare professionals from the American Heart Association/American Stroke Association. *Stroke* **2014**, *45*, 2532–2553. [CrossRef] [PubMed]
20. Cuccurullo, S.J.; Fleming, T.K.; Zinonos, S.; Cosgrove, N.M.; Cabrera, J.; Kostis, J.B.; Greiss, C.; Ray, A.R.; Eckert, A.; Scarpati, R.; et al. Stroke recovery program with modified cardiac rehabilitation improves mortality, functional and cardiovascular performance. *J. Stroke Cerebrovasc. Dis.* **2022**, *31*, 106322. [CrossRef] [PubMed]
21. Dobkin, B.H. Behavioral self-management strategies for practice and exercise should be included in neurological rehabilitation trials and care. *Curr. Opin. Neurol.* **2016**, *29*, 693–699. [CrossRef]
22. Nikolaev, V.A.; Nikolaev, A.A. Recent trends in telerehabilitation of stroke patients: A narrative review. *NeuroRehabilitation* **2022**, *51*, 1–22. [CrossRef]
23. Krawcyk, R.S.; Christoffersen, L.C.; Danielsen, A.K.; Kruuse, C. Motivators for physical activity in patients with minor stroke: A qualitative study. *Disabil. Rehabil.* **2023**, *45*, 277–285. [CrossRef]
24. Sammut, M.; Haracz, K.; English, C.; Shakespeare, D.; Crowfoot, G.; Nilsson, M.; Janssen, H. Participants' perspective of engaging in a gym-based health service delivered secondary stroke prevention program after TIA or mild Stroke. *Int. J. Environ. Res. Pub. Health* **2021**, *18*, 11448. [CrossRef] [PubMed]
25. Chen, T.; Zhang, B.; Deng, Y.; Zhang, J.C.; Song, F. Long-term unmet needs after stroke: Systematic review of evidence from survey studies. *BMJ Open* **2019**, *9*, e028137. [CrossRef] [PubMed]
26. Guo, Y.; Zhang, Z.; Lin, B.; Mei, Y.; Liu, Q.; Zhang, L.; Wang, W.; Li, Y.; Fu, Z. The unmet needs of community-dwelling stroke survivors: A systematic review of qualitative studies. *Int. J. Environ. Res. Pub. Health* **2021**, *18*, 2140. [CrossRef] [PubMed]

27. Australian Stroke Clinical Registry (AuSCR). Australian Stroke Clinical Registry: 2011 Annual Report. Available online: https://auscr.com.au/about/annual-reports/ (accessed on 11 August 2023).
28. Michie, S.; van Stralen, M.M.; West, R. The behaviour change wheel: A new method for characterising and designing behaviour change interventions. *Implement. Sci.* **2011**, *6*, 42. [CrossRef] [PubMed]
29. Whelton, P.K.; Carey, R.M. The 2017 Clinical Practice Guideline for High Blood Pressure. *JAMA* **2017**, *318*, 2073–2074. [CrossRef] [PubMed]
30. Heart Foundation. Waist Measurement. Available online: https://www.heartfoundation.org.au/bundles/your-heart/waist-measurement (accessed on 10 August 2023).
31. Bohannon, R. Six-minute walk test: A meta-analysis of data from apparently healthy elders. *Top Geriatr. Rehabil.* **2007**, *23*, 155–160. [CrossRef]
32. Casanova, C.; Celli, B.R.; Barria, P.; Casas, A.; Cote, C.; de Torres, J.P.; Jardim, J.; Lopez, M.V.; Marin, J.M.; de Oca, M.M.; et al. The 6-min walk distance in healthy subjects: Reference standards from seven countries. *Eur. Respir. J.* **2011**, *37*, 150–156. [CrossRef] [PubMed]
33. Jones, C.J.; Rikli, R.E.; Beam, W.C. A 30-s chair-stand test as a measure of lower body strength in community-residing older adults. *Res. Q. Exerc. Sport* **1999**, *70*, 113–119. [CrossRef]
34. Craig, C.L.; Marshall, A.L.; Sjostrom, M.; Bauman, A.E.; Booth, M.L.; Ainsworth, B.E.; Pratt, M.; Ekelund, U.L.; Yngve, A.; Sallis, J.F.; et al. International Physical Activity Questionnaire: 12-country reliability and validity. *Med. Sci. Sport. Exerc.* **2003**, *35*, 1381–1395. [CrossRef]
35. Jones, F.; Partridge, C.; Reid, F. The Stroke Self-Efficacy Questionnaire: Measuring individual confidence in functional performance after stroke. *J. Clin. Nurs.* **2008**, *17*, 244–252. [CrossRef]
36. Krupp, L.B.; LaRocca, N.G.; Muir-Nash, J.; Steinberg, A.D. The Fatigue Severity Scale: Application to patients with Multiple Sclerosis and Systemic Lupus Erythematosus. *Arch. Neurol.* **1989**, *46*, 1121–1123. [CrossRef]
37. Grace, J.; Mendelsohn, A.; Friedman, J.H. A comparison of fatigue measures in Parkinson's disease. *Park. Relat. Disord.* **2007**, *13*, 443–445. [CrossRef]
38. Bonner, N.S.; O'Halloran, P.D.; Bernhardt, J.; Cumming, T.B. Developing the Stroke Exercise Preference Inventory (SEPI). *PLoS ONE* **2016**, *11*, e0164120. [CrossRef]

healthcare

MDPI

Article

Co-Designed Cardiac Rehabilitation for the Secondary Prevention of Stroke (CARESS): A Pilot Program Evaluation

Sabah Rehman [1], Seamus Barker [1], Kim Jose [1], Michele Callisaya [1,2], Helen Castley [3], Martin G. Schultz [1], Myles N. Moore [1], Dawn B. Simpson [4], Gregory M. Peterson [5] and Seana Gall [1,6,*]

1 Menzies Institute for Medical Research, University of Tasmania, Hobart, TAS 7000, Australia; sabah.rehman@utas.edu.au (S.R.); seamus.barker@utas.edu.au (S.B.); kim.jose@utas.edu.au (K.J.); michele.callisaya@utas.edu.au (M.C.); myles.moore@utas.edu.au (M.N.M.)
2 Peninsula Clinical School, Monash University, Frankston, VIC 3199, Australia
3 Royal Hobart Hospital, Tasmanian Health Service, Hobart, TAS 7000, Australia; helen.castley@ths.tas.gov.au
4 College of Health, Medicine and Wellbeing, University of Newcastle, Callaghan, NSW 2308, Australia; dawn.simpson@newcastle.edu.au
5 School of Pharmacy and Pharmacology, University of Tasmania, Hobart, TAS 7005, Australia
6 Faculty of Medicine, Dentistry and Health Sciences, Monash University, Melbourne, VIC 3800, Australia
* Correspondence: seana.gall@utas.edu.au; Tel.: +61-3-6226-4728

Abstract: Structured health system-based programs, such as cardiac rehabilitation, may reduce the risk of recurrent stroke. This study aimed to co-design and evaluate a structured program of rehabilitation, developed based on insights from focus groups involving stroke survivors and health professionals. Conducted in Tasmania, Australia in 2019, the 7-week program comprised one hour of group exercise and one hour of education each week. Functional capacity (6 min walk test), fatigue, symptoms of depression (Patient Health Questionnaire), and lifestyle were assessed pre- and post-program, with a historical control group for comparison. Propensity score matching determined the average treatment effect (ATE) of the program. Key themes from the co-design focus groups included the need for coordinated care, improved psychosocial management, and including carers and peers in programs. Of the 23 people approached, 10 participants (70% men, mean age 67.4 ± 8.6 years) completed the program without adverse events. ATE analysis revealed improvements in functional capacity (139 m, 95% CI 44, 234) and fatigue (−5 units, 95% CI −9, −1), with a small improvement in symptoms of depression (−0.8 units, 95% CI −1.8, 0.2) compared to controls. The co-designed program demonstrated feasibility, acceptability, and positive outcomes, suggesting its potential to support stroke survivors.

Keywords: stroke; co-design; secondary prevention

1. Introduction

It is estimated that there are 29,000 strokes each year in Australia [1], with around 400,000 people in the community who have had a stroke [2]. At least 80% of stroke episodes are caused by modifiable risk factors [3]. Therefore, the control of risk factors in people who have had a stroke is important and is recognised in clinical guidelines for the management of stroke. For example, the Australian Stroke Foundation's Clinical Guidelines for the Management of Stroke recommend that "secondary prevention strategies should be considered for all patients with stroke or transient ischaemic attack (TIA) who are not receiving palliative care" [4]. Yet, the control of risk factors following stroke is disappointingly poor, including low smoking cessation [5], uncontrolled hypertension [6], and physical inactivity [7]. There is clear evidence for managing most stroke risk factors, which may include surgical and pharmacological interventions, along with lifestyle modifications. A 2023 overview of 15 systematic reviews of multimodal lifestyle-based interventions in people with stroke found moderate certainty evidence for lifestyle-based intervention, e.g., evidence they increased physical activity, and low certainty evidence for improved healthy eating and medication adherence [8]. Despite this evidence, at least 70% of stroke survivors in Australia report that they have unmet health needs, particularly in relation to secondary prevention [9], with 30% of people not receiving a formal discharge plan that included information and strategies to reduce their risk of another stroke [10].

One intervention that may improve secondary prevention of stroke is cardiac rehabilitation programs. These multimodal programs include the prescription of aerobic and resistance exercise and education to facilitate risk factor control and improved quality of life [11]. These programs are for people who have experienced or are at high risk of experiencing a cardiac event, thus the name refers to the patient group rather than the goal of improving cardiac function directly. In Australia, it is recommended that all cardiac patients be referred to these programs. Consequently, there are over 370 rehabilitation programs around Australia [12]. At face value, this type of program would appear to also address the needs of people with stroke in terms of risk factor management. However, in Australia [13] and other parts of the world [14], most cardiac rehabilitation programs do not include people with stroke, or they make up only a small percentage of users. The reasons for this are reported to include a lack of referrals, the complexity of including people with neurological deficits, potential safety risks (e.g., falls), and lack of resources [13–15]. Nonetheless, as a widely available, effective, embedded health system program, the potential adaptation and scale-up of cardiac rehabilitation programs to include stroke survivors is appealing.

Utilising cardiac rehabilitation programs to support secondary stroke prevention can be understood as a complex intervention [16] involving multiple interacting components that can be highly sensitive to the context of use. Changing the context from cardiac rehabilitation to a program for people with stroke requires an exploration of whether and how such a program should be adapted. Accordingly, the first aim of this project was to describe how to adapt cardiac rehabilitation as an intervention for secondary stroke prevention using co-design approaches among people who have had a stroke and health professionals. We hypothesized that it would be possible to adapt cardiac rehabilitation for people who have had a stroke using co-design processes. The second aim was to assess the feasibility of running the program through a pilot of the intervention, including evaluation of acceptability and association with health-related outcomes after stroke. We hypothesized that the program would be feasible and acceptable when pilot-tested within one health service.

2. Methods

The two aims of this project used distinct methods, which are outlined sequentially here: co-design, followed by delivery and evaluation of the pilot program.

2.1. Co-Design

2.1.1. Setting and Study Design

The aim of this study was to modify an existing cardiac rehabilitation program model for people with stroke at the Royal Hobart Hospital in Tasmania, Australia using the Promoting Action on Research Implementation in Health Services (PARIHS) framework in semi-structured focus groups to co-design the program [17].

2.1.2. Participants

Focus groups were conducted in June 2018 with people with lived experience of stroke and health professionals, separately. We aimed to have 8 to 10 participants per focus group, based on published recommendations [18], and the experienced qualitative researcher who facilitated the discussions. This size was deemed suitable to ensure diversity of opinion but also a manageable discussion between members. Participants with lived experience were recruited from the Stroke Foundation (an advocacy organisation) and the local Stroke Support Group. Health professionals from the local health network who provided care to people with stroke in the primary, acute, or rehabilitation settings were recruited for the additional focus group. People who coordinated an existing cardiac rehabilitation program in the health service were also included in this focus group. This study was approved by the Tasmanian Human Research Ethics Committee (H0017243), and all the participants provided written informed consent.

2.1.3. Process

The focus groups were held at the University of Tasmania. Background information about the management and secondary prevention of stroke, as well as an outline of existing cardiac rehabilitation programs, was provided. Workshops were facilitated by a senior qualitative researcher with experience leading focus groups. Discussion questions were prepared for each workshop by the research team and tailored to the perspectives of each group (Supplementary Table S1). Workshop discussions were audio-recorded, transcribed verbatim, and de-identified. Notes were taken during the workshops.

2.1.4. Analysis

All the data were imported into NVivo (Lumivero, Denver, CO, USA) before being read and coded by an experienced qualitative researcher (KJ). Inductive coding identified and categorised codes before identifying key themes via a thematic analysis [19].

2.2. Pilot Program Development, Delivery, and Evaluation

2.2.1. Program Development

Results of the thematic analysis, the existing local cardiac rehabilitation program, and clinical guidelines were used to design a 7-week, 2 h per week (1 h exercise, 1 h discussion) program (Figure 1). The program was delivered by a nurse, physiotherapist, and exercise physiologist, using existing resources developed by the Stroke Foundation for the education sessions [20].

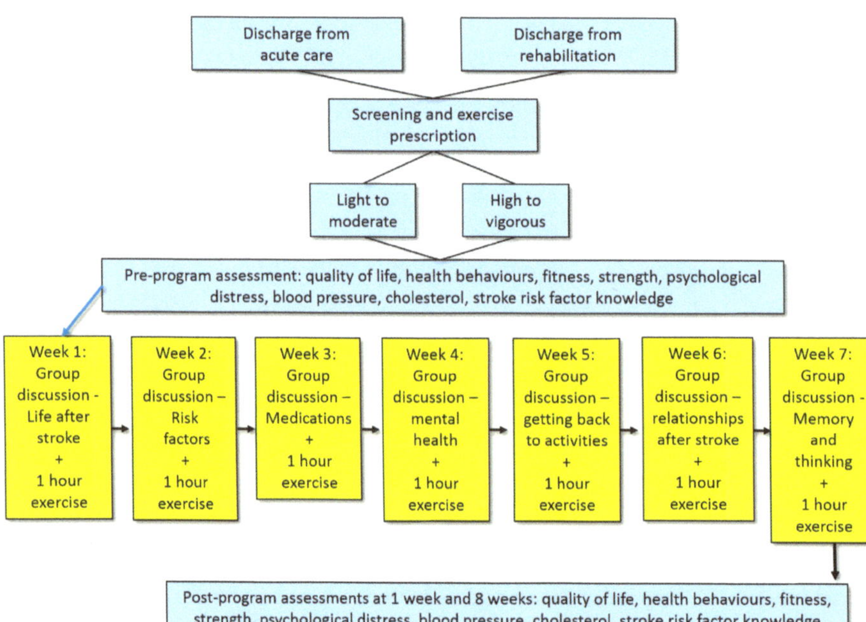

Figure 1. Co-designed CARESS program including screening, assessments, and content.

2.2.2. Program Delivery

Participants

The inclusion criteria were diagnosis of stroke, completed in-patient rehabilitation or discharged directly home from acute care at the Royal Hobart Hospital, and living at home. The Royal Hobart Hospital has the only stroke unit in the south of the state (population 250,000), with the statewide stroke protocol requiring all cases of stroke to be managed in that hospital. The exclusion criteria were moderate or severe dementia, and medically unstable or did not pass exercise screening (see below). We aimed for a sample size of 10 with two groups of 5 participants. This was for largely pragmatic reasons including the financial resources for the project and the size of the gym space available to conduct the group exercise.

Recruitment

Potential participants from the hospital were approached by research or clinical staff and provided a brief information sheet (see online supplement). The support persons of the individuals with stroke were also encouraged to consent and participate in the program. If interested in participating, participants underwent a pre-exercise screening assessment with a stroke neurologist [21]. If deemed only suitable for "sedentary" activity, the participant was excluded. Study staff then conducted cognitive screening using the Telephone Interview for Cognitive Status (TICS) [22], with those scoring <19 excluded. The pilot study was approved by the Tasmanian Human Research Ethics Committee (H0017731 and H27593). The participants provided written informed consent before participation.

Pre-Program and Follow-Up Assessments

The participants completed a detailed health assessment with the study nurse before the program, and then 1 and 6 weeks after the program. The assessment involved baseline measurement of lifestyle (diet, physical activity, and smoking), stroke knowledge, health-related quality of life (AQoL8D), psychological well-being (Patient Health Questionnaire), fatigue, and biomedical risk factors (e.g., functional capacity, blood pressure, weight, lipids—see Supplementary Table S2). If the participant elected to have a support person attend the education component of the program, the support person completed an abridged pre-program assessment. At 1 and 6 weeks, additional data were collected on satisfaction and the self-reported impact of the program. All the data were collected electronically in REDCap.

7-Week Program: Exercise Component

Individual exercise programs were planned by an exercise physiologist, physiotherapist, and, if necessary, a neurologist. Sessions comprised a 15 min warm-up, a 30 min low- to moderate-intensity aerobic and strength training exercise circuit, and a 15 min cool down. Full details are provided in the supplement (Supplementary Table S3). Heart rate and self-reported exertion were monitored during the exercise sessions [23]. Any adverse events during the exercise sessions were recorded using a standard form.

7-Week Program: Education Component

The study nurse led the education sessions (see Supplementary Table S4) using existing Stroke Foundation resources, which were adapted to the needs of the attendees. Open questions were used to facilitate discussion between group members. The sessions also encouraged the use of the Stroke Foundation's EnableMe website to identify and track goals for individual attendees.

2.2.3. Evaluation of Program Feasibility, Acceptability, and Effectiveness

We evaluated the program in terms of feasibility and acceptability, as well as a preliminary examination of the effectiveness of the program on health-related outcomes, acknowledging the small sample size of this pilot study.

Feasibility was assessed by the numbers screened, excluded, beginning, and finishing the program. Acceptability was examined using a descriptive analysis of survey questions related to the program at 1 week after the program concluded.

Evaluation of the potential effectiveness of the program on outcomes was examined using paired Student's *t*-tests or Fisher's exact tests to compare means or proportions between time points before and 6 weeks after the program. We also used a historical control group from an observational study of physical activity after stroke in 2015–16 in the same population to undertake exploratory analyses of program effectiveness [24]. Common outcomes between the studies were the 6 min walk test and the fatigue assessment scale. As the measure of symptoms of depression in the historical study differed from our study, the scores were converted to z scores for analysis. We estimated the average treatment effect (ATE) and average treatment effect on the treated (ATET) by propensity score matching (1:2) with age and sex using programs 'teffects' and 'psmatch'. Difference analyses were also used to estimate the effect of program participation by comparing the change in mean from baseline to follow-up between groups with propensity score matching. Complete case analysis was used. The analysis was performed using STATA 17 (StataCorp LLC, College Station, TX, USA).

3. Results

3.1. Program Co-Design

Nine participants attended the lived experience workshop (five people who were living with stroke, three spouses, and one person who had attended the local cardiac rehabilitation program), and eight people attended the health professional workshop (a pharmacist, a general practitioner, an aged care nurse, a neurologist, an exercise physiologist, a cardiac rehabilitation nurse, an occupational therapist, and a representative from the Heart Foundation).

The data produced through the two focus groups were combined for purposes of analysis. From the thematic analysis of the data, we identified two primary themes: 'existing post-stroke care' and 'adapted cardiac rehabilitation program considerations', along with subthemes, as described below.

3.1.1. Theme One: Existing Post-Stroke Care

Sub-Theme One: Isolation and Limited Support following Stroke

People with lived experience of stroke or cardiac disease and their supporters reported feeling isolated following discharge from the hospital system, and that ongoing support was lacking.

Health professionals highlighted delays for routine medical specialist follow-ups of up to three months due to waiting lists. Survivors of stroke were routinely provided with an information pack in the hospital with information developed by the Stroke Foundation. However, stroke survivors found this information overwhelming, given the acuity of their condition, and would have appreciated it if someone had discussed the information pack with them. Health professionals preferred to tailor information to the individual needs of each stroke survivor but reported that it was difficult to predict those needs during the period of hospitalisation.

Sub-Theme Two: Risk Factor Management

Survivors of stroke could not recall any specific discussions about managing risk factors that increased the risk of a subsequent stroke. Health professionals speculated that people with mild stroke or those who recovered fully might "trivialise their stroke" and return to previous lifestyle habits. Health professionals expressed concern that, after hospital discharge, consistency in the medical management of risk factors, such as high blood pressure, was made more difficult due to breakdowns in communication across the continuum of care. This continuum was complex for many people, involving transitions from the acute hospital to inpatient rehabilitation, and then to primary care in the community (under the auspices of a general practitioner).

3.1.2. Theme Two: Adapted CR Program Considerations

Sub-Theme One: Benefits

People with lived experience were overwhelmingly supportive of a program they could attend following stroke. The primary benefit they identified was meeting peers who had experienced stroke, as well as ameliorating isolation experienced after stroke. Health professionals recognised that "a support network is invaluable in the early recovery phase", although some were surprised that peer support was such a strong focus for people following a stroke. Survivors of stroke and their caregivers valued a point of human contact in a program who could answer any questions.

Sub-Theme Two: Processes

The processes associated with cardiac rehabilitation, such as referral pathways, which would need to be adapted to suit people with stroke, were discussed. Concerns were raised regarding not overburdening stroke survivors too soon after their stroke, as well as not conflicting with a process of stroke rehabilitation taking place in hospital or community settings. Participants suggested that the timing of referral to the program would need to be carefully considered to optimally fit within the overall continuum of care of the stroke survivor. One suggestion, by a health professional, was for referral to take place after discharge from the stroke rehabilitation process. Another suggested that a referral mechanism was needed that accounted for the vast number of points within the continuum of care from which a referral to the program could potentially come. The need to promote the program to referrers, as well as stroke survivors, was emphasised.

Another process that was discussed was that of assessment and the need for appropriate program inclusion and exclusion criteria. Additionally, it was suggested that the prescription of a tailored, rather than generic, exercise program would require an assessment of the specific physical issues of the individual stroke survivor by an appropriate allied health professional.

Sub-Theme Three: Format

People with lived experience of stroke were emphatic that any group needed to be "very informal" and focused on life experiences and peer-to-peer learning, rather than didactic in style. People with lived experience of stroke suggested that having written materials to take home with them would assist in retaining information, acknowledging that their cognitive function and memory could be compromised following stroke. Educational material would ideally be developed by a multidisciplinary team, who may not need to be involved after the development phase. The inclusion of *carers* in the education component was acknowledged as important by health professionals, survivors of stroke, and the carers themselves, who were also seeking sources of peer support. In terms of length, it was suggested that six weeks (the length of the current cardiac rehabilitation program at the hospital) would be too short to effect behaviour change, and so a longer program, potentially including intermittent follow-up, was favoured. It was suggested that nurses could be program facilitators but with professional input for the exercise component from physiotherapists or exercise physiologists. In terms of participants, people with lived experience of stroke advocated that stroke survivors with mobility limitations could attend the program. Health professionals suggested that clustering participants into cohorts, based on shared functional impacts, or age, could allow a "targeted approach to the program", but there was no consensus reached on this point. People with lived experience suggested that the program could serve as a common point of case coordination and provide referrals, as needed, to other services.

Sub-Theme Four: Content

People with lived experience of stroke or cardiac disease felt that the inclusion of exercise in the rehabilitation program was "a terrific idea". Health professionals, however, raised concerns regarding the variability of physical function following stroke, and about exercise prescription. One concern was not wanting to provide exercises that were different to those being prescribed by the providers of stroke rehabilitation, due to the potential to confuse the patient or work at cross-purposes. One health professional felt that "targeted therapy" should be the purview of stroke rehabilitation, not a modified cardiac rehabilitation program. In contrast, another health professional felt stroke survivors should be prescribed an individualised program, despite the challenges of delivering that with supervision in a group environment. This issue also prompted the suggestion that exercise-focused allied health professionals would need to be involved in the program.

People with lived experience of stroke and health professionals identified the importance of addressing the impact of stroke on mental health and how this can, in turn, impact recovery. Stroke survivors suggested that this topic was not well covered during hospital admission despite its importance, and so should be included in a stroke-adapted cardiac rehabilitation program. People with lived experience of stroke also suggested that a modified cardiac rehabilitation program should emphasise that stroke is a "chronic disease" with effects that can last "the rest of your life".

A person who had previously completed the local cardiac rehabilitation program described how it covered "cardio health", including the role of smoking, drinking, obesity, and genetics. These were considered suitable topics for the lifestyle education component by people with lived experience, although they preferred an informal, peer-to-peer format.

3.2. Program Delivery and Evaluation

Of the 23 people approached to participate in the study, 10 (43%) participated in two groups of 5 people (Figure 2). Only two participants invited a support person to participate in the program. Only one support person completed both the baseline and follow-up assessments, so the results are not presented here. The reasons for non-participation included returning to work, non-response to contact, and not being interested in participating. Completion of each week of the program varied between 100% and 60% across the two groups. The characteristics of the participants are shown in Table 1.

Table 1. Characteristics of participants at baseline (n = 10) in the CARESS program.

	n/Mean	%/sd
Age (years) mean (SD)	66.5	9.12
Sex		
Men	7	70
Women	3	30
Type of stroke		
Ischaemic	10	100
Haemorrhagic	-	
Time from stroke (weeks)	12.47	6.98
BMI	29.8	5.63
Lifetime smoking > 100 cigarettes		
No	3	30
Yes	7	70
Current smoker		
No	10	100
Yes	0	0
History of hypertension		
No	1	10
Yes	9	90

Table 1. *Cont.*

	n/Mean	%/sd
Hypercholesterolaemia		
No	3	30
Yes	7	70
Diabetes		
No	9	90
Yes	1	10
Atrial fibrillation		
No	9	90
Yes	1	10

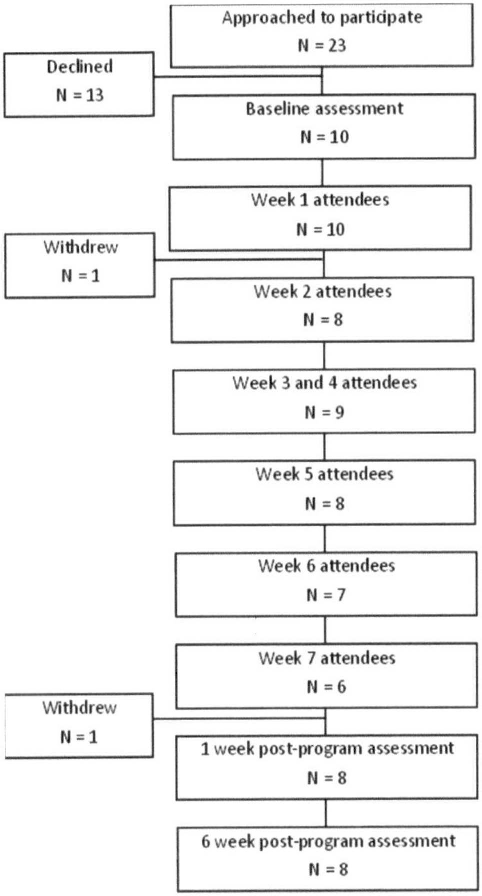

Figure 2. Flow chart of participation in CARESS pilot program.

Satisfaction and impact were rated highly by participants at 1 week after program completion (n = 8, 80% completed assessment, Table 2). All the participants recommended the program to others and agreed/strongly agreed that the program helped them to learn about their health and encouraged them to take better care of themselves and make lifestyle changes.

Table 2. Satisfaction and impact of CARESS program reported 1 week after completion.

Satisfaction with Program	N	Mean (SD)/%
How would you rate this program? (1 = worst possible program, 10 = best possible program)	8	8.6 (0.77)
Would you recommend this program to other people who have had a stroke?		
Yes	8	100%
No	0	0%
Overall, how satisfied were you with the program? (1= very satisfied, 5 = very unsatisfied)	8	1.12 (0.35)
Impact of program		
The program helped me to understand my health issues (1 = strongly agree, 5 = strongly disagree)	8	1.37 (0.51)
Strongly agree/agree	8	100%
Disagree/strongly disagree	0	0
The program helped me to learn ways to take better care of myself (1 = strongly agree, 5 = strongly disagree)	8	1.25 (0.46)
Strongly agree/agree	8	100%
Disagree/strongly disagree	0	0

Knowledge about stroke increased from baseline to follow-up at 1 or 6 weeks after program completion (Supplementary Table S5). For example, the proportion correctly reporting stroke risk factors increased from baseline to 1 and 6 weeks, including for high blood pressure (20% baseline, 88% 6-week follow-up); smoking (50% baseline; 63% 6-week follow-up); and overweight (40% baseline; 63% 6-week follow-up). Compared to before the program, a greater proportion of people also identified the FAST signs and stated they would call an ambulance if having stroke symptoms.

There was some evidence that the program was associated with positive improvements in health outcomes (Table 3). In analyses comparing baseline to 6 weeks after the program, some positive changes in quality of life, fatigue, symptoms of depression, functional capacity, and fruit and vegetable intake were observed, although these did not reach statistical significance. There was a slight increase in systolic and diastolic blood pressures but no change in total cholesterol, body mass index or grip strength from baseline to follow-up.

Table 3. Comparison of functional capacity, fatigue, and symptoms of depression between CARESS program participants (n = 7) and historical controls (n = 14) with propensity score matching on age and sex.

	Average Treatment Effects Analysis		Difference-in-Differences (DID) Analysis				
			Program Participants		Historical Controls		
	ATE (95% CI)	ATET (95% CI)	Baseline Mean (95% CI)	Follow-Up Difference Mean (95% CI)	Baseline Mean (95% CI)	Follow-Up Difference Mean (95% CI)	DiD (95% CI)
6 min walk test (meters)	139 (44, 234) *	117 (−25, 262)	350 (153, 547)	117 (−69, 304)	337.3 (209, 466)	66 (−10, 143)	51 (−215, 317)
Fatigue	−5 (−9, −1) *	−4 (−9, 2)	22 (13, 30)	−4 (−9, 2)	19 (13, 25)	2 (−4, 7)	−5 (16, 5)
Symptoms of depression z-scores	−0.8 (−1.8, 0.2)	−0.5 (−1.3, 0.4)	−0.1 (−1.1, 1.1)	−0.7 (−1.3, −1.5)	−0.4 (−0.7, −0.1)	0.1 (−0.4, 0.8)	−0.9 (−2.2, 0.5)

* $p < 0.05$.

The program findings were also compared to a historical control group of 31 people from an observational study in the same region (see online Supplementary Table S6 for characteristics). Propensity score matching with age and sex was performed to compare the outcomes of program participants (n = 7) with historical controls (n = 14). These analyses demonstrated that the program participants had improvements in functional capacity on the 6 min walk test, fatigue levels, and depression symptoms compared to the historical controls (Table 4).

Table 4. Health outcomes before and 6 weeks after the CARESS program.

	Baseline		6-Week Follow-Up		
Outcome Measure	**n/Mean**	**%/sd**	**n/Mean**	**%/sd**	***p*-Value**
Quality of Life (AQoL) utility score	0.74	0.21	0.84	0.12	0.25
Balance test mean (SD)	24.7	3.40	22.3	5.18	0.26
Symptoms of depression (z-score) mean (SD)	0.11	1.1	−0.65	1.1	0.19
Fatigue score mean (SD)	22.1	8.38	18.87	4.51	0.34
6 min walk test (meters) mean (SD)	397.67	169.68	490.12	124.01	0.22
Fruit and vegetable intake per day					0.18
0–1 servings	0	0	0	0	
2–3 servings	10	100	6	75	
4 or more servings	0	0	2	25	
Physical activity MET (min/week)	3326.5	4692.77	3174.85	3562.45	0.94
Body mass index	30.86	6.36	30.79	6.03	0.88
Grip strength					
Right	31.42	13.00	32.22	12.55	0.55
Left	26.39	11.44	26.46	13.86	0.97
Total cholesterol (mmol/L)	3.1	0.44	3.1	0.82	0.88
Systolic blood pressure (mmHg)	128.4	15.1	138.8	18.0	0.21
Diastolic blood pressure (mmHg)	78.8	15.5	83.7	12.4	0.48

4. Discussion

We successfully co-designed and piloted a modified cardiac rehabilitation program to enhance risk factor management after stroke. In accordance with the evidence base and the co-design process, the exercise completed in our program was tailored and delivered by allied health professionals who progressed the exercise over the program. It was designed to result in physiological changes that modify known risk factors. Similarly, the education and discussion in the program were designed to begin behavioural changes and improve psychological well-being. The program was feasible and acceptable in a non-randomised pilot study based in a single tertiary hospital. The exploratory analyses showed potentially positive changes in health outcomes 6 weeks after the program when compared to a historical control group.

Compared with pre-program participation, small but positive associations with improved quality of life, fatigue, symptoms of depression, functional capacity, and stroke knowledge were found. Importantly, we were able to use a historical control group to show that changes in fatigue, depression symptoms, and functional capacity were greater than those seen in the usual recovery phase without program participation [24]. Our findings, albeit in a small sample from one hospital network, are supported by a growing body of literature demonstrating the benefits of similar, multimodal programs on a range of cardiovascular risk factors [25–29]. Recent cohort studies provide preliminary evidence that a modified cardiac rehabilitation program can decrease mortality, hospital readmissions, and subsequent strokes among stroke survivors [30,31]. Participation in these types of programs has been shown to increase participants' self-efficacy, coping and resilience, albeit in cardiac populations [32,33], which potentially has a compounding effect on both cardiovascular health and general well-being, resulting in greater outcomes than the sum of the individual components.

An important feature of the program was the use of co-design, including people with lived experience of stroke and health professionals. Co-design assisted with practical aspects of program design and delivery and provided insights into the potential wider benefits of such a program. Among people with lived experience of stroke, a strong rationale for this type of group program was that it could ameliorate isolation, provide a source of peer support, and be a centralised point of contact for the stroke survivor. The co-design process was confirmatory in terms of discussion highlighting the fragmented care people with stroke were receiving when returning to the community, the lack of guidance on risk factors and the importance of other aspects of recovery, including mental health, which has also been found in quantitative studies [9,10].

Given the strong rationale for this type of program, including existing evidence of effectiveness, the next steps could be a hybrid implementation and effectiveness trial [34]. The very high rating of program satisfaction, attendance, and perceived impact support this approach. One reason for us proposing this type of program and working together with the existing team who deliver a similar program to people with cardiac disease was that, theoretically, implementation should be more straightforward. However, as noted by others, many barriers exist to the implementation of new programs as well as the integration of people with stroke into existing programs [15,35]. Among these barriers, funding for such a program is particularly problematic. While all hospital networks with stroke units fund comprehensive rehabilitation services focused on recovery of function, we are aware of very few that fund this type of program focused on more holistic aspects of 'recovery'. It appears inequitable to have hundreds of state-funded services across the country seemingly directed at all cardiac patients while, for people with stroke, it is only those with physical limitations—approximately 50%—who can access state-funded care through rehabilitation services. Difficulties related to the division of care between hospitals, which are state-funded, and primary or community care, which is federally funded, likely contribute to this issue [36].

The limitations of the pilot study include the small number of participants from a single centre. This was overcome to some extent by using the historical control group to compare outcomes over time. The characteristics of the sample show they were younger, more often male and with worse co-morbidities than other similar post-stroke populations [37]. The study was based at one hospital site, limiting external validity; however, it is the only hospital with a stroke unit in the region, meaning the patients who attend that hospital are representative of the broader community. The co-design process included people with lived experience and health professionals guided by an experienced facilitator; however, the groups were small and, if repeated with further groups, may have yielded different results. The study was conducted prior to the COVID-19 pandemic. Care for people with stroke, and other conditions, within the hospital system has changed considerably since then, with face-to-face and group programs suspended [38]. We did not have a comprehensive assessment of all important outcomes for people who have had a stroke. For example, we assessed symptoms of depression but not other psychological factors such as stress, anxiety, or coping. While we intended to recruit support people, only one such person participated, so we could not do any meaningful analyses. However, the inclusion of support people was noted to be important during the co-design, so future studies or programs should include this group to potentially assist with the high burden they experience [39]. The main strengths of the study were the use of co-design and the leveraging of an existing model of health care within the hospital system.

5. Conclusions

We found that a co-designed program in one hospital for people after stroke modelled on cardiac rehabilitation was feasible, acceptable, and associated with small but positive changes in outcomes important for people after stroke. Future studies should focus on expanding the evidence base for the effectiveness and implementation of such programs.

Supplementary Materials: The following supporting information can be downloaded at: https://www.mdpi.com/article/10.3390/healthcare12070776/s1, Table S1, questions used for co-design workshops; Table S2, assessments undertaken before, 1 week, and 6 weeks after the program; Table S3, recommended aerobic and resistance training exercises in CARESS program; Table S4, group discussion topics informed by co-design workshops; Table S5, stroke knowledge before and after

CARESS program completion; Table S6, characteristics of historical control group. References [40–46] are cited in the supplementary materials.

Author Contributions: Conceptualization, M.C., H.C., M.G.S., M.N.M., G.M.P. and S.G.; methodology, M.C., H.C., M.G.S., M.N.M., G.M.P. and S.G.; formal analysis, S.R., S.B. and K.J.; investigation, S.B., M.N.M., D.B.S. and G.M.P.; data curation, H.C., M.N.M. and D.B.S.; writing—original draft, S.R., S.B., K.J. and S.G.; writing—review and editing, S.R., S.B., K.J., M.C., H.C., M.G.S., M.N.M., D.B.S., G.M.P. and S.G.; supervision, S.G.; project administration, M.N.M. and D.B.S.; funding acquisition, M.C., H.C., M.G.S., G.M.P. and S.G. All authors have read and agreed to the published version of the manuscript.

Funding: This study was funded by the Royal Hobart Hospital Research Foundation through an starter grant (GNT 18-103); Synergies to Prevent Stroke (STOPstroke), funded by the National Health and Medical Research Council (GNT1182071) and the National Heart Foundation of Australia Future Leader Fellowship to SLG (GNT102061).

Institutional Review Board Statement: The studies were conducted in accordance with the Declaration of Helsinki and approved by the Tasmanian Human Research Ethics Committee (H0017243, approval date, 6 June 2018; H0017731, approval date 10 December 2018; H0027593, approval date 4 November 2022).

Informed Consent Statement: Written informed consent was obtained from the patient(s) to publish this paper.

Data Availability Statement: The data presented in this study are available on request from the corresponding author.

Acknowledgments: We gratefully acknowledge Ken Walsh from the University of Tasmania, who designed and ran the co-design workshops. We also thank Sue Sanderson, the co-ordinator of the Cardiac Rehabilitation Service for the Royal Hobart Hospital.

Conflicts of Interest: The authors declare no conflict of interest.

References

1. Australian Institute of Health and Welfare. *Estimating the Incidence of Stroke and Acute Coronary Syndrome Using the National Integrated Health Services Information Analysis Asset, Catalogue Number CDK 21*; Australian Institute of Health and Welfare: Canberra, Australia, 2022.
2. Australian Institute of Health and Welfare. *Heart, Stroke and Vascular Disease: Australian Facts*; Australian Institute of Health and Welfare: Canberra, Australia, 2023.
3. O'Donnell, M.J.; Chin, S.L.; Rangarajan, S.; Xavier, D.; Liu, L.; Zhang, H.; Rao-Melacini, P.; Zhang, X.; Pais, P.; Agapay, S.; et al. Global and regional effects of potentially modifiable risk factors associated with acute stroke in 32 countries (INTERSTROKE): A case-control study. *Lancet* **2016**, *388*, 761–775. [CrossRef] [PubMed]
4. Stroke Foundation. Living Clinical Guidelines for Stroke Management. 2023. Available online: https://informme.org.au/guidelines/living-clinical-guidelines-for-stroke-management (accessed on 31 January 2024).
5. Gall, S.L.; Dewey, H.M.; Thrift, A.G. Smoking cessation at 5 years after stroke in the North East Melbourne Stroke Incidence Study. *Neuroepidemiology* **2009**, *32*, 196–200. [CrossRef] [PubMed]
6. Gall, S.L.; Thrift, A.G. Control of hypertension 5 years after stroke in the North East Melbourne Stroke Incidence Study (NEMESIS). *Hypertension* **2006**, *48*, 260–265.
7. Simpson, D.; Callisaya, M.L.; English, C.; Thrift, A.G.; Gall, S.L. Self-reported exercise prevalence and determinants in the long term after stroke: The North East Melbourne Stroke Incidence Study. *J. Stroke Cerebrovasc. Dis.* **2017**, *26*, 2855–2863. [CrossRef] [PubMed]
8. Hall, P.; Lawrence, M.; Blake, C.; Lennon, O. Interventions for behaviour change and self-management of risk in stroke secondary prevention: An overview of reviews. *Cerebrovasc. Dis.* **2023**, *53*, 1–13. [CrossRef] [PubMed]
9. Olaiya, M.T.; Cadilhac, D.A.; Kim, J.; Nelson, M.R.; Srikanth, V.K.; Andrew, N.E.; Thrift, A.G. Long-term unmet needs and associated factors in stroke or TIA survivors: An observational study. *Neurology* **2017**, *89*, 68–75. [CrossRef] [PubMed]
10. Stroke Foundation. *National Stroke Audit—Acute Services Report 2023*; Stroke Foundation: Melbourne, Australia, 2023.
11. Woodruffe, S.; Neubeck, L.; Clark, R.A.; Gray, K.; Ferry, C.; Finan, J.; Sanderson, S.; Briffa, T.G. Australian Cardiovascular Health and Rehabilitation Association (ACRA) core components of cardiovascular disease secondary prevention and cardiac rehabilitation 2014. *Heart Lung Circ.* **2015**, *24*, 430–441. [CrossRef] [PubMed]
12. Heart Foundation. Cardiac Services Directory. 2024. Available online: https://www.heartfoundation.org.au/bundles/support/cardiac-services-directory (accessed on 5 January 2024).

13. Howes, T.; Mahenderan, N.; Freene, N. Cardiac Rehabilitation: Are People with Stroke or Transient Ischaemic Attack Being Included? A Cross-Sectional Survey. *Heart Lung Circ.* **2020**, *29*, 483–490. [CrossRef] [PubMed]
14. Toma, J.; Hammond, B.; Chan, V.; Peacocke, A.; Salehi, B.; Jhingan, P.; Marzolini, S. Inclusion of People Poststroke in Cardiac Rehabilitation Programs in Canada: A Missed Opportunity for Referral. *CJC Open* **2020**, *2*, 195–206. [CrossRef]
15. Jeffares, I.; Merriman, N.A.; Doyle, F.; Horgan, F.; Hickey, A. Inclusion of stroke patients in expanded cardiac rehabilitation services: A cross-national qualitative study with cardiac and stroke rehabilitation professionals. *Disabil. Rehabil.* **2022**, *44*, 3610–3622. [CrossRef]
16. Craig, P.; Dieppe, P.; Macintyre, S.; Michie, S.; Nazareth, I.; Petticrew, M. Developing and evaluating complex interventions: The new Medical Research Council guidance. *BMJ* **2008**, *337*, a1655. [CrossRef] [PubMed]
17. Kitson, A.; Harvey, G.; McCormack, B. Enabling the implementation of evidence based practice: A conceptual framework. *Qual. Health Care* **1998**, *7*, 149–158. [CrossRef]
18. Jenny, K. Qualitative Research: Introducing focus groups. *BMJ* **1995**, *311*, 299.
19. Braun, V.; Clarke, V. Is thematic analysis used well in health psychology? A critical review of published research, with recommendations for quality practice and reporting. *Health Psychol. Rev.* **2023**, *17*, 695–718. [CrossRef] [PubMed]
20. Stroke Foundation. Life after Stroke Fact Sheets. 2024. Available online: https://strokefoundation.org.au/what-we-do/for-survivors-and-carers/after-stroke-factsheets (accessed on 24 February 2024).
21. Exercise and Sports Science Australia. Pre-Exercise Screening Systems. 2024. Available online: https://www.essa.org.au/Public/Public/ABOUT_ESSA/Pre-Exercise_Screening_Systems.aspx (accessed on 1 March 2019).
22. Brandt, J.; Spencer, M.; Folstein, M. The Telephone Interview for Cognitive Status. *Cogn. Behav. Neurol.* **1988**, *1*, 111–118.
23. Borg, G. *Borg's Perceived Exertion and Pain Scales*; Human Kinetics: Champaign, IL, USA, 1998.
24. Simpson, D.B.; Breslin, M.; Cumming, T.; de Zoete, S.; Gall, S.L.; Schmidt, M.; English, C.; Callisaya, M.L. Go home, sit less: The impact of home versus hospital rehabilitation environment on activity levels of stroke survivors. *Arch. Phys. Med. Rehabil.* **2018**, *99*, 2216–2221. [CrossRef]
25. Kirk, H.; Kersten, P.; Crawford, P.; Keens, A.; Ashburn, A.; Conway, J. The cardiac model of rehabilitation for reducing cardiovascular risk factors post transient ischaemic attack and stroke: A randomized controlled trial. *Clin. Rehabil.* **2014**, *28*, 339–349. [CrossRef] [PubMed]
26. Boyne, P.; Welge, J.; Kissela, B.; Dunning, K. Factors Influencing the Efficacy of Aerobic Exercise for Improving Fitness and Walking Capacity after Stroke: A Meta-Analysis with Meta-Regression. *Arch. Phys. Med. Rehabil.* **2017**, *98*, 581–595. [CrossRef]
27. Wang, C.; Redgrave, J.; Shafizadeh, M.; Majid, A.; Kilner, K.; Ali, A.N. Aerobic exercise interventions reduce blood pressure in patients after stroke or transient ischaemic attack: A systematic review and meta-analysis. *Br. J. Sport. Med.* **2019**, *53*, 1515–1525. [CrossRef]
28. Saunders, D.H.; Sanderson, M.; Hayes, S.; Johnson, L.; Kramer, S.; Carter, D.; Jarvis, H.; Brazzelli, M.; Mead, G.E. Physical Fitness Training for Patients with Stroke. *Stroke* **2020**, *51*, e299–e300. [CrossRef]
29. MacKay-Lyons, M.; Gubitz, G.; Giacomantonio, N.; Wightman, H.; Marsters, D.; Thompson, K.; Thornton, M. Program of Rehabilitative Exercise and Education to Avert Vascular Events After Non-Disabling Stroke or Transient Ischemic Attack (PREVENT Trial): A Randomized Controlled Trial. *Neurorehabil. Neural Repair.* **2022**, *36*, 119–130. [CrossRef] [PubMed]
30. Cuccurullo, S.J.; Fleming, T.K.; Kostis, W.J.; Greiss, C.; Gizzi, M.S.; Eckert, A.; Ray, A.R.; Scarpati, R.; Cosgrove, N.M.; Beavers, T.; et al. Impact of a Stroke Recovery Program Integrating Modified Cardiac Rehabilitation on All-Cause Mortality, Cardiovascular Performance and Functional Performance. *Am. J. Phys. Med. Rehabil.* **2019**, *98*, 953–963. [CrossRef] [PubMed]
31. Cuccurullo, S.J.; Fleming, T.K.; Zinonos, S.; Cosgrove, N.M.; Cabrera, J.; Kostis, J.B.; Greiss, C.; Ray, A.R.; Eckert, A.; Scarpati, R.; et al. Stroke Recovery Program with Modified Cardiac Rehabilitation Improves Mortality, Functional & Cardiovascular Performance. *J. Stroke Cerebrovasc. Dis.* **2022**, *31*, 106322. [PubMed]
32. Bagheri, H.; Shakeri, S.; Nazari, A.M.; Goli, S.; Khajeh, M.; Mardani, A.; Vlaisavljevic, Z. Effectiveness of nurse-led counselling and education on self-efficacy of patients with acute coronary syndrome: A randomized controlled trial. *Nurs. Open* **2022**, *9*, 775–784. [CrossRef] [PubMed]
33. McKenzie, K.M.; Park, L.K.; Lenze, E.J.; Montgomery, K.; Rashdi, S.; Deych, E.; Stranczek, N.A.; McKenzie, E.J.; Rich, M.W.; Barry, V.G.; et al. A prospective cohort study of the impact of outpatient Intensive Cardiac Rehabilitation on depression and cardiac self-efficacy. *Am. Heart J. Plus* **2022**, *13*, 100100. [CrossRef]
34. Curran, G.M.; Bauer, M.; Mittman, B.; Pyne, J.M.; Stetler, C. Effectiveness-implementation hybrid designs: Combining elements of clinical effectiveness and implementation research to enhance public health impact. *Med. Care* **2012**, *50*, 217. [CrossRef] [PubMed]
35. Marzolini, S. Including Patients with Stroke in Cardiac Rehabilitation: Barriers and Facilitators. *J. Cardiopulm. Rehabil. Prev.* **2020**, *40*, 294–301. [CrossRef] [PubMed]
36. Australian Institute of Health and Welfare. *Australia's Health 2018. Australia's Health Series no. 16. AUS 221—'How Does Australia's Health System Work?'*; Australian Institute of Health and Welfare: Canberra, Australia, 2018; Chapter 2.
37. Machado, N.; Williams, G.; Olver, J.; Johnson, L. Is early initiated cardiorespiratory fitness training within a model of stroke-integrated cardiac rehabilitation safe and feasible? *J. Stroke Cerebrovasc. Dis.* **2024**, *33*, 107493. [CrossRef]
38. Australian Stroke Coalition. *The Impact of COVID-19 and Long COVID on Stroke Risk and Australian Stroke Services*; Australian Stroke Coalition: Melbourne, Australia, 2023.

39. Tziaka, E.; Tsiakiri, A.; Vlotinou, P.; Christidi, F.; Tsiptsios, D.; Aggelousis, N.; Vadikolias, K.; Serdari, A. A Holistic Approach to Expressing the Burden of Caregivers for Stroke Survivors: A Systematic Review. *Healthcare* **2024**, *12*, 565. [CrossRef]
40. Leppala, J.; Lagstrom, H.; Kaljonen, A.; Laitinen, K. Construction and evaluation of a self-contained index for assessment of diet quality. *Scand. J. Public Health* **2010**, *38*, 794–802. [CrossRef]
41. Craig, C.L.; Marshall, A.L.; Sjostrom, M.; Bauman, A.E.; Booth, M.L.; Ainsworth, B.E.; Pratt, M.; Ekelund, U.L.; Yngve, A.; Sallis, J.F.; et al. International physical activity questionnaire: 12-country reliability and validity. *Med. Sci. Sport. Exerc.* **2003**, *35*, 1381–1395. [CrossRef]
42. Richardson, J.; Iezzi, A.; Khan, M.A.; Maxwell, A. Validity and reliability of the Assessment of Quality of Life (AQoL)-8D multi-attribute utility instrument. *Patient* **2014**, *7*, 85–96. [CrossRef]
43. Cumming, T.B.; Mead, G. Classifying post-stroke fatigue: Optimal cut-off on the Fatigue Assessment Scale. *J. Psychosom. Res.* **2017**, *103*, 147–149. [CrossRef]
44. Towfighi, A.; Ovbiagele, B.; El Husseini, N.; Hackett, M.L.; Jorge, R.E.; Kissela, B.M.; Mitchell, P.H.; Skolarus, L.E.; Whooley, M.A.; Williams, L.S.; et al. Poststroke depression: A scientific statement for healthcare professionals from the American Heart Association/American Stroke Association. *Stroke* **2017**, *48*, e30–e43. [CrossRef]
45. Dyer, N.; Sorra, J.S.; Smith, S.A.; Cleary, P.D.; Hays, R.D. Psychometric properties of the Consumer Assessment of Healthcare Providers and Systems (CAHPS®) Clinician and Group Adult Visit Survey. *Med. Care* **2012**, *50*, S28–S34. [CrossRef]
46. Hickey, A.; Holly, D.; McGee, H.; Conroy, R.; Shelley, E. Knowledge of Stroke Risk Factors and Warning Signs in Ireland: Development and Application of the Stroke Awareness Questionnaire (SAQ). *Int. J. Stroke* **2011**, *7*, 298–306. [CrossRef] [PubMed]

healthcare

MDPI

Article

Mediation Role of Behavioral Decision-Making Between Self-Efficacy and Self-Management Among Elderly Stroke Survivors in China: Cross-Sectional Study

Xiaoxuan Wang [1], Hu Jiang [1], Zhixin Zhao [1], Noubessi Tchekwagep Kevine [1], Baoxia An [2], Zhiguang Ping [3], Beilei Lin [1,*] and Zhenxiang Zhang [1,*]

1 Nursing and Health School, Zhengzhou University, Zhengzhou 450001, China; wangxiaoxuan222666@163.com (X.W.); kevine3noubessi@gmail.com (N.T.K.)
2 Henan Huaxian People Hospital, Anyang 456400, China
3 College of Public Health, Zhengzhou University, Zhengzhou 450001, China
* Correspondence: linbeilei@zzu.edu.cn (B.L.); zhangzx6666@zzu.edu.cn (Z.Z.); Tel.: +86-0371-86565001 (B.L.); +86-0371-86565001 (Z.Z.)

Abstract: Background: Identifying the factors that impact self-management is crucial, as elderly stroke survivors frequently face challenges in self-management. Self-efficacy and behavioral decision-making are reported as influencing factors of self-management, but their relationship within the elderly population remains unconfirmed. This study aimed to explore whether self-efficacy impacts self-management through the mediating role of behavioral decision-making among elderly stroke survivors. **Methods:** A cross-sectional design and convenience sampling method were used in this study. A total of 291 elderly stroke survivors were recruited from a tertiary hospital in Henan Province, China, between March and July of 2024. Questionnaires were distributed to collect sociodemographic, self-efficacy, behavioral decision-making, and self-management data. A path analysis and correlation analysis were used to analyze the data. This study adhered to the Strengthening the Reporting of Observational Studies in Epidemiology (STROBE) guidelines. **Results:** Elderly stroke survivors reported having a moderate level of self-management. There was a positive correlation between self-efficacy, behavioral decision-making, and self-management (all $p < 0.01$). The mediation model indicated that behavioral decision-making mediated the association of self-efficacy and self-management in the regression model (95% *CI* 0.03 to 0.14), and the effect value was 0.08. It was also confirmed that behavioral decision-making mediated the impact of self-efficacy and self-management, accounting for 25.81% of the total effect. **Conclusion:** Self-efficacy is not solely a key factor influencing self-management in elderly stroke survivors, but it also improves their self-management behaviors by facilitating behavioral decision-making. As a result, healthcare professionals should consider self-efficacy and behavioral decision-making as crucial elements for assessing elderly stroke survivors during discharge and follow-up.

Keywords: stroke; self-efficacy; behavioral decision-making; self-management

1. Introduction

The latest Global Burden of Disease (GBD) report indicates that the number of global stroke cases has surpassed a notably high 93 million [1]. China has the largest number of stroke survivors in this statistic, and the number of stroke survivors exceeds 28 million [1]. Among these stroke survivors, a substantial proportion, accounting for 50.81%, is over 60 years old [2]. In other words, the proportion of elderly stroke survivors in China exceeds more than 14 million. Furthermore, with the continuous acceleration of the aging population in the past decade in China, the number of elderly stroke survivors has been increasing [3]. Therefore, it is pertinent for researchers to focus on elderly stroke survivors.

The advancement in medical care and healthcare has led to the early detection and rapid treatment of stroke, thus reducing morbidity and mortality rates among stroke survivors. However, most stroke survivors, especially the elderly with multiple chronic diseases, cognitive impairment, and poor daily living activity, often face significant challenges in disease management and rehabilitation after returning home [4,5]. In addition, advanced age has also been proven to be a risk factor for post-stroke depression [6] and post-stroke fatigue [7]. Therefore, we may deduce that disease management for elderly stroke survivors is quite challenging.

Self-management has been identified as a crucial model for elderly care [8]. The components of self-management post-stroke have been delineated as follows: disease management, safe medication practices, diet management, daily living management, rehabilitation exercises, and so on [9]. However, a previous study has found that elderly stroke survivors have a lower level of self-management [10]. Exploring the factors influencing self-management among elderly stroke survivors is essential for designing interventions to improve their self-management.

Self-efficacy refers to an individual's judgment of their own ability to organize and execute the action processes required to achieve specific behavioral goals [11]. Stroke survivors with higher self-efficacy tend to have stronger motivation and engage in self-management more effectively [12]. Given that elderly stroke survivors often experience diminished physical function and lower self-efficacy compared with younger patients [13], the relationship between self-efficacy and self-management is particularly critical.

Additionally, behavioral decision-making is another important factor influencing stroke self-management. The process of behavioral change relies on scientific decision-making [14]. Behavioral decision-making is an interdisciplinary concept that originated from the behavioral decision theory established by Edwards in the 1950s [15]. Our research team previously explored the behavioral decision-making of stroke survivors [16], defining stroke behavioral decision-making as the process by which stroke survivors, under the influence of social, economic, and cultural environments, comprehensively weigh their own needs, expectations, and environmental factors. Guo et al. [17] indicated that elderly stroke survivors rarely make proactive rehabilitation decisions in the early stages of recovery.

A meta-analysis has found that self-efficacy is an important variable in health decision-making [18]. Our research group previously integrated a literature review, qualitative research, and theoretical analysis to preliminarily construct a situational theoretical Recurrence Risk Perception and Behavioral Decision Model in stroke survivors [16], which was in alignment with a subsequent study [19]. This model can guide how behavioral surveys are conducted among stroke survivors. It found that stroke survivors undergo a series of internal decision-making processes when they decide to adopt healthy behaviors. Moreover, the process of behavioral decision-making is affected by self-efficacy [16]. Therefore, we speculate that the self-efficacy of elderly stroke survivors will influence self-management by affecting behavioral decision-making. Previous studies have only explored the relationships between two variables [12,18,20]. However, the relationship between these three variables is not yet clear, especially in the population of elderly stroke survivors. Therefore, our study aimed to explore the relationships between self-efficacy, behavioral decision-making, and self-management among elderly stroke survivors, guided by the stroke behavioral decision-making model. In addition, this study will provide new perspectives for developing behavioral management measures for elderly stroke survivors. The research hypotheses are as follows, as shown in Figure 1:

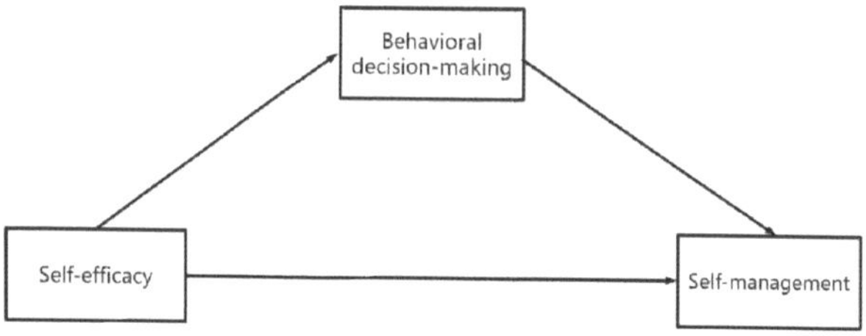

Figure 1. The hypothesis model of self-efficacy, behavioral decision-making, and self-management in elderly stroke survivors.

Hypothesis 1. *Self-efficacy is positively correlated with self-management.*

Hypothesis 2. *Self-efficacy is positively associated with decision-making.*

Hypothesis 3. *Behavioral decision-making positively and significantly relates to self-management.*

Hypothesis 4. *Behavioral decision-making partially mediates the relationships between self-efficacy and self-management.*

2. Materials and Methods

2.1. Design

This was a cross-sectional study, and convenience sampling was used. We followed the guidelines for Strengthening the Reporting of Observational Studies in Epidemiology (STROBE, see Supplementary Materials).

2.2. Sample

This study was conducted among hospitalized stroke survivors at a tertiary hospital in Luoyang, Henan Province, China. Eligible elderly stroke survivors who complied with this study's inclusion criteria were invited to participate in this voluntary study. Inclusion criteria for elderly stroke survivors comprised the following: (a) over 60 years old; (b) diagnosed with stroke by MRI or CT [21]; (c) in the stages of recovery from stroke; and (d) exhibited normal language abilities (Token Test score $\geq$ 17) and cognitive function (Mini-Mental State Examination, MMSE score $\geq$ 27). Exclusion criteria for elderly stroke survivors comprised the following: (a) having severe cardiac, liver, or renal dysfunction or other malignant tumors or (b) having a history of serious mental illness or a family history of serious mental illness.

According to Liu [22], the sample size was 5–10 times greater than the number of independent variables. There were 26 variables included in this study, which were as follows: 12 general information questions, 7 dimensions of the stroke self-management scale, 2 dimensions of the stroke self-efficacy questionnaire, and 4 dimensions of the behavioral decision-making scale for stroke survivors. The modified Rankin scale was also used. Considering that 10% of questionnaires were invalid, the minimum sample size of this study was 288 stroke survivors; hence, a sample size of 291 met the requirement for testing the hypothesis models.

2.3. Measurements

2.3.1. General Information Questionnaire

A demographic and disease-specific data questionnaire was designed and used to collect information on gender, age, marriage, residential area, working state, educational level, number of strokes, duration of stroke, family history of stroke, type of stroke, number of chronic diseases, and activity of daily living (ADL).

2.3.2. The Modified Rankin Scale (MRS)

The modified Rankin scale was developed by Rankin [23] in 1957 for assessing the neurological recovery of stroke survivors. It consists of six levels with a total score ranging from 0 to 5, where a score of 0 indicates no symptoms and no assistance required, while a score of 5 signifies severe disability and complete dependence on others for assistance. A score less than 3 indicates a favorable prognosis, and a score of 3 or above suggests a poor prognosis [24]. The Cronbach's alpha value of this scale is 0.773.

2.3.3. The Stroke Self-Management Scale (SSMS)

The stroke self-management scale was developed by Wang et al. [25] in 2013. It includes 7 dimensions and 50 items, which are disease management (11 items), safe medication management (5 items), dietary management (8 items), daily living management (8 items), emotion management (5 items), social functioning and interpersonal management (6 items), and rehabilitation exercise management (7 items). It is a 5-point Likert scale. The total score ranges from 50 to 250 points. Higher scale scores mean higher levels of self-management. The Cronbach's alpha value of the SSMS is 0.874.

2.3.4. The Stroke Self-Efficacy Questionnaire (SSEQ)

The stroke self-efficacy questionnaire was developed by Jones et al. [26] in 2008. This questionnaire comprises 2 dimensions: movement (8 items) and self-management (5 items). Each item is rated on an 11-point Likert scale ranging from 0 ('little confidence') to 10 ('strong confidence'). Li [27] revised the SSEQ into a Chinese version and deleted 2 items in 2015. The total score ranges from 0 to 110 points. Higher scale scores mean higher levels of self-efficacy. The Cronbach's alpha value of the SSEQ is 0.969.

2.3.5. The Behavioral Decision-Making Scale for Stroke Patients

The behavioral decision-making scale for stroke patients was developed by Lin et al. [28] in 2022. It is divided into four dimensions and consists of 29 items: behavioral change motivation (10 items), behavioral change intention (9 items), decision-making factors (5 items), and decisional balance (5 items). It is a 5-point Likert scale ranging from 1 ('little agreement') to 5 ('strong agreement'). The total score ranges from 30 to 150 points. The higher the score, the higher the level of behavioral decision-making in stroke survivors, and the easier it is to trigger healthy behavioral decisions, resulting in healthy behaviors. The Cronbach's alpha value of this scale is 0.934.

2.4. Data Collection

Data collection spanned from 10 March 2024 to 15 July 2024. This research involved two trained assistants who were responsible for enrolling stroke survivors for in-person interviews. Patient identification was facilitated through medical records and hospital databases, with confirmation by the principal investigator. For this pre-testing phase, 5 stroke survivors who had only completed elementary school were selected. The assistants meticulously checked the questionnaires for any ambiguities or points needing clarification. Their insights led to modifications to ensure clear understanding and accurate responses to the survey questions in the main study. Prospective participants were briefed on this study's objectives and provided with informed consent before participation. Upon granting written approval of the survey, 300 individuals received a set of questionnaires to complete.

2.5. Ethical Considerations

The experimental protocol in this study was approved by the Zhengzhou University ethics committee in China (approval number: ZZURIB2021-115) in 2021, and all methods were conducted following relevant guidelines and regulations. All participants gave written informed consent.

2.6. Data Analysis

A statistical analysis was conducted using SPSS version 26.0, focusing on descriptive statistics. Samples with missing data exceeding 10% were discarded. Upon conducting the Kolmogorov–Smirnov test, it was determined that the scores of self-management in this research did not adhere to a normal distribution. Consequently, these non-normally distributed figures were characterized using the median and the interquartile range. For categorical data, representation was conducted through counts and their corresponding percentages. The Mann–Whitney U test and the Kruskal–Wallis test were used to assess differences in self-management across demographic characteristics. Spearman correlation was used to examine the associations between self-efficacy, behavioral decision-making, and self-management. Model 4 in the SPSS 26.0 macros program PROCESS compiled by Hayes [29] was used to construct the mediation model with 5000 bootstrap samples.

3. Results

3.1. Common Method Bias

The results showed that 16 factors with an eigenvalue greater than 1 were co-precipitated, and the variance explained by the first factor was 24.91%, which was less than the critical standard of 40%, indicating that the common method deviation of this study was not significant.

3.2. Demographic Characteristics

This study recruited 300 stroke survivors, and nine questionnaires were excluded due to non-response to some questions. A total of 291 elderly stroke survivors were included, resulting in a final valid return rate of 97%. More than 67.01% of elderly stroke survivors were men. Only 58 (11.2%) survivors in the sample had a university degree or more. In addition, more than half (59.45%) of elderly stroke survivors had at least one chronic disease comorbidity. Comparative analyses of self-management based on demographic characteristics showed no statistically significant differences in self-management scores with respect to marriage, educational level, duration of stroke, family history of stroke, mRS, and ADL. Furthermore, gender, residential area, working state, the number of strokes, the type of stroke, and the number of chronic diseases were found to have statistically significant differences in terms of self-management scores. A comparison of the scales' scores of survivors who had a stroke with different characteristics is shown in Table 1.

Table 1. Differences in terms of self-management in demographic factors of elderly stroke survivors ($n = 291$).

Variables	Category	*n* (%)	Self-Management [M(P25, P75)]	Z/H
Gender	Men	195 (67.01)	174 (157, 193)	−2.504 *
	Women	96 (32.99)	187.5 (161.25, 209.5)	
Marriage	Married	259 (89.00)	180 (157, 198)	−0.006
	Divorced	32 (11.00)	174 (158, 203)	
Residential area	Rural	108 (37.11)	191 (165, 209.5)	−4.288 ***
	Urban	183 (62.89)	170 (156, 191.25)	
Working state	Unemployed	105 (36.08)	184 (163, 201.75)	12.514 **
	Pensioner	84 (28.87)	189.5 (149.25, 211.75)	
	Working	102 (35.05)	164.5 (157, 190.25)	
Educational level	Primary or below	112 (38.49)	171 (156, 191)	−0.010
	Junior high school	78 (26.80)	177 (156, 201)	
	High school	79 (27.15)	186 (161, 198)	
	University or above	22 (7.56)	208 (182.25, 225.25)	
Number of strokes	1	156 (53.60)	188 (162, 200)	9.117 *
	2	95 (32.65)	165 (156, 191)	
	3 or more	40 (13.75)	169 (144, 192)	
Duration of stroke	<3 months	55 (18.90)	188 (159, 208)	3.988
	3 months~	131 (45.02)	176 (160, 193)	
	1 year~	44 (15.12)	172.5 (146.75, 199.75)	
	3 years or more	61 (20.96)	182 (156.25, 212)	
Family history of stroke	Yes	58 (19.93)	181 (146.75, 205)	−0.344
	No	233 (80.07)	177 (159, 197.75)	
Type of stroke	Ischemic	239 (82.13)	177 (157, 196)	−2.043 *
	Hemorrhagic	52 (17.87)	189 (162, 208)	
mRS (scores)	<3	243 (83.51)	184 (158, 198)	−1.708
	≥3	48 (16.49)	172 (153.25, 185)	
Number of chronic diseases	1	16 (5.50)	191 (159.5, 193.75)	15.343 ***
	2	173 (59.45)	172 (156, 192.5)	
	3	56 (19.24)	175 (156.25, 201.5)	
	4 or more	46 (15.81)	199 (175.5, 212)	
ADL	40~	9 (3.09)	176 (151.5, 207)	−0.010
	60~	282 (96.91)	178.5 (158, 198)	

Note: * $p < 0.05$, ** $p < 0.01$, *** $p < 0.001$.

3.3. Correlations Among the Main Variables

Spearman's correlation analysis was used to investigate the correlations among the three variables of self-efficiency, behavioral decision-making, and self-management. The results showed that self-efficacy was significantly positively correlated with behavioral decision-making ($r = 0.355$, $p < 0.01$) and self-management ($r = 0.408$, $p < 0.01$). Furthermore, behavioral decision-making was significantly positively correlated with self-management ($r = 0.366$, $p < 0.01$).

3.4. Mediation Model

According to the procedure and steps of mediating effect testing by Wen et al. [30], firstly, we examined the predictive effects of self-efficacy on self-management. Then, we used the bootstrap method (with 5000 resamples) to test the mediating role of behavioral decision-making. We controlled for some general demographic factors (such as gender, residential area, working state, number of strokes, type of stroke, and number of chronic diseases). Self-efficacy was positively related to self-management ($\beta = 0.31$, $t = 6.50$, $p < 0.001$). After adding a mediating variable, self-efficacy ($\beta = 0.23$, $t = 4.75$, $p < 0.001$) and behavioral decision-making ($\beta = 0.23$, $t = 4.80$, $p < 0.001$) were positively correlated with self-management. The results are shown in Table 2. Figure 2 presents the influencing paths of the mediation model.

Table 2. Testing the mediation effects of behavioral decision-making in terms of the relationship between self-efficiency and self-management.

Regression Equation		Global Fit Index			Significance of Regression Coefficient	
Outcome variable	Predictor variable	R	R^2	F	B (95% CI)	t
Self-management	Gender	0.51	0.26	14.21	0.16 (−0.05, 0.37)	1.51
	Residential area				0.34 (0.14, 0.54)	3.33 **
	Working state				−0.17 (−0.29, −0.05)	−2.88 **
	Number of strokes				−0.14 (−0.28, −0.01)	−2.02 *
	Type of stroke				0.20 (−0.05, 0.46)	1.58
	Number of chronic diseases				0.18 (0.06, 0.30)	2.92 **
	Self-efficacy				0.31 (0.22, 0.41)	6.50 ***
Behavioral decision-making	Gender	0.41	0.17	14.98	0.28 (0.03, 0.53)	2.19 *
	Residential area				0.36 (0.12, 0.60)	2.94 **
	Working state				−0.01 (−0.15, 0.13)	−0.16
	Number of strokes				0.18 (0.01, 0.35)	2.12 *
	Type of stroke				0.22 (−0.09, 0.52)	1.41
	Number of chronic diseases				−0.13 (−0.27, 0.02)	−1.73
	Self-efficacy				0.34 (0.23, 0.46)	5.98 ***
Self-management	Gender	0.56	0.32	16.28	0.10 (−0.11, 0.30)	0.94
	Residential area				0.26 (0.06, 0.46)	2.58 *
	Working state				−0.17 (−0.28, −0.06)	−2.94 **
	Number of strokes				−0.19 (−0.32, −0.05)	−2.68 **
	Type of stroke				0.15 (−0.09, 0.40)	1.23
	Number of chronic diseases				0.21 (0.09, 0.33)	3.51 **
	Self-efficacy				0.23 (0.14, 0.33)	4.75 ***
	Behavioral decision-making				0.23 (0.14, 0.33)	4.80 ***

Note: * $p < 0.05$, ** $p < 0.01$, *** $p < 0.001$. Gender, residential area, working state, number of strokes, type of stroke.

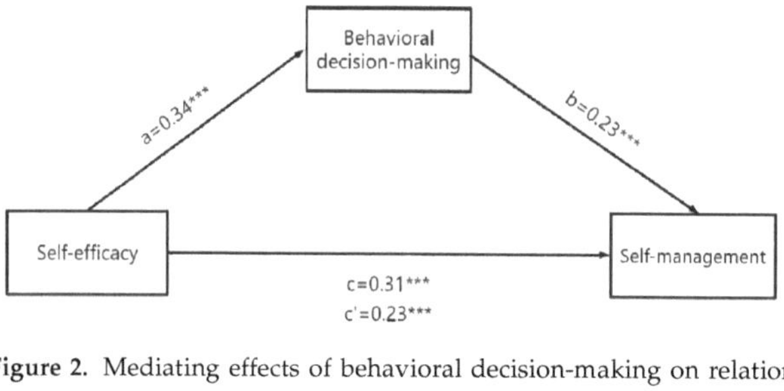

Figure 2. Mediating effects of behavioral decision-making on relationship between self-efficacy and self-management (*** $p < 0.001$). Numbers associated with a, b, c, and c′ are unstandardized regression coefficients. c: total effects of self-efficacy on self-management; c′: direct effects of self-efficacy on self-management.

To ensure the accuracy of the test, the 95% *CI* of the mediating effects of behavioral decision-making was 0.03 to 0.14, which does not contain 0, indicating that the mediating effects of behavioral decision-making between self-efficacy and self-management were established, and the effects accounted for 25.81%.

4. Discussion

This study reported on the influencing factors of self-management among elderly stroke survivors and the relationships between these factors. To the best of our knowledge, this is the first study to examine the relationships between self-efficacy, behavioral decision-making, and self-management. Furthermore, our study expanded the application scope of the behavioral decision-making model for stroke and validated its applicability within the elderly stroke survivor population.

Also, the findings of our study indicated that the self-management levels of elderly stroke survivors were moderately high, which was consistent with previous research [31]. Among them, the daily living management scores for stroke survivors were relatively high, while the scores for rehabilitation exercise management and disease management were relatively low. This may be because the vast majority (96.91%) of stroke survivors in our study had relatively high ADL scores, allowing them to achieve a high level of self-care in their daily lives. As a result, their daily living management was not significantly affected by stroke. On the contrary, disease management requires elderly stroke survivors to quickly adapt to the role of a patient and be able to persist in disease monitoring and management. However, elderly stroke survivors often experience a decline in memory and cognitive functions [32,33] due to factors like age, which may lead to forgetfulness or the insufficient mastery of disease monitoring skills in tasks such as blood pressure and blood sugar monitoring. In addition, a previous longitudinal study in China found that physical activity emerged as a significant predictor of decreased daily living activities among older adults [34], which was consistent with our study. However, elderly stroke survivors are a high-risk population for frailty [35], falls [36], and sarcopenia [37]. Risk factors such as frailty and falls can severely impact the ADL of elderly stroke survivors, thereby reducing their self-efficacy and self-management. Therefore, health professionals should implement the assessment of these weakness and risk factors in elderly stroke survivors. They should also provide these individuals with proper guidance and health education to help them prevent incidents such as falls while participating in exercise and disease management.

Our study indicated that self-efficacy can positively affect self-management among elderly stroke survivors. This result is consistent with previous research results [12,38,39]. The reasons for this may be that elderly stroke survivors with higher self-efficacy have intrinsic motivation, thus having more confidence to engage in self-management behaviors [12]. According to the Health Action Process Approach (HAPA) theory [40], self-efficacy is a crucial aspect in all stages of behavior changes, whether in the context of the emergence of behavioral intentions, the execution of behavior, or overcoming difficulties in the process of behavior. Elderly stroke survivors often have poorer physical function and less confidence in stroke management and rehabilitation. In other words, self-efficacy plays a more significant role in the rehabilitation process among elderly stroke survivors. Consequently, healthcare professionals should incorporate self-efficacy into a multifaceted evaluation framework for elderly stroke survivors to better grasp their disease conditions.

Moreover, our study found that the relationship between self-efficacy and self-management was also influenced by a mediator, namely behavioral decision-making. In other words, elderly stroke survivors with higher self-efficacy were shown to have a higher level of behavioral decision-making, which improved their engagement in self-management more effectively. This might be because elderly stroke survivors with higher self-efficacy have more control over their condition [12], which in turn allows them to have stronger behavioral motivation and intention when making decisions regarding self-management behaviors. Specifically, elderly stroke survivors are better able to juggle their own needs and make decisions that are in their best interest, thereby adopting self-management behaviors more effectively. The role of behavioral decision-making among stroke survivors has been confirmed in previous studies [17,41]. Guo et al. [17] found that the difficulty of behavioral decision-making is a barrier to prompting stroke survivors to engage in self-management behaviors.

However, behavioral decision-making is an extremely complex process [42]. After being discharged and returning home, elderly stroke survivors are often overprotected by caregivers [43] due to their advanced age. This reduces the autonomy and initiative of elderly stroke survivors in making their own decisions. Therefore, autonomy is paramount in behavioral decision-making among elderly stroke survivors and in turn crucial for their behavioral changes. Considering the decline in physical and cognitive abilities of elderly stroke survivors, to ensure efficient decision-making, the assistance of healthcare professionals and family members should be utilized while protecting the decision-making autonomy of elderly stroke survivors. Shared decision-making (SDM) is a patient-centered model in which doctors and patients share information, discuss options, and make decisions together based on mutual respect and equality [44]. This approach aims to better meet patients' needs and improve their treatment experience. American cardiovascular societies have all endorsed shared decision-making [45]. Healthcare professionals and family members should fully take into consideration the preferential needs of elderly stroke survivors and collaborate synergistically with them to make the most suitable health decisions [46]. Patient Decision Aids (PDAs) [47] are evidence-based tools that provide patients with decision-relevant information, assist them in weighing the pros and cons, and help them in making informed decisions. Healthcare professionals can design various decision aids, such as question prompt lists [48], to help elderly stroke survivors make careful decisions and reduce decisional conflict. However, it should be noted that the surveyed carried out by He et al. [20] included 229 stroke survivors and found that elderly stroke survivors have a higher level of behavioral decision-making compared to middle-aged and younger stroke survivors. Although this may not directly align with our conventional understanding and even though the sample size of this study was not large, this is indeed an objective result. Future research could consider conducting multicenter, large-sample surveys to assess the behavioral decision-making levels of elderly stroke survivors.

4.1. Clinical Implications

This study offers a new perspective on stroke behavior management. Firstly, the role of self-efficacy in promoting self-management deserves attention. For elderly stroke survivors, the establishment of self-efficacy may be more challenging. According to self-efficacy theory [49], successful experiences are one of the most important ways to gain self-efficacy. Therefore, healthcare professionals may consider setting gradual rehabilitation goals tailored to the conditions of elderly stroke survivors, allowing them to build confidence through successful management. Additionally, the significant role of behavioral decision-making among elderly stroke survivors was proven in our study. Hence, healthcare professionals should convey to the families of elderly stroke survivors the importance of patients' independent ability to make decisions with the help of family members [50].

4.2. Limitations

This study has certain limitations. Firstly, it is a cross-sectional study, so we cannot establish causal relationships between variables. Additionally, the elderly stroke survivors included in this study had a relatively high ADL level. This may, to some extent, contribute to Type I errors. Typically, most elderly stroke survivors experience significant functional impairments following a stroke, resulting in decreased ADL levels and compromised self-management abilities. Therefore, the generalizability of our study's findings is limited and cannot be extended to elderly stroke survivors with lower ADL levels. Moreover, although this study adequately considered potential influencing factors, there are some unique factors affecting the self-management of older adults that were not fully considered, such as falls and frailty related to the decline in physical function in old age. Future research could focus on the impact of these factors on the self-efficacy and self-management of elderly stroke survivors. Lastly, this study concentrated on how the inherent characteristics of elderly stroke survivors affect their self-management; thus, all the factors examined pertain to the survivors themselves. Individual behavior is also influenced by family and societal factors [31]. Consequently, future research will incorporate family and social elements pertaining to elderly stroke survivors to investigate the multifaceted influences on behavioral management.

5. Conclusions

This study explored the impact of self-efficacy, behavioral decision-making, and self-management on stroke survivors. In summary, self-efficacy and behavioral decision-making are significantly related to self-management. Behavioral decision-making played a mediation role in the relationship between self-efficacy and self-management among elderly stroke survivors. Furthermore, this study indicated that elderly stroke survivors were more likely to adopt behavioral decision-making to improve self-management when they have higher self-efficacy. These findings suggest a new perspective for healthcare professionals in elderly stroke behavior management. While enhancing the self-efficacy levels of elderly stroke survivors, it is also necessary to consider how to assist them in making behavioral decisions that align with their health rights and interests.

Supplementary Materials: The following supporting information can be downloaded at https://www.mdpi.com/article/10.3390/healthcare13070704/s1, Table S1: The Strengthening the Reporting of Observational Studies in Epidemiology (STROBE) guideline statement—a checklist of items.

Author Contributions: Conceptualization, Z.Z. (Zhenxiang Zhang) and B.L.; Methodology, Z.Z. (Zhenxiang Zhang) and B.L.; Formal Analysis, X.W. and Z.P.; Investigation, X.W. and H.J.; Writing—Original Draft Preparation, X.W. and H.J.; Writing—Review and Editing, X.W., H.J., Z.Z. (Zhixin Zhao), and N.T.K.; Visualization, X.W.; Supervision, B.A.; Project Administration, Z.Z. (Zhenxiang Zhang) and B.L.; Funding Acquisition, Z.Z. (Zhenxiang Zhang) and B.L. All authors have read and agreed to the published version of the manuscript.

Funding: This work was supported by The National Natural Science Foundation of China Foundation Project (72174184) and China Postdoctoral Science Foundation (2023M743197). A funding institution provided financial support for the design and collection, data analysis, and article publication stages of this study.

Institutional Review Board Statement: The Zhengzhou University ethics committee in China approved all study procedures (approval number: ZZURIB2021-115, 1 November 2021).

Informed Consent Statement: Informed consent was obtained from all participants involved in this study.

Data Availability Statement: The data supporting the findings of this study are available on request from the corresponding author. The data are not publicly available due to privacy or ethical restrictions.

Acknowledgments: We express our gratitude to the stroke survivors who participated in this study.

Conflicts of Interest: The authors declare no competing interests.

References

1. GBD 2019 Stroke Collaborators. Global, Regional, and National Burden of Stroke and Its Risk Factors, 1990–2019: A Systematic Analysis for the Global Burden of Disease Study 2019. *Lancet. Neurol.* **2021**, *20*, 795–820. [CrossRef]
2. Ma, Q.; Li, R.; Wang, L.; Yin, P.; Wang, Y.; Yan, C.; Ren, Y.; Qian, Z.; Vaughn, M.G.; McMillin, S.E.; et al. Temporal Trend and Attributable Risk Factors of Stroke Burden in China, 1990–2019: An Analysis for the Global Burden of Disease Study 2019. *Lancet. Public Health* **2021**, *6*, e897–e906. [CrossRef]
3. Report on Stroke Prevention and Treatment in China Writing Group. Brief report on stroke prevention and treatment in China, 2021. *Chin. J. Cerebrovasc. Dis.* **2023**, *20*, 783–793. [CrossRef]
4. de Graaf, J.A.; Schepers, V.P.M.; Nijsse, B.; van Heugten, C.M.; Post, M.W.M.; Visser-Meily, J.M.A. The Influence of Psychological Factors and Mood on the Course of Participation up to Four Years after Stroke. *Disabil. Rehabil.* **2022**, *44*, 1855–1862. [CrossRef] [PubMed]
5. Reistetter, T.; Hreha, K.; Dean, J.M.; Pappadis, M.R.; Deer, R.R.; Li, C.-Y.; Hong, I.; Na, A.; Nowakowski, S.; Shaltoni, H.M.; et al. The Pre-Adaptation of a Stroke-Specific Self-Management Program Among Older Adults. *J. Aging Health* **2023**, *35*, 632–642. [CrossRef] [PubMed]
6. Liu, L.; Li, X.; Marshall, I.J.; Bhalla, A.; Wang, Y.; O'Connell, M.D.L. Trajectories of Depressive Symptoms 10 Years after Stroke and Associated Risk Factors: A Prospective Cohort Study. *Lancet* **2023**, *402* (Suppl. 1), S64. [CrossRef]
7. Alghamdi, I.; Ariti, C.; Williams, A.; Wood, E.; Hewitt, J. Prevalence of Fatigue after Stroke: A Systematic Review and Meta-Analysis. *Eur. Stroke J.* **2021**, *6*, 319–332. [CrossRef]
8. Ory, M.G.; Ahn, S.; Towne, S.D.; Smith, M.L. Chronic Disease Self-Management Education: Program Success and Future Directions. In *Geriatrics Models of Care: Bringing "Best Practice" to an Aging America*; Malone, M.L., Capezuti, E.A., Palmer, R.M., Eds.; Springer International Publishing: Cham, Switzerland, 2015; pp. 147–153. ISBN 978-3-319-16068-9. [CrossRef]
9. Tomás, C.C.; Oliveira, E.; Sousa, D.; Uba-Chupel, M.; Furtado, G.; Rocha, C.; Teixeira, A.; Ferreira, P.; Alves, C.; Gisin, S.; et al. Proceedings of the 3rd IPLeiria's International Health Congress: Leiria, Portugal. 6–7 May 2016. *BMC Health Serv. Res.* **2016**, *16* (Suppl. 3), 200. [CrossRef]
10. Wang, L.; Pan, Q.; Zhou, J.; Yu, Q.; Zeng, W.; Zhang, M.; Guo, M. Status and influencing factors of health self-management in elderly stroke patients in Wuhan. *Chin. J. Gerontol.* **2017**, *37*, 4658–4660. [CrossRef]
11. Bandura, A. Social Cognitive Theory: An Agentic Perspective. *Annu. Rev. Psychol.* **2001**, *52*, 1–26. [CrossRef]
12. Szczepańska-Gieracha, J.; Mazurek, J. The Role of Self-Efficacy in the Recovery Process of Stroke Survivors. *Psychol. Res. Behav. Manag.* **2020**, *13*, 897–906. [CrossRef] [PubMed]
13. Brouwer-Goossensen, D.; van Genugten, L.; Lingsma, H.F.; Dippel, D.W.J.; Koudstaal, P.J.; den Hertog, H.M. Self-Efficacy for Health-Related Behaviour Change in Patients with TIA or Minor Ischemic Stroke. *Psychol. Health* **2018**, *33*, 1490–1501. [CrossRef] [PubMed]
14. Kelly, M.P.; Barker, M. Why Is Changing Health-Related Behaviour so Difficult? *Public Health* **2016**, *136*, 109–116. [CrossRef]
15. Edwards, W. Behavioral Decision Theory. *Annu. Rev. Psychol.* **1961**, *12*, 473–498. [CrossRef]
16. Lin, B.; Jin, Y.; Mei, Y.; Zhang, W.; Zhang, Z.; Wang, W.; Xue, L.; An, B. Preliminary Construction of Recurrence Risk Perception and Behavioral Decision Model in Stroke Patients. *Mil. Nurs.* **2024**, *41*, 1–5.
17. Guo, Z.; Zeng, S.; Ling, K.; Chen, S.; Yao, T.; Li, H.; Xu, L.; Zhu, X. Experiences and Needs of Older Patients with Stroke in China Involved in Rehabilitation Decision-Making: A Qualitative Study. *BMC Med. Inform. Decis. Mak.* **2024**, *24*, 330. [CrossRef]
18. Sheeran, P.; Maki, A.; Montanaro, E.; Avishai-Yitshak, A.; Bryan, A.; Klein, W.M.P.; Miles, E.; Rothman, A.J. The Impact of Changing Attitudes, Norms, and Self-Efficacy on Health-Related Intentions and Behavior: A Meta-Analysis. *Health Psychol.* **2016**, *35*, 1178–1188. [CrossRef]
19. Jin, Y.; Zhang, Z.; Cadilhac, D.A.; Qiu, Y.; Zhang, W.; Mei, Y.; Ping, Z.; Zhang, L.; Lin, B. Developing a Chain Mediation Model of Recurrence Risk Perception and Health Behavior Among Patients With Stroke: A Cross-Sectional Study. *Asian Nurs. Res.* **2024**, *18*, 384–392. [CrossRef]
20. He, F.; Lin, B.; Liu, X.; Zhang, Z.; Wang, J. Current situation of the health behavioral decision making in ischemic stroke patients and its influencing factors analysis. *Chin. J. Nurs.* **2024**, *59*, 2222–2229. [CrossRef]
21. Neurology, C.; Society, C. Diagnostic Criteria of Cerebrovascular Diseases in China (Version 2019). *Chin. J. Neurol.* **2019**, *9*, 710–715. [CrossRef]
22. Liu, N. The Sample Size Estimation in Quantitative Nursing Research. *Chin. J. Nurs.* **2010**, *45*, 378e80. [CrossRef]
23. Rankin, J. Cerebral Vascular Accidents in Patients over the Age of 60: I. General Considerations. *Scott. Med. J.* **1957**, *2*, 127–136. [CrossRef] [PubMed]
24. Fan, Y.; Ji, X.; Lan, L. The Application of mRS in the Methods of Outcome Assessment in Chinese Stroke Trials. *Chin. J. Nerv.Ment. Dis.* **2015**, *41*, 412–415. [CrossRef]

25. Wang, Y. Construction and Application of Self-Management Intervention Project for Patients After Stroke. Master's Thesis, Chengdu University of Traditional Chinese Medicine, Chengdu, China, 2013.
26. Jones, F.; Partridge, C.; Reid, F. The Stroke Self-Efficacy Questionnaire: Measuring Individual Confidence in Functional Performance after Stroke. *J. Clin. Nurs.* **2008**, *17*, 244–252. [CrossRef]
27. Li, H.; Fang, L.; Bi, R.; Cheng, H.; Huang, J.; Feng, L. The reliability and validity of the Chinese version of Stroke Self Efficacy Questionnaire. *Chin. J. Nurs.* **2015**, *50*, 790–794. [CrossRef]
28. Lin, B.; Zhang, Z.; Mei, Y.; Wang, W.; Wang, P.; Tang, Q.; Guo, J.; Zhang, W. Development and psychometric test of the Behavioral Decision-making Scale for Stroke Patients. *Chin. J. Nurs.* **2022**, *57*, 1605–1610. [CrossRef]
29. Hayes, A. Introduction to Mediation, Moderation, and Conditional Process Analysis. *J. Educ. Meas.* **2013**, *51*, 335–337. [CrossRef]
30. Wen, Z.; Ye., B. Different Methods for Testing Moderated Mediation Models: Competitors or Backups? *Acta Psychol. Sin.* **2014**, *46*, 714–726. [CrossRef]
31. Shuqi, H.; Siqin, L.; Xiaoyan, W.; Rong, Y.; Lihong, Z. The Risk Factors of Self-Management Behavior among Chinese Stroke Patients. *Int. J. Clin. Pract.* **2023**, *2023*, 4308517. [CrossRef]
32. Gil-Salcedo, A.; Dugravot, A.; Fayosse, A.; Jacob, L.; Bloomberg, M.; Sabia, S.; Schnitzler, A. Long-Term Evolution of Functional Limitations in Stroke Survivors Compared with Stroke-Free Controls: Findings from 15 Years of Follow-Up Across 3 International Surveys of Aging. *Stroke* **2022**, *53*, 228–237. [CrossRef]
33. Dhana, K.; Aggarwal, N.T.; Beck, T.; Holland, T.M.; Dhana, A.; Cherian, L.J.; Desai, P.; Evans, D.A.; Rajan, K.B. Lifestyle and Cognitive Decline in Community-Dwelling Stroke Survivors. *J. Alzheimers Dis.* **2022**, *89*, 745–754. [CrossRef]
34. Wang, L.-Y.; Chen, H.-X.; Zhu, H.; Hu, Z.-Y.; Zhou, C.-F.; Hu, X.-Y. Physical Activity as a Predictor of Activities of Daily Living in Older Adults: A Longitudinal Study in China. *Front. Public Health* **2024**, *12*, 1444119. [CrossRef]
35. Dohle, E.; Lewis, B.; Agarwal, S.; Warburton, E.A.; Evans, N.R. Frailty Reduces Penumbral Volumes and Attenuates Treatment Response in Hyperacute Ischemic Stroke. *Age Ageing* **2024**, *53*, afae266. [CrossRef] [PubMed]
36. Samuelsson, C.M.; Hansson, P.-O.; Persson, C.U. Determinants of Recurrent Falls Poststroke: A 1-Year Follow-up of the Fall Study of Gothenburg. *Arch. Phys. Med. Rehabil.* **2020**, *101*, 1541–1548. [CrossRef] [PubMed]
37. Su, Y.; Yuki, M.; Otsuki, M. Prevalence of Stroke-Related Sarcopenia: A Systematic Review and Meta-Analysis. *J. Stroke Cerebrovasc. Dis.* **2020**, *29*, 105092. [CrossRef] [PubMed]
38. Vaughn, R.M.; Gangwani, R.; Mark, J.I.; Fletcher, K.; Baratta, J.M.; Cassidy, J.M. Predictive Utility of Self-Efficacy in Early Stroke Rehabilitation. *Top. Stroke Rehabil.* **2024**, *30*, 1–9. [CrossRef]
39. Liu, Q.; Jin, Y.; Wang, Y.; Feng, J.; Qiao, X.; Ji, L.; Si, H.; Bian, Y.; Wang, W.; Yu, J.; et al. Association between Self-Efficacy and Self-Management Behaviours among Individuals at High Risk for Stroke: Social Support Acting as a Mediator. *J. Clin. Nurs.* **2023**, *32*, 71–82. [CrossRef]
40. Schwarzer, R. Self-Efficacy in the Adoption and Maintenance of Health Behaviors: Theoretical Approaches and a New Model. In *Self-Efficacy: Thought Control of Action*; Hemisphere Publishing Corp: Washington, DC, USA, 1992; pp. 217–243, ISBN 978-1-56032-269-6. [CrossRef]
41. Holder, C.; Krishnamurthi, R.; Theadom, A. Exploring Facilitators and Barriers to Long-Term Behavior Change Following Health-Wellness Coaching for Stroke Prevention: A Qualitative Study Conducted in Auckland, New Zealand. *Brain Behav.* **2023**, *13*, e2671. [CrossRef]
42. Juavinett, A.L.; Erlich, J.C.; Churchland, A.K. Decision-Making Behaviors: Weighing Ethology, Complexity, and Sensorimotor Compatibility. *Curr. Opin. Neurobiol.* **2018**, *49*, 42–50. [CrossRef]
43. Guo, Z.; Zeng, S.; Ling, K.; Chen, S.; Yao, T.; Li, H.; Xu, L.; Zhu, X. A Qualitative Study on the Experience of Rehabilitation Decision-Making in Semi-disabled Elderly Patients with Stroke. *J. Chengdu Med. Coll.* **2024**, *19*, 342–346.
44. Légaré, F.; Witteman, H.O. Shared Decision Making: Examining Key Elements and Barriers to Adoption into Routine Clinical Practice. *Health Aff.* **2013**, *32*, 276–284. [CrossRef]
45. MacDonald, B.J.; Turgeon, R.D. Incorporation of Shared Decision-Making in International Cardiovascular Guidelines, 2012–2022. *JAMA Netw. Open* **2023**, *6*, e2332793. [CrossRef]
46. Armstrong, M.J. Shared Decision-Making in Stroke: An Evolving Approach to Improved Patient Care. *Stroke Vasc. Neurol.* **2017**, *2*, 84–87. [CrossRef] [PubMed]
47. Elwyn, G.; Laitner, S.; Coulter, A.; Walker, E.; Watson, P.; Thomson, R. Implementing Shared Decision Making in the NHS. *BMJ* **2010**, *341*, c5146. [CrossRef] [PubMed]
48. Lukasczik, M.; Wolf, H.D.; Vogel, H. Development and Initial Evaluation of the Usefulness of a Question Prompt List to Promote Patients' Level of Information about Work-Related Medical Rehabilitation: A Pilot Study. *Front. Rehabil. Sci.* **2024**, *5*, 1266065. [CrossRef]

49. Nasiri, M.; Jafari, Z.; Rakhshan, M.; Yarahmadi, F.; Zonoori, S.; Akbari, F.; Moghimi, E.S.; Amirmohseni, L.; Abbasi, M.; Sharstanaki, S.K.; et al. Application of Orem's Theory-Based Caring Programs among Chronically Ill Adults: A Systematic Review and Dose-Response Meta-Analysis. *Int. Nurs. Rev.* **2023**, *70*, 59–77. [CrossRef]
50. Fang, Y.; Tao, Q.; Zhou, X.; Chen, S.; Huang, J.; Jiang, Y.; Wu, Y.; Chen, L.; Tao, J.; Chan, C.C. Patient and Family Member Factors Influencing Outcomes of Poststroke Inpatient Rehabilitation. *Arch. Phys. Med. Rehabil.* **2017**, *98*, 249–255.e2. [CrossRef]

healthcare

MDPI

Project Report

"When the Word Is Too Big, It's Just Too Hard": Stroke Survivors' Perspectives About Health Literacy and Delivery of Health Information †

Dana Wong [1], Lauren M. Sanders [2,3], Alison Beauchamp [4], Claire Formby [5], Emma E. Smith [1,6], Creina Hansen [2], Kathryn McKinley [7,8], Karella De Jongh [9] and Karen Borschmann [9,10,*]

1 School of Psychology and Public Health, La Trobe University, Bundoora, VIC 3086, Australia; d.wong@latrobe.edu.au (D.W.); e.smith5@latrobe.edu.au (E.E.S.)
2 Department of Neurosciences, St Vincent's Hospital Melbourne, Fitzroy, VIC 3065, Australia; creina.hansen@svha.org.au (C.H.)
3 Department of Medicine, Melbourne Medical School, University of Melbourne, Parkville, VIC 3010, Australia
4 School of Rural Health, Monash University, Warragul, VIC 3820, Australia; alison.beauchamp@monash.edu
5 Health Independence Program, St Vincent's Hospital Melbourne, Fitzroy, VIC 3065, Australia; claire.formby@svha.org.au
6 School of Psychological Sciences, University of Melbourne, Parkville, VIC 3010, Australia
7 Allied Health, Northern Health, Epping, VIC 3076, Australia; kathryn.mckinley@nh.org.au
8 Speech Pathology, St Vincent's Hospital Melbourne, Fitzroy, VIC 3065, Australia
9 Allied Health, St Vincent's Hospital Melbourne, Fitzroy, VIC 3065, Australia
10 The Florey Institute, University of Melbourne, Heidelberg, VIC 3084, Australia
* Correspondence: karenb@unimelb.edu.au

† The paper is an extended version of our paper "When the Word is Too Big, It's Just Too Hard: How can Clinicians Support Patients' Health Literacy to Improve Recovery after Stroke?" published in Proceedings of the Stroke 2023—The Combined Stroke Society of Australasia and Smart Strokes Nursing and Allied Health Scientific Meeting, Melbourne, Australia, 22–25 August 2023.

Abstract: Background: Health literacy can impact comprehension, recall, and implementation of stroke-related information, especially in the context of cognitive and communication impairments, cultural-linguistic diversity, or ageing. Yet there are few published lived experience perspectives to inform tailoring of health information. **Objectives:** We aimed to (i) explore perspectives about the impact of health literacy on information needs and preferences of stroke survivors with diverse characteristics; and (ii) identify ways to better tailor information delivery for stroke survivors with low health literacy. **Methods:** This qualitative study was conducted using the Ophelia (Optimising Health Literacy and Access) methodology. First, health literacy information was collected from participants. Hierarchical cluster analysis was used to identify different health literacy profiles within the participant sample. Four profiles were identified, from which four case vignettes were created. Second, focus groups and interviews were conducted to explore the health information needs and preferences of the case vignettes. Qualitative data were analysed with reflexive thematic analysis. **Results:** Nineteen people participated (median (IQR) age = 65 (49, 69), 10 (53%) female); five used interpreters. Participants represented diverse socioeconomic, cultural, and stroke-related characteristics, and generally had low health literacy. Four qualitative themes were generated highlighting the impact of *Individual knowledge, capacity, and beliefs about stroke and health services* on people's capacity to engage with stroke-related information; *Tailoring and personalisation of information delivery* to the patient's knowledge, capacity, and beliefs; *Having a support network to rely on*; and patients *Feeling like I am in safe hands* of clinicians and services. **Conclusions:** Findings provide several important directions for improving accessible stroke information delivery suitable for people with all levels of health literacy, and to optimise patient understanding, recall, and implementation of healthcare information.

 https://doi.org/10.3390/healthcare13050541

Keywords: stroke; health literacy; organisational literacy; Ophelia methodology; health information; cognitive impairment; communication disability; cultural and linguistic diversity

1. Introduction

Low health literacy, defined as people's ability to seek, understand, engage with, and implement health information, is surprisingly prevalent in the general community. Only 41% of Australian adults have sufficient health literacy to understand and use health information [1,2]. Low health literacy is particularly common in people with older age, limited education, and in some culturally and linguistically diverse (CALD) populations AIHW [2,3]. One in two people with stroke experience cognitive impairment and one in four have communication impairments [4]. This can further compromise health literacy and affect comprehension, recall, and effective implementation of health-related information [5,6]. With low health literacy impacting poorer stroke outcomes including medication adherence, general health status, and hospital readmission [7], it is incumbent on health practitioners to provide appropriate health information to support stroke recovery

Organisational literacy, or the health literacy environment, is the degree to which organisations can acknowledge and accommodate variations in patient health literacy and thereby support patients to manage their health and navigate the health system. Proponents of improving organisational literacy, rather than attempting to improve health literacy, support a "universal precautions" approach to heath communication. Such an approach requires habitual use of clear communications to improve accessibility of health information for all people with stroke, regardless of their health literacy [8]. This shifts the onus of responsibility from the marginalised patient to that of the health service to provide appropriately tailored stroke care [9]. Health services have a responsibility to support health literacy [10]; however, to date there is limited evidence that this occurs consistently in clinical practice. A recent qualitative study of Australian stroke clinicians found that only 60% had received training to support their communication with people with aphasia [11], and there are gaps between clinicians' theoretical understanding of information provision and their actual practice [12]. Although there are lived experience-informed guidelines for the provision of information for people with stroke [13], adult learning principles are not always applied by health professionals when providing information [14], and the reading level of many stroke education materials is too high [15].

Poor organisational health literacy can lead to poor experiences of healthcare and poor outcomes post-stroke [2]. Therefore, it is incumbent upon stroke services to improve their awareness of and responsiveness to low health literacy in their service users. To do this, it is important to include the voices of people with lived experience of stroke to ensure that service improvements reflect the values and needs of patients. In particular, it is important to include the voices of people with cognitive and communication difficulties, limited education, and those from CALD backgrounds, given their increased likelihood of low health literacy and their frequent exclusion from stroke research [16].

Our study had two main aims. Firstly, we aimed to explore stroke survivors' perspectives on health literacy and how it may impact the information needs and preferences of people with stroke, including people typically under-represented in stroke research. Secondly, we aimed to identify targets or directions for improving organisational literacy—i.e., ways to enable stroke services to better tailor information delivery to stroke survivors with low health literacy, and therefore support their patients to understand and use stroke information to optimise their outcomes.

2. Materials and Methods

This qualitative study was conducted in two stages using the Ophelia (Optimising Health Literacy and Access) methodology [17]. In Stage 1, health literacy information was collected from participants to create case vignettes that represented their common characteristics. In Stage 2, focus groups and interviews were conducted about the health information needs and preferences of the people described in the case vignettes. This article is a revised and expanded version of a paper entitled "When the Word is Too Big, it's Just Too Hard: How can Clinicians Support Patients' Health Literacy to Improve Recovery after Stroke?", which was presented at Stroke 2023, Melbourne, Australia, in August 2023 [18].

2.1. Participants

Inclusion criteria for the study were community-dwelling adults (≥18 years old) with stroke or transient ischemic attack who attended St Vincent's Hospital Melbourne (SVHM) outpatient stroke clinic between January 2021 and February 2022. SVHM is a public tertiary hospital in inner Melbourne that caters to a broad demographic of the local multicultural community.

Clinic lists were screened by clinician researchers (CF and LS) and consecutive, eligible participants were invited to participate via a telephone call or discussion during a stroke clinic appointment. Purposeful recruitment was undertaken to include people whose preferred language was not English (especially people from Vietnamese background as this population was a common user group of interpreter services at SVHM). Potential participants identified as likely to have aphasia, cognitive impairment, or low English literacy were offered an Assisted Communication or Easy English version of the Patient Information and Consent Form, with use of interpreters when required. Participants were made aware that this research was being conducted with aim of improving stroke services at SVHM. Further information about the research teams' interest in the topic was discussed according to patient interest. Participant recruitment was limited by strict and prolonged COVID-19 related lockdowns in Melbourne during the data collection period.

2.2. Materials and Procedures

Materials were developed and pilot tested by the multidisciplinary research team, who had extensive research and clinical experience in stroke recovery, supported communication (for post-stroke aphasia and cognition difficulties), health literacy, and interpreter services, and lived experience of stroke.

2.2.1. Stage 1

Electronic health records were reviewed to collect patient data relating to demographics (gender, age, languages spoken, highest level of education, birth country, living arrangements, carer support), clinical details of stroke including any description or assessment of language impairment, communication support needs and cognition, and global disability (modified Rankin score, mRS). Education level was classified as follows: did not complete primary school, completed primary school, completed secondary school, certificate/apprenticeship/diploma, degree, or post-graduate qualification. Observed communication or cognition impairments were also noted during participant interviews that were conducted by researcher CF, an experienced stroke clinician.

Socioeconomic status was categorised based on postcode of home address using the Index of Relative Socio-economic Advantage and Disadvantage, (1 = most disadvantaged, 5 = most advantaged) ABS [19]. Lower scores indicate relatively greater disadvantage and a lack of advantage in general. For example, an area could have a low score if there are many households with low incomes, or many people in unskilled occupations, and a few households with high incomes, or few people in skilled occupations.

Structured interviews, developed collaboratively by the research team, were conducted to collect information not available in medical records, and participant data relating to health literacy, global disability (modified Rankin score, mRS), stroke-related information needs, and knowledge of stroke and secondary stroke prevention. Interviews were undertaken in person, via telephone or via telehealth, depending on patient preference and COVID-19 pandemic restrictions. Interviews were conducted by author CF (an experienced stroke clinician and researcher) between December 2021 and March 2022. Interpreters were used as required. Participants were offered breaks during the interview and interviews were conducted across two sessions, if needed.

Formal cognitive assessment using the Oxford Cognitive Screen (Australian version, OCS-AU) was planned; however, due to challenges with telehealth administration during the pandemic, this was not conducted.

Health literacy was evaluated using the Health Literacy Questionnaire (HLQ) [20] and the Brief Health Literacy Screening Tool (BRIEF) [21]. The HLQ measures health literacy across nine independent scales, each measuring a different aspect of health literacy. The HLQ is considered highly reliable (composite reliability ranges from 0.8 to 0.9) [22] and is widely used, including in populations with cardiovascular disease [23]. Five HLQ scales were used for this study: Scale 2, Having sufficient information to manage my health; Scale 3, Actively managing my health; Scale 4, Social support for health; Scale 6, Ability to actively engage with healthcare providers; and Scale 7, Navigating the healthcare system. Scales 2, 3, and 4 are answered using a 4-point Likert scale (range 1–4) and scales 6 and 7 answered using a 5-point Likert scale (range 1–5). The Brief Health Literacy Screening Tool (BRIEF) [24] is a 4-item measure (range 1–20) that captures people's functional health literacy (i.e., the ability to read and understand written information). The instrument has been widely used across different health conditions, including stroke [25].

2.2.2. Stage 2

Using HLQ data collected in Stage 1, four different groupings ("clusters") of participants were identified, each representing a different health literacy profile within the sample (see Section 2.3 for detail). Brief case vignettes were then developed representing the four participant clusters. An example vignette is contained in Table 1; the remaining three vignettes are Supplementary Files. The vignettes were then used to guide discussions in the Stage 2 focus groups and interviews.

Participants were invited to attend small focus groups. Focus groups were conducted in June 2022 via Zoom by DW (experienced clinical neuropsychologist, group facilitator, and qualitative researcher), AB (experienced health literacy researcher), and CF (clinician researcher), all of whom are female. Each group commenced with a brief introduction about the interviewing team and the aims of the project, which were (1) to improve the way stroke services were delivered at both SVHM and more broadly, and (2) to make it easier for survivors of stroke to understand and use information about their health. Participants were also provided with the opportunity to introduce themselves. Using PowerPoint slides and a verbal description, participants were presented with 1–2 vignettes (see Table 1) which best represented the experiences of the group. Participants were then asked a series of questions about how stroke services could meet the needs of the "character" in the vignette. Questions included (i) "Does this sound like someone you know, or something you may have experienced?", (ii) "What things might make it difficult for [character] to find, understand, and use information about [their] stroke?", (iii) "What strengths does she have to help her make changes?", and (iv) "What could our health service do to make things easier/better for [character]?" The group facilitators encouraged all participants to share their views and ensured that everyone had the chance to do so either verbally or in the Zoom chat. Communication support strategies, such as slowed pace of speech, repetition, paraphrasing, and reflective summaries of participants' comments to confirm their meaning, were used by facilitators as required. Interviewers made notes during discussions, and a summary of participant comments was then shown on a slide for participants to confirm that the summary accurately described their views.

Table 1. Case vignette example: Character "Mai".

Description
Mai is a 75-year-old woman who moved to Australia in the 1970s. She was born in Vietnam and only speaks Vietnamese. She did not complete high school and worked in a factory for most of her life. Mai's husband died two years ago. Her main support is now her daughter who lives close by but works long hours and has two small children. Because of the COVID-19 pandemic, Mai was unable to have visitors while she was in hospital after her stroke. She found this very scary and a lot of the time was unsure what was happening. Her daughter spoke to the doctors each day, but she is not sure what they spoke about. None of the doctors or nurses could speak Vietnamese, nor was she offered an interpreter, so she was unable to ask any questions. The Vietnamese language leaflets she was given did not always make sense to her.
Mai has a good GP who speaks Vietnamese. This helps Mai trust him in discussing her problems. Her daughter cannot always come to Mai's specialist appointments with her. She likes appointments where she has an interpreter—this means she can ask questions. She prefers to hear spoken information rather than have it in writing, as she is not a confident reader. It also gives her chance to socialise. Since having her stroke, she does not very often see people from her community.
Mai takes lots of medications and had lots of tests after her stroke. She is not sure what they are all for, but the doctor told her they are important. Her doctors have told her to exercise more and change her diet. Mai likes the food she cooks and walks round the block every other day. She does not think she needs to change this, as she is taking the tablets the doctor told her to.

For participants who indicated that participation in focus groups was too challenging, individual semi-structured interviews were undertaken via Zoom or telephone by author CF with an interpreter when required. Duration ranged from 15 to 60 min. For telephone interviews, a spoken description of the vignettes was provided and similar questions to that of the focus groups described above used as prompts to elicit information.

Audio from each focus group and interview was recorded and transcribed verbatim. If the participant did not wish to be recorded, a written summary of their interview was taken.

2.3. Data Analysis

2.3.1. Stage 1

Data related to individual participants' demographics, health literacy, and stroke-related information needs were analysed descriptively. STATA version 15 [26] and SPSS version 22 [27] were used for analyses of quantitative data. A p-value of <0.05 was assumed for statistical significance. Hierarchical cluster analysis was used to identify different health literacy profiles within the patient sample using Ward's method for linkage [28]. Based on previous work [17], a range of cluster solutions of between 2 and 8 clusters was pre-determined. Selection of the most appropriate cluster solution was based on two criteria: first, whether the standard deviation within each scale within each cluster was below 0.6; and second, whether distinct patterns of HLQ scale scores were seen between clusters. Demographic, clinical, and health data were reported for each cluster, providing a detailed picture of a "typical" person within that cluster.

2.3.2. Stage 2

The focus groups and interviews were transcribed and analysed using reflexive thematic analysis [29,30]. A critical realist approach to analysis was taken, seeking to understand the meaning participants made of their experiences (via the case vignettes) and the influence of broader social and structural contexts, within the shared context of engaging with health services following a stroke. Data were coded through a process of familiarisation (rereading the transcripts several times), then generating initial codes based on both verbatim utterances and underlying patterns and concepts, and constantly revisiting the transcripts as the codes were refined. Generation and refinement of codes was conducted by researcher ES (research assistant with Honours-level training in psychology) in consultation with DW, using NVivo 1.7.1. The research team (CF, CH, DW, ES, KB) then collaboratively grouped the codes and generated themes during a Zoom meeting using Ideaflip online software (ideaflip.com). Themes were defined and labelled, and relationships between themes were explored together as a team.

3. Results

3.1. Stage 1

Nineteen participants completed structured interviews in Stage 1. Participants were interviewed via telephone (n = 16) in their homes or local communities, face to face (n = 2) in the stroke clinic or via Zoom (n = 1) in their home. Interpreters were utilised in five interviews. Family members were present for all face to face, Zoom, and interpreter interviews. It is unknown if anyone else was present during telephone calls conducted in English.

Participant characteristics are shown in Table 2. The median (IQR) age of participants was 65 (49, 69) years, 10 (53%) were female and 9 (47%) were male, and 9 (47%) completed education beyond high school. Eleven participants (58%) resided in areas of the highest socioeconomic category, and two (11%) resided in the lowest category. Eleven participants (58%) were born in Australia, and the remainder in Asia or Europe. Five participants (26%) spoke Vietnamese, and all used interpreters during their interviews. The remaining 14 people were interviewed in English without interpreters. The median time post-stroke was 9.5 months (IQR 6, 14). As mentioned, cognitive assessment could not be completed, and medical records generally had no record of cognitive status. Cognitive impairment was noted for six (32%) participants; three of these by the researcher based on clinical impression, and three by the family (clinical impression was more difficult for these participants due to use of an interpreter). Seven (37%) participants had mild communication impairments at the time of stroke (NIHSS 1–3 for aphasia or dysarthria). All participants completed the interviews independently, without carer support or personalised communication support.

HLQ data approximated normal distribution, and homogeneity of variance was not violated. Mean HLQ scores are shown in Table 3. For scales 2, 3, and 4 (maximum possible score 4.00), the lowest score was seen for scale 2, Having sufficient information to manage my health (mean score 2.67, SD 0.76). For scales 6 and 7 (maximum possible score 5.00), the lowest mean score was for scale 7, Navigating the healthcare system (mean score 3.38, SD 1.01). For the BRIEF, median score was 12 (inter-quartile range 8, 19) from a possible range of 4–20.

Table 2. Participant characteristics.

ID	Age Bracket, Gender, Born in/Outside Australia [a]	Highest Education	SES [b]	Months Since Stroke	Stroke Type (Oxford)	Stroke Severity (NIHSS) [c]	mRS [d]	Communication/Cognitive Impairment [e]
1 *	60–69, M, Australia	Degree	5	9	Right PACI	5	1	0
2 *	60–69, M, Outside Australia	High school	4	6	Right TACI	5	2	NIHSS 1—mild aphasia; cognitive impairment
3 *	20–29, F, Australia	Certificate/ apprenticeship/diploma	2	10	Right POCI	1	1	0
4	60–69, M, Outside Australia	Certificate/ apprenticeship/diploma	2	5	Right PACI	1	1	NIHSS 1—dysarthria
5 *	40–49, F, Australia	Degree	5	8	Right PACI with haemorrhagic transformation	2	0	0
6 *	70–79, F, Australia	Primary school	5	14	Left haemorrhage	2	2	Cognitive impairment
7 *	50–59, M, Australia	Post-graduate	5	16	Left POCI	1	1	0
8	50–59, M, Australia	High school	5	15	Left PACI	1	2	0
9*	60–69, F, Outside Australia	Degree	3	8	Left POCI	1	2	0
10	60–69, F, Australia	High school	5	4	Left PACI	3	1	0
11 *	40–49, F, Australia	Certificate/ apprenticeship/diploma	1	4	Left TACI	1	1	NIHSS 1—mild aphasia; Cognitive impairment
12	70–79, M, Outside Australia	Primary school	5	9	Bilateral POCI	1	1	Cognitive impairment
13 *	60–69, F, Outside Australia	Degree	1	12	Left POCI	5	1	Cognitive impairment
14	80–89, M, Outside Australia	Primary school	5	11	Left POCI	5	2	Cognitive impairment
15	60–69, F, Outside Australia	Primary school	5	8	Right PACI	5	1	0

Table 2. *Cont.*

ID	Age Bracket, Gender, Born in/Outside Australia [a]	Highest Education	SES [b]	Months Since Stroke	Stroke Type (Oxford)	Stroke Severity (NIHSS) [c]	mRS [d]	Communication/Cognitive Impairment [e]
16	60–69, M, Australia	Primary school	2	10	Left and right POCI	1	3	NIHSS 1—aphasia
17 *	30–39, M, Australia	Primary school	4	61	Left haemorrhage	5	3	NIHSS 2—aphasia
18	40–49, F, Australia	Degree	5	6	Left haemorrhage	1	2	NIHSS 3—aphasia
19	70–79, F, Outside Australia	Primary school	5	14	Right LACI	5	4	NIHSS 1—mild aphasia

Note: * Completed Stage 1 and 2 of research project; [a] demographic information is reported broadly (age bracket, born in/outside Australia) to preserve participant confidentiality;

[b] SES = socio-economic status (SES) quintile based on postcode of home address; [c] National Institutes of Health Stroke Scale (NIHSS) at time of hospital admission, scored by researcher from medical record review; [d] mRS = modified Rankin score, established at time of research interview; [e] communication and cognition impairments were classified from medical record review and clinical impression of participant during interview, by experienced stroke researcher (CF), and cognitive impairment reported by the family was also noted for participants who were interviewed with an interpreter. LACI = lacunar infarct. TACI = total anterior circulation infarct. PACI = partial anterior circulation infarct. POCI = posterior circulation infarct

Table 3. Health literacy scores for the sample.

Health Literacy Scale	Mean (Standard Deviation)
HLQ scale 2: Having sufficient information to manage my health	2.67 (0.76)
HLQ scale 3: Actively managing my health	3.05 (0.72)
HLQ scale 4: Social support for health	3.24 (0.80)
HLQ scale 6: Ability to actively engage with healthcare providers	3.53 (1.02)
HLQ scale 7: Navigating the healthcare system	3.38 (1.01)
BRIEF Health Literacy Screener; median (inter-quartile range)	12 (8, 19)

From the cluster analysis of HLQ data, four distinct profiles were identified, representing a diversity of health literacy strengths and weaknesses, as shown in Table 4.

Table 4. Cluster analysis, reporting HLQ and BRIEF scores only.

<table>
<tr><th>Cluster Number</th><th>% of Sample</th><th>Having Sufficient Information</th><th>Actively Managing Health</th><th>Social Support for Health</th><th>Active Engages with Health Providers</th><th>Navigating Health Services</th><th>BRIEF HLST Score</th></tr>
<tr><td>1</td><td>47%</td><td>3.19</td><td>3.49</td><td>3.73</td><td>3.80</td><td>3.76</td><td>17.0</td></tr>
<tr><td colspan="8">This cluster represents nearly half the sample. People in this cluster have reasonably good health literacy overall, but are not completely confident they know all they need to about what happens next after the stroke. Because of limited experience with the health system prior to their stroke, they find it hard to know what services are available, and also what questions they should ask the specialist—this may be because they lack confidence to discuss concerns with them.</td></tr>
<tr><td>2</td><td>5%</td><td>1.00</td><td>1.40</td><td>1.00</td><td>5.00</td><td>5.00</td><td>13.0</td></tr>
<tr><td colspan="8">This was the smallest cluster in the sample. People in this cluster tend to have little support from family or friends to help with their health, and have large gaps in their knowledge, which may make it difficult to set goals, make plans, and work out how to look after themselves post-stroke. They have no problems talking with providers and being quite assertive in that relationship, and are also able to advocate for themselves in relation to obtaining the right healthcare. However, their BRIEF score is low, which means they may struggle to understand patient education materials, possibly contributing to a perception that they do not have enough information about their condition.</td></tr>
<tr><td>3</td><td>21%</td><td>1.94</td><td>3.05</td><td>3.10</td><td>4.05</td><td>3.88</td><td>7.8</td></tr>
<tr><td colspan="8">People in this cluster have very large gaps in their knowledge, and feel they are lacking information about their condition. They are quite keen to take responsibility for their health, so providing information that they understand may be very helpful. Their BRIEF score is very low, so it may be that the information they receive is not comprehensible for them. They have quite good social support for health. They also feel reasonably confident in talking with providers and asking questions, and do have some understanding of the health services available to them.</td></tr>
<tr><td>4</td><td>26%</td><td>2.65</td><td>2.60</td><td>2.92</td><td>2.32</td><td>1.97</td><td>20.0</td></tr>
<tr><td colspan="8">People in this cluster have gaps in their knowledge and do not feel the information they are given is right for them, which may impact on their ability and motivation to manage their health (their "engagement"). They report only moderate social support for health. People in this cluster are very passive in their interaction with health providers and have limited knowledge of how the healthcare system works and where to find the right providers.</td></tr>
</table>

3.2. Stage 2

Ten participants from the Stage 1 cohort participated in Stage 2. Nine people declined to participate in Stage 2 (carer responsibilities n = 1; time constraints n= 4; no longer wished to participate n= 1; new illness n = 1; unable to be contacted n = 2). Of those who participated in Stage 2, 6 (60%) were female and 4 (40%) male, median (IQR) age = 57 (38, 65); time since stroke = 10 (7, 14) months, and 7 (70%) completed education beyond high school). One participant in Stage 2 spoke Vietnamese and completed the interview with an interpreter. Four people (40%) were identified as having cognitive impairment, and three (30%) had communication impairment. The rates of cognitive and communication impairments noted in the group of people who did not complete Stage 2 were 2/9 (22%) and 4/9 (44%), respectively.

Two 90 min focus groups were undertaken, each with three participants. Four individual interviews were undertaken via telephone (n = 3) or Zoom (n = 1). Due to time constraints and the rich discussion generated by the vignettes, no participants were presented with all four vignettes. All focus group participants were presented with one vignette. Two interview participants were presented with one vignette, one interview participant was presented with two vignettes, and one participant did not wish to hear the vignette and was interviewed about their own experiences. One participant did not wish to be recorded, so instead a summary of their interview was written by the researcher. Despite the attrition between Stage 1 and 2 of the study, we deemed theoretical sufficiency [31] to be achieved after 10 interviews.

Reflexive Thematic Analysis Findings

As depicted in Figure 1, four themes and one subtheme were generated about health literacy needs and preferences of stroke survivors, and how cognitive difficulties, communicative difficulties, and culture may affect these needs and preferences. The first theme, "Individual knowledge, capacity, and beliefs about stroke and health services", considers the individual characteristics, history, and worldview of the patient, and the subtheme, "Systemic and societal context influencing individual stroke literacy", considers the influence of the patient's context on their individual knowledge, capacity, and beliefs about stroke and health services. The second theme, "Tailoring and personalisation of information delivery", considers the characteristics of the healthcare information presented to the patient, its delivery to the patient, and the value of tailoring information and delivery to the patient based on their knowledge, capacity, and beliefs. The third theme, "Having a support network to rely on", considers the multifaceted roles of support people in facilitating access to healthcare information and supporting patients to implement healthcare recommendations. The final theme, "Feeling like I am in safe hands", considers the extent to which the patient trusts and is confident in the quality of care they receive from clinicians and services. Feeling in safe hands is influenced by the patient's knowledge, capacity, and beliefs (Theme 1), the extent to which information delivery is tailored to their needs (Theme 2), and the interactions of their support network, clinicians, and services (Theme 3). Each of these themes influences understanding, recall, and implementation of healthcare information by the patient.

Theme 1: Individual knowledge, capacity, and beliefs about stroke and health services. This theme pertains to the influence of individual knowledge, beliefs, strengths, and challenges on how patients make sense of their stroke journey and health information. This theme also contains a subtheme, *Systemic and societal context influencing individual stroke literacy.* Table 5 describes the key concepts reflected in Theme 1 and its subtheme, and provides illustrative quotes.

Theme 2: Tailoring and personalisation of information delivery. This theme highlights the importance of delivering healthcare information in a manner that is relevant and meaningful for each individual patient. There is no "one size fits all" approach, so healthcare providers need to use a range of strategies to meet the needs and preferences of individual patients. As outlined in Table 6, participants stressed the importance of tailoring information delivery to their needs, knowledge, capacity, and beliefs. When materials, resources, and information delivery are appropriate to the needs and capacity of the stroke survivor, they support the understanding, recall, and implementation of healthcare information. Specific suggestions made by participants for support materials and information delivery methods are listed in Table 7.

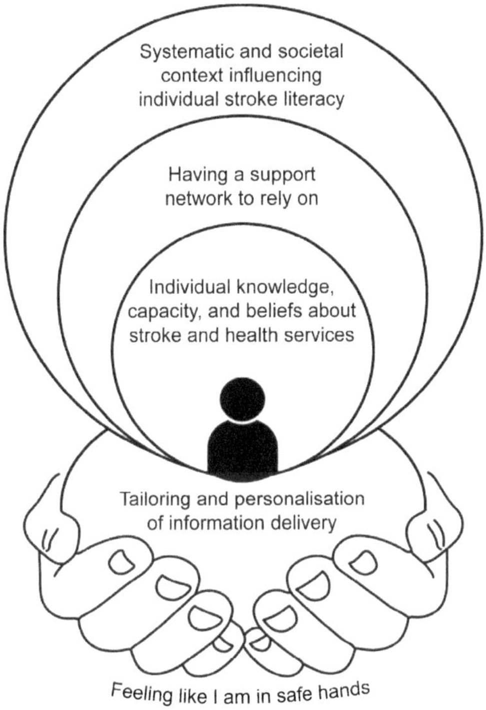

Figure 1. Schematic of the themes and relationship between them.

Table 5. Descriptions of key concepts and illustrative quotes for Theme 1, "Individual knowledge, capacity, and beliefs about stroke and health" and its subtheme, "Systemic and societal context influencing individual stroke literacy".

Concept Reflected in Theme	Description	Quotes
Prior knowledge of stroke	Prior knowledge of stroke and experience navigating healthcare services helped participants to understand what was happening to them, "how things work" and to access appropriate support. Not having prior knowledge about stroke made it more difficult for participants to understand health information.	*Doctors just assume that you know [there are a range of stroke outcomes]. I felt very confused when I was in hospital because of that… I didn't know the repercussions of a stroke. I didn't know what happens afterwards. I didn't know any of that.*—P9
Individual capacity to engage with healthcare information	Individual capacity was central to how participants understood, recalled, and implemented healthcare information. Capacity was affected by stroke-related characteristics such as changes to cognitive function (memory, attention, planning) and motor ability, as well as demographic factors such as language spoken at home. Emotional responses to stroke such as frustration and feeling scared and incapable also impacted participants' capacity to advocate for themselves and engage with healthcare information. For instance, some participants reported that fear of appearing "stupid" made them feel less comfortable asking questions of their healthcare provider.	*[responding to case vignette] She already feels a bit worried about asking questions that might be silly, and that will put her on the back foot a little bit more.*—P5

Table 5. *Cont.*

Concept Reflected in Theme	Description	Quotes
Psychological factors	Individual psychological factors which participants considered to enhance understanding and implementation of healthcare information included high levels of confidence, optimism, tolerance of uncertainty, and being in a state of readiness to change.	*[responding to case vignette] He's been told over and over a thousand times [to make lifestyle changes], but unless you acknowledge it and are ready, it's not going to make any difference.*—P11
Subtheme: Systemic and societal context influencing individual stroke literacy	This subtheme highlights the influence of prevailing social and cultural narratives on individual knowledge, capacity, and beliefs. These narratives appeared to influence participants' experience of stroke, their stroke literacy, and how actively they sought support. Several participants described stigma and mystery surrounding stroke, which influenced how easily they understood information presented to them, and how they responded to the signs of their own stroke.	*I didn't know I had stroke. I didn't go to the doctor for four days afterwards because no one told me that this was a stroke.*—P9
Stigma and mystery around stroke	Stigma and mystery surrounding stroke also influenced participants' expectations for their post-stroke lives. Several participants mentioned that prior to their stroke they held the belief that people "become a vegetable" following a stroke. Having an expectation that people who have had a stroke are unable to be helped, are not worth helping, or will be given up on by society was thought to influence patient engagement with healthcare information.	*Sometimes people think that having a stroke is like, it's the end of the world. It's not, but it makes people feel like that's it. You become a vegetable, you can't do anything for yourself.*—P9

Table 6. Descriptions of key concepts and illustrative quotes for Theme 2, "*Tailoring and personalisation of information delivery*".

Concept Reflected in Theme	Description	Quotes
Feeling overwhelmed and confused	Many participants reported feeling confused by the way information was presented to them, or overwhelmed by too much information at once.	*When the word is too big, it's just too hard.*—P17 *Sometimes when you're given information, you get confused, it jumbles up in your brain. . .you feel like an idiot because, oh, you should know that, but it's just confused.*—P9
The value of accessible information delivery	A frequent suggestion was to supplement spoken information with visual information (including using videoconference rather than telephone for telehealth interactions), experiential learning, and to offer accessible take-home materials.	*It sometimes depends on what's being learned, but sometimes it's easy to do things in real life and being shown things in real life that you're trying to do. . . or you need someone there with you to explain it first for something that you're looking at for the first ever time.*—P5 *The simpler, the message the better. . .We don't need to know all the technicalities of stroke, we just need to know what to do and what [are] the impacts.*—P1
Having resources available and explained	Participants appreciated having standard resources such as the My Stroke Journey pack. Many participants identified that it was helpful for a clinician to step them through the resource so that they knew which parts were relevant and how they might apply that information in their lives.	*The human experience of learning is important rather than just being given things to read.*—P7

Table 6. *Cont.*

Concept Reflected in Theme	Description	Quotes
The value of interpreters and translations	For participants who did not understand English well, translators and translated materials were essential to understanding healthcare information.	P13: *I can't read English.* Interviewer: *I hear that they gave you documents in English, which is very unhelpful because you can't read it.* P13: *Yes.*
Clinician support and strategies to enhance understanding and recall	Participants used a variety of strategies to enhance their understanding and recall, including taking notes and recording appointments, and using the Internet to supplement supplied information between appointments. However, not all participants had the capacity to use such strategies following their stroke. For instance, one participant had difficulty using their hand to write. Proactive behaviour by the healthcare provider, such as checking patient comprehension and providing take-home written information and resources, was appreciated by participants. Active, regular monitoring and being sent reminders about upcoming appointments were also identified as assisting with recall and implementation of health information.	*I'm supposed to get my bloods done every six months. I don't like going. . .but [the GP] will nag me until I go.*—P9
Obtaining the information that is needed	Participants also highlighted the importance of tailoring information to their specific circumstances and knowledge. This included assisting them to identify achievable goals, and taking into account their primary concerns, their understanding of what happened to them, and other important aspects of their world. For instance, participants commonly identified the prevention of future stroke as a primary concern. Not having sufficient understanding of the cause of their stroke caused considerable worry. In some instances, this worry undermined healthcare information. One participant expressed anxiety about advice to return to exercise, knowing that high blood pressure had contributed to their stroke.	*I was exercising when it happened. If I exercised to that point, is it going to happen again? Was there something that I was doing that made that happen?*—P5

Theme 3: Having a support network to rely on. This theme identifies the importance of having access to friends, family, and services to assist in understanding, recalling, and implementing healthcare information. As shown in Table 8, supportive friends and family were crucial allies for participants at every stage of the stroke journey, from the acute stage to ongoing chronic care. They helped the participants to feel cared for, that there was someone with whom to share the difficult experiences, and that empowered them to understand and respond to health information together.

Theme 4: Feeling like I am in safe hands. This theme highlights the importance of having access to effective healthcare services, feeling confident in the quality of care, and feeling safe to speak up and ask questions. When patients feel they are in safe hands, they believe that their healthcare team is competent, trustworthy, and has their best interests at heart, and that they are working together in alliance. This enables participants to better engage with health information. Table 9 describes key concepts important for "feeling like I am in safe hands".

Table 7. Recommendations from participants about tailoring and personalising delivery of information for people with stroke.

	Patient Characteristics to Consider
1.	Are there motor and mobility challenges (including writing)?
2.	Are there speech and communication difficulties?
3.	Are there cognitive difficulties including attention, planning, and memory?
4.	What is their language ability?
5.	What is their prior knowledge?
6.	Who is the audience? The patient? Their support people?
7.	What support do they have to engage with the information? Family? Friends? Other support?
8.	What information is most important at this stage in their journey?
	Information Delivery and Resources
1.	Tailor information to patient concerns and goals
2.	Include practical information to inform day-to-day decisions
3.	Encourage questions
4.	Ask the patient to summarise what has been discussed to gauge understanding (teach-back)
5.	Make translations and translators available
6.	Turn on video for telehealth calls and support information delivery with visual cues
7.	Be proactive in offering to take notes and provide take-home materials
8.	Deliver the information in a number of formats, e.g., talking and writing notes
9.	Keep written information simple; avoid jargon, use plain English, consider resources in Easy English
10.	In written materials, highlight the main points with good design and use dot points
11.	Use diagrams and pictures to supplement written information
12.	Consider sharing document summaries or "fact sheets" that highlight the key messages
13.	Offer audio and video take-home materials, not just written materials
14.	Offer high-quality, reliable Internet resources (that are flagged as being from a trustworthy source)

Table 8. Descriptions of key concepts and illustrative quotes for Theme 3, "*Having a support network to rely on*".

Concept Reflected in Theme	Description	Quotes
Family and friends as interpreters/translators and advocates	Supportive friends and family assisted in interpreting information for participants in a way they could understand. In some instances, friends and family translated information into the participant's preferred language. Family and friends played an important advocacy role for participants within healthcare settings, helping the participants' needs and preferences to be heard. Supportive friends and family assisted in managing healthcare concerns, such as treatment adherence, and ensuring participants attended appointments.	*When the doctors tell me what to do I can't understand. . .I'll try to listen and try take in everything they say, but I can't do that. . . but by my friend to explain it a little different, then I get it.*—P17

Table 8. *Cont.*

Concept Reflected in Theme	Description	Quotes
Lacking access to close others is a barrier	Not having access to supportive family and friends was described as a major barrier to navigating the complexity of the healthcare system, understanding, recalling and implementing healthcare information, and feeling supported in recovery. One participant noted that not being able to take support people to appointments due to COVID-19 restrictions was difficult. Another participant noted that living in a different city to their family negatively impacted their sense of agency, access to services, and ability to implement healthcare advice.	*At the time when my blood pressure become very high, then I find that difficult because I'm on my own.*—P13
Having access to different kinds of support	Several participants stressed that it was important for patients to know they can bring support people to appointments, and that when family or friends were not available to support and advocate for patients, a professional advocate could fill this role. Accessing peer support from other stroke survivors was helpful for some participants. These participants found it beneficial to engage with people who understood their experiences and could offer practical guidance to navigate their new post-stroke reality.	*If you got someone, you feel much comfortable and much better off than on your own.*—P2
Feeling isolated versus connected	Several participants mentioned that friendships and acquaintances dropped away following their stroke, perhaps because of stigma surrounding stroke and low stroke literacy in the community. Feeling connected with others gave a sense of being part of a support network. The Stroke Foundation "Enable Me" newsletter, which contains stories and advice about life after stroke, was highlighted as being useful and reaffirming.	*After you've had a stroke… I found that people don't want to talk to you about it…I don't think it's [that] they don't want to know. I think they just don't know what to say.*—P9 *Every week they email you a newsletter. It does make a difference actually because you see other people's stories in there and you don't feel alone.*—P9

Table 9. Descriptions of key concepts and illustrative quotes for Theme 4, *"Feeling like I am in safe hands"*.

Concept Reflected in Theme	Description	Quotes
Feeling safe to speak up and ask questions	Participants described the importance of feeling like they could ask questions and clarify information if they did not understand.	*If you are seeing a doctor that you feel safe and comfortable with… you're more likely to speak up and say that you don't understand. Whereas, if it's a doctor that comes in… speaking very fluently in their medical terminology, you might go, "Okay, yes, thank you," and just walk out of there with no idea. If you feel safe and comfortable, you might be more likely to say, "I have no idea what you said".*—P11

Table 9. *Cont.*

Concept Reflected in Theme	Description	Quotes
Person-centred care is crucial	Being seen as a person rather than a condition was of central importance to participants. Having a caring, collaborative relationship that centred patient goals, strengths, and capacities enhanced the feeling of being seen as a "whole person". Features of collaborative relationships included being included in decision making, creating a safe environment, not assuming prior knowledge of stroke, and having sufficient time to ensure patients understand information and can ask questions. This also helped to build confidence in the treating team, foster trust in the information supplied, and enhanced the feeling of being in safe hands.	*At the time when I was in hospital… I actually felt like people were making decisions around me and not including me.*—P9
Not feeling rushed	Many participants reported that interactions with healthcare providers felt rushed. Feeling rushed discouraged participants from asking questions and exacerbated stroke-related cognitive difficulties.	*I feel sometimes rushed… When things are rushed…it becomes anxious and then you forget everything.*—P6
Coordinated care and consistent messages	Participants reported feeling in safe hands when their care was well coordinated. This included how well individual practitioners appeared to coordinate patient information and progress, such as following up on test results, making monitoring appointments, and making referrals to additional services. It also included the coordination of the broader healthcare team in sharing reports and test results where appropriate, and providing consistent messaging to the patient. Participants reported being particularly confused when multiple members of a team gave them different information during their hospital stay.	*All the medical terminology and getting information from this person, that person, and just information overload.*—P11
Having access to appropriate healthcare	Being linked in with suitable healthcare professionals was also an important part of feeling in safe hands. Participants who lived regionally, who did not have strong social support, or who spoke a language other than English had difficulty accessing appropriate medical and support services.	*Because I'm rural…when I went to ED [Emergency Department] with my stroke, I was left in ED for six hours before I even got a bed… [in that time] I could have driven to Melbourne and potentially been getting treated.*—P11
Having a trusted point of contact	Participants appreciated help accessing additional support such as from the Stroke Foundation, and acknowledged the important role of GPs and social workers in helping to make these connections. Some participants suggested that having a trusted point of contact they could get in touch with to ask questions between appointments would be useful and reassuring.	*I had help from a social worker. That was the best thing because he made me aware of the services that were around. If they hadn't done that, I'd still be sitting here thinking, "Well, I don't know how to do this".*—P9

4. Discussion

Using the novel Ophelia (Optimising Health Literacy and Access) methodology, the aim of this study was to explore perspectives on the associations between health literacy and the information needs and preferences of stroke survivors, and identify targets or directions for improving organisational health literacy to better tailor information delivery. Our participants, including people typically under-represented in stroke research (i.e., those from CALD backgrounds, and with cognitive and communication impairments), provided rich insights into the impact of health literacy on their ability to seek, understand, engage with, and act on health information. Four themes were generated in discussions about the four case vignettes used to describe typical health literacy profiles. The first theme highlighted the impact of *Individual knowledge, capacity, and beliefs about stroke and health services* on their capacity to engage with stroke-related information. The second theme, *Tailoring and personalisation of information delivery*, pointed to the importance of accessible healthcare information delivered in a manner that is tailored to the patient's knowledge, capacity, and beliefs—rather than adopting a "one-size-fits-all" approach. Thirdly, *Having a support network to rely on* emphasised the multifaceted roles of family and other support people in facilitating access to, comprehension of, and implementation of healthcare information. Finally, *Feeling like I am in safe hands* described the importance of patient trust and confidence in the quality of care they receive from clinicians and services. Our findings provide several important directions for improving organisational literacy to optimise understanding, recall, and implementation of healthcare information by the patient, and therefore their healthcare experiences and outcomes.

Health literacy scores of participants in Stage 1 were generally low. Participants were fairly typical of SVHM patients, with 42% born outside Australia and 26% speaking a language other than English (i.e., Vietnamese), requiring an interpreter. During the study year, 48% of all patients admitted to the stroke unit at SVHM were born in a country other than Australia (compared with 31% nationally) and 18% spoke languages other than English (compared with 8% nationally) [32]. Despite most participants being more than six months post-stroke, health literacy scores were lowest for "having sufficient information to manage my health" and "navigating the healthcare system". This is consistent with previous research where stroke survivors and care givers report receiving an inadequate amount of information, or receiving information at an inappropriate time, or stroke survivors not recalling information provided [33].

These findings reinforce the need for clinicians to consider all the factors that impact healthcare communication, including health literacy, preferred language, older age, cognition, aphasia and other communication disability, and available support when developing and delivering health information. The subset of participants who completed Stage 2, several of whom had lived experience of these issues, were able to provide simple practical recommendations for clinicians to support people with such challenges (listed in Table 3). They suggested comprehensive consideration of patient characteristics that are likely to impact understanding of and engagement with health information (to address the issues raised in Theme 1); tailoring of information using communication support strategies such as the use of pictures, videos, and gesture to support text and spoken language; and providing notes, handouts, and resource links for patients to refer to outside of clinical appointments (Theme 2). These recommendations are consistent with strategies used in evidence-based cognitive rehabilitation programs [34,35], aphasia-friendly written education materials [36,37], and healthcare communication post-stroke [38].

Efforts to tailor information to patients' individual health literacy require clinicians to assess and understand, rather than assume, their patients' prior knowledge, capacity, and beliefs about stroke and health services. Assessment of health literacy goes beyond standard stroke assessment tools, but can be achieved fairly quickly by asking questions such as "What do you understand about stroke?" Similarly, assessment of cognitive and communication support needs is often overlooked in standard stroke care [39,40] and is not captured by commonly used tools that assess functional outcomes such as the modified Rankin scale [41]. In our attempts to purposively recruit participants with cognitive and communication impairments for this study, we found that mRS scores were not helpful indicators of these difficulties, and there was typically limited identification of cognitive or communication issues in health records. This suggests that indicators of challenges to health literacy may be "flying under the radar", precluding the opportunity to adequately tailor healthcare communication.

Medical, nursing, and allied health professionals also require training and competencies in how to adapt their communication for people with cognitive impairment [35] and aphasia [42]. Examples of free training include Stroke Foundation [43] and Aphasia Institute [44]. This is often overlooked in training programs [38]. Simply presenting standard information is not sufficient for patients to understand and implement it. Developing clear competency frameworks and associated training protocols to support communication of health information for people with low health literacy is a priority for future research. These protocols should also encourage clinicians to develop a communication style that engenders trust and confidence in their patients. "Feeling like they are in safe hands" (Theme 4) was considered critical by our participants for supporting their engagement with health information and feeling safe to ask questions.

Given the importance of support networks in facilitating access to healthcare information (as reflected in Theme 3), stroke survivors who do not have family members or close others available to support them require clinicians to take extra steps to ensure they understand and feel safe. The subtheme we identified on the *Systemic and societal context influencing individual stroke literacy* also highlights that improving stroke literacy and reducing stigma in the broader community is likely to positively impact people's experiences of stroke. This points to the importance of community awareness initiatives, not just about early stroke signs (e.g., F.A.S.T) but also campaigns that include information about life after stroke, especially "invisible" difficulties such as fatigue, cognitive impairment, depression, and anxiety, which are commonly overlooked and misunderstood [39,40]. Including people with lived experience as partners in teams dedicated to health service design and public health campaigns can be an effective strategy that enables the needs of people with stroke to be considered.

Limitations

Our findings should be considered in the context of several limitations. Firstly, there was almost 50% participant attrition between Stage 1 and 2 of the project, particularly of people born outside Australia who spoke Vietnamese and required an interpreter. Of interest, a larger proportion of people who completed both stages were noted to have cognitive impairment than those who did not complete Stage 2 (40% vs. 22%), but fewer had communication impairment (30% vs. 44%), though numbers were small. There were several stated reasons for not participating in Stage 2, but these did not always reflect the extra challenge involved in participating in research for those who do not speak English, which may have formed a barrier to participation even if not directly stated. Notably, Vietnamese-speaking participants tended to prefer face-to-face interviews, but this was not an option throughout a substantial proportion of the data collection period due to pandemic-related restrictions. This meant that while participants from CALD backgrounds were well represented in Stage 1 (and therefore in the case vignettes), they were not as well represented in the focus groups and interviews, so their perspectives on the delivery of health information for the characters in those vignettes were not as prominent. While we deemed theoretical sufficiency to have been reached after 10 interviews, it remains possible that richer information could be gleaned with a more diverse sample. Future research should address this issue, which should be more feasible outside the context of restrictions preventing face-to-face appointments. Additionally, participants were recruited from one stroke unit in Melbourne, Australia. Perspectives of stroke survivors from other regions of Australia and from different CALD communities around the world would be valuable to include in future research.

While there were concerted efforts to recruit people with cognitive and communication impairments, we hoped to recruit more. These efforts were hampered by the lack of information about cognitive and language abilities in health records. Cognitive and language screening, with clear reporting of any impairments in health records, would be a helpful addition to standard stroke care. We originally planned to conduct formal cognitive assessment with participants; however, this plan was revised in the context of pandemic-related lockdowns, given the challenges of assessing cognition via telehealth. While various sources of information were used to identify possible cognitive impairments, the lack of a consistent formal assessment of cognition limited our understanding of participants' cognitive capabilities and thus the generalisability of results. Future research should incorporate cognitive and language screening to facilitate purposive recruitment as well as characterise samples and ensure inclusion of people with cognitive and communication impairments in stroke research [16]. At a minimum, screening of self-reported cognitive status (thinking and memory) and its impact on daily life is feasible. The extent and impact of language difficulties can be rated by trained examiners using AusTOMs ratings.

5. Conclusions

Our study provides valuable perspectives from stroke survivors about the impact of health literacy on their needs and preferences about the delivery of health information. Listening to the voices of those who are typically under-represented has allowed us to identify key improvements that would improve stroke service delivery. These include considering health literacy levels of patient populations when developing stroke information resources, and assessment of individuals' cognitive and communication support needs as standard practice. Training is necessary to support clinician and researcher competencies in tailored healthcare communication. Community awareness initiatives are recommended to improve stroke literacy in the general population. These improvements are feasible—for example, in response to our findings, the stroke team at SVHM ran clinician workshops on health literacy and have adjusted their service model to ensure responsivity to low health literacy. It will be important to evaluate the impact of these and similar other service improvements. Greater awareness of and response to health literacy in stroke services has the potential to improve patient experiences and outcomes of stroke care.

Supplementary Materials: The following supporting information can be downloaded at: https://www.mdpi.com/article/10.3390/healthcare13050541/s1, Case Vignettes.

Author Contributions: Conceptualisation: K.B., L.M.S., D.W., A.B., K.D.J., K.M. and C.H.; methodology: K.B., L.M.S., D.W. and A.B.; formal analysis: A.B., C.F., D.W. and E.E.S.; investigation: C.F., A.B. and D.W.; data curation: C.F. and K.B.; writing: D.W., K.B. and E.E.S.; writing—review and editing: all authors; supervision: K.B., L.M.S. and D.W.; project administration: K.B. and C.F.; funding acquisition, K.B. and L.M.S. All authors have read and agreed to the published version of the manuscript.

Funding: This work was supported by the St Vincent's Hospital (Melbourne) Research Endowment Fund under grant number 91960.

Institutional Review Board Statement: The study was conducted in accordance with the Declaration of Helsinki, and approved by the Ethics Committee of St. Vincent Hospital Melbourne [HREC 140/21], approved on 18 October 2021.

Informed Consent Statement: Informed consent was obtained from all subjects involved in the study.

Data Availability Statement: Data can be made available upon reasonable request to the authors.

Acknowledgments: We thank participants and their supporters, and Allied Health and stroke team members who contributed to this study.

Conflicts of Interest: The authors declare no conflicts of interest.

Abbreviations

The following abbreviations are used in this manuscript:

BRIEF	Brief Health Literacy Screening Tool
CALD	culturally and linguistically diverse
HLQ	Health Literacy Questionnaire
mRS	modified Rankin score
Ophelia Methodology	Optimising Health Literacy and Access Methodology

References

1. Australian Bureau of Statistics [ABS]. *Health Literacy*; ABS cat. no. 4233.0; ABS.: Canberra, Australia, 2009.
2. Australian Institute of Health and Welfare [AIHW]. *Australia's Health 2018*; AIHW: Darlinghurst, Australia, 2018.
3. Sorensen, K.; Van den Broucke, S.; Fullam, J.; Doyle, G.; Pelikan, J.; Slonska, Z.; Brand, H.; (HLS-EU) Consortium Health Literacy Project European. Health literacy and public health: A systematic review and integration of definitions and models. *BMC Public Health* **2012**, *12*, 80. [CrossRef] [PubMed]
4. Weterings, R.P.; Kessels, R.P.; de Leeuw, F.E.; Piai, V. Cognitive impairment after a stroke in young adults: A systematic review and meta-analysis. *Int. J. Stroke* **2023**, *18*, 888–897. [CrossRef] [PubMed]
5. Liu, Y.B.; Chen, Y.L.; Xue, H.P.; Hou, P. Health Literacy Risk in Older Adults with and Without Mild Cognitive Impairment. *Nurs. Res.* **2019**, *68*, 433–438. [CrossRef] [PubMed]
6. Evans, F.A.; Wong, D.; Lawson, D.W.; Withiel, T.D.; Stolwyk, R.J. What are the most common memory complaints following stroke? A frequency and exploratory factor analysis of items from the Everyday Memory Questionnaire-Revised. *Clin. Neuropsychol.* **2020**, *34*, 498–511. [CrossRef]
7. Bushnell, C.; Arnan, M.; Han, S. A new model for secondary prevention of stroke: Transition coaching for stroke. *Front. Neurol.* **2014**, *5*, 219. [CrossRef]
8. Coleman, C.; Birk, S.; DeVoe, J. Health Literacy and Systemic Racism-Using Clear Communication to Reduce Health Care Inequities. *JAMA Intern. Med.* **2023**, *183*, 753–754. [CrossRef]
9. Hart, M.; Santos, A.D.; Leclair, L.; Jones, B.; Ranta, A. Improving Indigenous Stroke Outcomes by Shifting Our Focus from Health to Cultural Literacy. *Curr. Neurol. Neurosci. Rep.* **2024**, *25*, 3. [CrossRef]
10. Australian Commission on Safety and Quality in Health Care [ACSQHC]. *National Statement on Health Literacy—Taking Action to Improve Safety and Quality*; ACSQHC: Sydney, Australia, 2014.
11. Giummarra, M.J.; Power, E.; Stolwyk, R.; Crotty, M.; Parsons, B.; Lannin, N.A.; Shweta Kalyani, K. Health services for young adults with stroke: A service mapping study over two Australian states. *Health Soc. Care Community* **2024**, *2024*, 8762322. [CrossRef]
12. Roy, D.; Gasquoine, S.; Caldwell, S.; Nash, D. Health Professional and Family Perceptions of Post-Stroke Information. *Nurs. Prax. New Zealand* **2015**, *31*, 7–24. [CrossRef]
13. Forster, A.; Brown, L.; Smith, J.; House, A.; Knapp, P.; Wright, J.J.; Young, J. Information provision for stroke patients and their caregivers. *Cochrane Database Syst. Rev.* **2012**, *11*, Cd001919. [CrossRef]
14. Lynch, E.A.; Nolan, J.; Bulto, L.N.; Mitchell, J.; McGrath, A.; Lane, S.; Harvey, G.; Cadilhac, D.A.; Harling, R.; Godecke, E. Is learning being supported when information is provided to informal carers during inpatient stroke rehabilitation? A qualitative study. *Disabil. Rehabil.* **2024**, *46*, 3913–3921. [CrossRef]
15. Aran, N.; Tregobov, N.; Kooij, K.; Harris, D.; Goel, G.; Poureslami, I. Health literacy and health outcomes in stroke management: A systematic review and evaluation of available measures. *J. Humanit. Soc. Sci.* **2022**, *5*, 172–191.
16. Shiggins, C.; Ryan, B.; Dewan, F.; Bernhardt, J.; O'Halloran, R.; Power, E.; Lindley, R.I.; McGurk, G.; Rose, M.L. Inclusion of People With Aphasia in Stroke Trials: A Systematic Search and Review. *Arch. Phys. Med. Rehabil.* **2024**, *105*, 580–592. [CrossRef] [PubMed]
17. Beauchamp, A.; Batterham, R.W.; Dodson, S.; Astbury, B.; Elsworth, G.R.; McPhee, C.; Jacobson, J.; Buchbinder, R.; Osborne, R.H. Systematic development and implementation of interventions to OPtimise Health Literacy and Access (Ophelia). *BMC Public Health* **2017**, *17*, 230. [CrossRef] [PubMed]
18. Wong, D.; Smith, E.; Beauchamp, A.; Formby, C.; Sanders, L.; De Jongh, K.; Hansen, C.; McKinley, K.; Cording, A.; Borschmann, K. When the Word is Too Big, it's Just Too Hard: How can Clinicians Support Patients' Health Literacy to Improve Recovery after Stroke? In Proceedings of the Stroke 2023, Melbourne, Australia, 22–25 August 2023; pp. 3–78.

19. Australian Bureau of Statistics [ABS]. Socio-Economic Indexes for Areas (SEIFA). Available online: https://www.abs.gov.au/statistics/people/people-and-communities/socio-economic-indexes-areas-seifa-australia/latest-release (accessed on 8 December 2024).
20. Osborne, R.H.; Batterham, R.W.; Elsworth, G.R.; Hawkins, M.; Buchbinder, R. The grounded psychometric development and initial validation of the Health Literacy Questionnaire (HLQ). *BMC Public Health* **2013**, *13*, 658. [CrossRef]
21. Chew, L.D.; Bradley, K.A.; Boyko, E.J. Brief questions to identify patients with inadequate health literacy. *Fam. Med.* **2004**, *36*, 588–594.
22. Elsworth, G.R.; Beauchamp, A.; Osborne, R.H. Measuring health literacy in community agencies: A Bayesian study of the factor structure and measurement invariance of the health literacy questionnaire (HLQ). *BMC Health Serv. Res.* **2016**, *16*, 508. [CrossRef]
23. Aaby, A.; Friis, K.; Christensen, B.; Rowlands, G.; Maindal, H.T. Health literacy is associated with health behaviour and self-reported health: A large population-based study in individuals with cardiovascular disease. *Eur. J. Prev. Cardiol.* **2017**, *24*, 1880–1888. [CrossRef]
24. Haun, J.; Luther, S.; Dodd, V.; Donaldson, P. Measurement variation across health literacy assessments: Implications for assessment selection in research and practice. *J. Health Commun.* **2012**, *17* (Suppl. 3), 141–159. [CrossRef]
25. Towfighi, A.; Cheng, E.M.; Ayala-Rivera, M.; Barry, F.; McCreath, H.; Ganz, D.A.; Lee, M.L.; Sanossian, N.; Mehta, B.; Dutta, T.; et al. Effect of a coordinated community and chronic care model team intervention vs usual care on systolic blood pressure in patients with stroke or transient ischemic attack: The SUCCEED randomized clinical trial. *JAMA Netw. Open* **2021**, *4*, e2036227. [CrossRef]
26. StataCorp. *Stata Statistical Software: Release 15*; StataCorp LP: College Station, TX, USA, 2017.
27. IBM Corp. *IBM SPSS Statistics for Windows*; IBM Corp: Armonk, NY, USA, 2013.
28. Batterham, R.W.; Buchbinder, R.; Beauchamp, A.; Dodson, S.; Elsworth, G.R.; Osborne, R.H. The OPtimising HEalth LIterAcy (Ophelia) process: Study protocol for using health literacy profiling and community engagement to create and implement health reform. *BMC Public Health* **2014**, *14*, 694. [CrossRef] [PubMed]
29. Braun, V.; Clarke, V. Using thematic analysis in psychology. *Qual. Res. Psychol.* **2006**, *3*, 77–101. [CrossRef]
30. Braun, V.; Clarke, V. One size fits all? What counts as quality practice in (reflexive) thematic analysis? *Qual. Res. Psychol.* **2020**, *18*, 328–352. [CrossRef]
31. Braun, V.; Clarke, V. To saturate or not to saturate? Questioning data saturation as a useful concept for thematic analysis and sample-size rationales. *Qual. Res. Sport Exerc. Health* **2021**, *13*, 201–216. [CrossRef]
32. Breen, S.; Cadilhac, D.A.; Lannin, N.A.; Kim, J.; Dalli, L.; Anderson, C.S.; Kilkenny, M.; Shehata, S.; Faux, S.; Dewey, H.; et al. *The Australian Stroke Clinical Registry Annual Report 2018*; The Florey Institute of Neuroscience and Mental Health: Heidelberg, Australia, 2019; p. 70.
33. Crocker, T.F.; Brown, L.; Lam, N.; Wray, F.; Knapp, P.; Forster, A. Information provision for stroke survivors and their carers. *Cochrane Database Syst. Rev.* **2021**, *11*, CD001919. [CrossRef]
34. Withiel, T.D.; Wong, D.; Ponsford, J.L.; Cadilhac, D.A.; New, P.; Mihaljcic, T.; Stolwyk, R.J. Comparing memory group training and computerized cognitive training for improving memory function following stroke: A phase II randomized controlled trial. *J. Rehabil. Med.* **2019**, *51*, 343–351. [CrossRef]
35. Wong, D.; Pike, K.; Stolwyk, R.; Allott, K.; Ponsford, J.; McKay, A.; Longley, W.; Bosboom, P.; Hodge, A.; Kinsella, G.; et al. Delivery of neuropsychological interventions for adult and older adult clinical populations: An Australian expert working group clinical guidance paper. *Neuropsychol. Rev.* **2023**, *34*, 985–1047. [CrossRef]
36. Rose, T.A.; Worrall, L.E.; Hickson, L.M.; Hoffmann, T.C. Aphasia friendly written health information: Content and design characteristics. *Int. J. Speech Lang. Pathol.* **2011**, *13*, 335–347. [CrossRef]
37. Rose, T.; Worrall, L.; McKenna, K. The effectiveness of aphasia-friendly principles for printed health education materials for people with aphasia following stroke. *Aphasiology* **2003**, *17*, 947–963. [CrossRef]
38. Lamborn, E.; Carragher, M.; O'Halloran, R.; Rose, M.L. Optimising Healthcare Communication for People with Aphasia in Hospital: Key Directions for Future Research. *Curr. Phys. Med. Rehabil. Rep.* **2024**, *12*, 89–99. [CrossRef]
39. Grech, M.; Withiel, T.; Klaic, M.; Fisher, C.A.; Simpson, L.; Wong, D. Characterisation of young stroke presentations, pathways of care, and support for 'invisible' difficulties: A retrospective clinical audit study. *Brain. Impair.* **2024**, *25*, IB23059. [CrossRef] [PubMed]
40. Humphrey, S.; Pike, K.; Long, B.; Ma, H.; Bourke, R.; Wright, B.; Wong, D. "I felt like I was not a priority": A qualitative study of the lived experience of ischaemic stroke patients treated with endovascular clot retrieval and intravenous thrombolysis. *Neuropsychol. Rehabil.* 2025, *under review*.
41. Kapoor, A.; Lanctôt, K.L.; Bayley, M.; Kiss, A.; Herrmann, N.; Murray, B.J.; Swartz, R.H. "Good outcome" isn't good enough: Cognitive impairment, depressive symptoms, and social restrictions in physically recovered stroke patients. *Stroke* **2017**, *48*, 1688–1690. [CrossRef] [PubMed]

42. Burton, B.; Isaacs, M.; Brogan, E.; Shrubsole, K.; Kilkenny, M.F.; Power, E.; Godecke, E.; Cadilhac, D.A.; Copland, D.; Wallace, S.J. An updated systematic review of stroke clinical practice guidelines to inform aphasia management. *Int. J. Stroke* **2023**, *18*, 1029–1039. [CrossRef]
43. Stroke Foundation. Working Effectively with People with Lived Experience to Design, Conduct and Promote Stroke Research. 2025. Available online: https://informme.org.au/learning-modules/working-effectively-with-people-with-lived-experience-to-design-conduct-and-promote-stroke-research (accessed on 18 February 2025).
44. Aphasia Institute. Introduction to Supported Conversation for Adults with Aphasia (SCA™) eLearning Module. 2025. Available online: https://www.aphasia.ca/health-care-providers/education-training/online-options/ (accessed on 18 February 2025).

healthcare

MDPI

Article

Prepare: Improving End-of-Life Care Practice in Stroke Care: Insights from a National Survey and Semi-Structured Interviews

C. Elizabeth Lightbody [1,*], Clare Gordon [1], Christopher Burton [2], Catherine Davidson [1], Damian Jenkinson [3], Aasima Saeed Patel [4], Freja Jo Petrie [1], Alison Rouncefield-Swales [5], Nikola Sprigg [6], Katherine Stewart [7], Mehrunisha Suleman [8,9], Caroline Leigh Watkins [1], Clare Thetford [1] and PREPARE Study Research Team [†]

1 School of Nursing and Midwifery, University of Central Lancashire, Preston PR1 2HE, UK; cgordon8@uclan.ac.uk (C.G.); clwatkins@uclan.ac.uk (C.L.W.); cthetford@uclan.ac.uk (C.T.)
2 Dean of Health Sciences, University of East Anglia, Norwich NR4 7TJ, UK; chris.burton@uea.ac.uk
3 University Hospitals Dorset, Bournemouth BH7 7DW, UK; damian.jenkinson@uhd.nhs.uk
4 Research Facilitation and Delivery Unit, University of Central Lancashire, Preston PR1 2HE, UK; apatel212@uclan.ac.uk
5 Research and Evaluation, The Institute for Research in Schools, London SW7 5HD, UK; alisonrouncefieldswales@researchinschools.org
6 School of Medicine, Faculty of Medicine & Health Sciences, University of Nottingham, Nottingham NG8 1BB, UK; nikola.sprigg@nottingham.ac.uk
7 Lancashire Teaching Hospitals NHS Foundation Trust, Preston PR2 9HT, UK; katherine.stewart@lthtr.nhs.uk
8 The Ethox Centre, University of Oxford, Oxford OX3 7DQ, UK; mehrunisha.suleman@ethox.ox.ac.uk
9 Global Studies Center, Gulf University for Science and Technology, Kuwait City 32093, Kuwait
* Correspondence: celightbody@uclan.ac.uk
† Membership of the PREPARE Study Research Team is provided in the Acknowledgments.

Abstract: Background: Stroke has high mortality. Challenges in providing end-of-life care include uncertainty among healthcare professionals about when to start care. While generic tools and guidelines exist, which outline components of quality end-of life care, they may not fully address stroke's unpredictable trajectories, complicating care planning. **Objective:** To enhance understanding of end-of-life care post-stroke. **Methods:** We undertook an explanatory sequential mixed methods approach, including a cross-sectional survey and semi-structured interviews. All 286 United Kingdom (UK) National Health Service (NHS) hospitals providing inpatient stroke care were approached for participation in an on-line cross-sectional survey. The survey of healthcare professionals from UK stroke units was used to map current stroke end-of-life care and models of care. Fourteen staff who completed the survey and agreed to a future interview were purposively selected. The semi-structured interviews with healthcare professionals involved in delivering end-of-life care post-stroke were conducted and interpreted using the Theoretical Domains Framework. We aimed to enhance our understanding of the experiences, expectations, challenges and barriers in providing end-of-life care post-stroke, including effective clinical decision-making. **Results:** Across 108 responding survey sites, 317 responses were received. Results showed a lack of structured tools and approaches, an absence of stroke-specific guidance and variable delivery of end-of-life care post-stroke. Thirteen staff (nurses, occupational therapists, medical stroke consultants, and a speech and language therapist) agreed to be interviewed. The data provided a fuller understanding of the context within which end-of-life care post-stroke is delivered. The varied challenges faced include: uncertain prognosis, complex decision-making process, varying skill levels, staffing levels, the hospital environment, emotional strain on both families and staff, inequitable access to specialist palliative care, and difficulties associated with different models of care (stroke service structures and cultural context). **Conclusions:** Provision of end-of-life care post-stroke is complex, challenging, uncertain, and inconsistent. There is limited evidence or guidance to support healthcare professionals. There is a need for implementation support, which includes education, to better enable quality and more consistent end-of-life care post-stroke. Further research is required to assess interventions that can support end-of-life care post-stroke to aid clinicians in providing quality palliative care for stroke patients.

Keywords: stroke; end-of-life care; experiences; survey

1. Introduction

Stroke is a major cause of death, with 13% of patients dying in hospital (this figure is much higher in some types of stroke [1]) and 25–30% of survivors dying within a year [2]. In England, stroke-related deaths total 32,000 annually [3].

Unpredictable trajectories of stroke complicate care planning [4,5]. The abruptness with severe stroke from normal function to sudden death restricts opportunities for advance care planning. Others may have an erratic trajectory of prologued declines with recovery, meaning the timing of death is less certain than other conditions, such as cancer. All these factors contribute to uncertainty when planning care. The absence of stroke-specific end-of-life care guidelines further complicates management. Unlike cancer, which has well-established palliative care pathways, stroke lacks standardised protocols to guide decision-making in the transition to end-of-life care [6]. As a result, healthcare professionals often rely on generic end-of-life frameworks, which are less able to account for the complexity of stroke and the impact of stroke on symptom management. Many stroke patients also experience communication difficulties, fluctuating consciousness, or cognitive impairments [7,8], challenging shared decision-making. This uncertainty leads to inconsistent care and difficulty aligning treatment with patient and family expectations [9]. An audit in a large NHS Trust highlighted limited access to specialist palliative care, with most discussions occurring with families rather than patients and only two-thirds of patients having individualised care plans.

National Health Service (NHS) and government publications outline what quality end-of-life care should look like [10–14]. The National Clinical Guideline for Stroke [15] makes several recommendations about what should be available, as well as key considerations, but acknowledges gaps in research on implementation. The Guideline [15] is clear that stroke teams must increase their awareness and expertise in end-of-life care and recognise that this is a core part of their role. However, research on end-of-life care in stroke remains limited, as clinical focus is on acute treatment and rehabilitation.

Several studies have described stroke end-of-life care needs [16–20]. An international review on end-of-life care post-stroke [21] reported poor symptom control, insufficient emotional care, family difficulties accessing information about the patient's condition, and inadequate support. From an organisational perspective, the stroke service structure and cultural context as a place where end-of-life care is delivered, including staffing, skills, and logistical issues, needs to be examined.

Aim: To enhance understanding of the experiences, expectations, challenges, and barriers in providing end-of-life care post-stroke, including clinical decision-making.

2. Methods

2.1. Design

We undertook an explanatory sequential mixed methods approach, conducting a cross-sectional survey and semi-structured interviews with NHS staff members providing end-of-life care post-stroke. End-of-life care is generally defined as care in the final 12 months of life [22–24], but in this study, end-of-life care is defined as care for patients at risk of dying within 30 days of hospital admission post-stroke as 11–30% of people die within 30 days [25]. The study was reviewed by the NRES Committee North West—Greater Manchester South Research Ethics Committee and received a favourable opinion.

2.2. Participant Selection

All 286 UK hospitals providing inpatient stroke care were identified through the Royal College of Physicians' Sentinel Stroke National Audit Programme (SSNAP) and the Scottish Stroke Care Audit. The named hospital contact for the audit was sent an email asking if the hospital was willing to participate. Hospitals were sent three email reminders to confirm participation. Both audits reported 100% participation. When the hospital confirmed willing to participate, researchers contacted the stroke unit coordinator/ward sister/charge nurse or stroke clinical lead for permission to send an email inviting 3–4 stroke clinicians from each site to complete a survey. Eligible staff included physicians, allied health team leader, stroke nurses, and palliative care leads. Ineligible staff were those not directly involved in end-of-life care decision-making or care delivery. An online survey link was provided, with an option for a paper copy. The first section of the online questionnaire contained the study participant information sheet, with checkboxes to confirm they had read and understood the information sheet; they could withdraw at any time and their contact information and responses would be kept confidential. The participant was unable to proceed unless these checkboxes were completed. Consent was implied by completing the survey.

In terms of interview participants, five sites representing different service configurations/taxonomies (size, type, end-of-life care champion/ Clinical lead and access to end-of-life care specialist). Up to three staff who completed the survey and agreed to a future interview were purposively selected based on factors such as seniority and job role to ensure that diverse experiences were represented within this study. A sampling grid was used to ensure representativity, and those willing to participate signed a pre-interview consent form.

3. Data Collection

3.1. Survey

A bespoke online survey was developed by the research team, reviewed by expert clinicians in the Research Management Group (RMG), and piloted with clinicians to assess question clarity, response options, and participant acceptability. The survey had eight sections and 41 questions covering several areas: respondent, hospital and stroke service characteristics, use of end-of-life guidance, care responsibilities, environment, education, training, and factors influencing end-of-life care in acute stroke. Responses included free-text (qualitative) and categorical (quantitative) data. Completion time was estimated at 30 min. The survey was distributed using Qualtrics.

3.2. Interviews

The semi-structured interview guide was informed by the survey findings, with input from the RMG and Patient and Public Involvement Group. The guide was shaped by the Theoretical Domains Framework (TDF) [26] which is a synthesis of theories primarily focussing on behaviour change. The guide was used to explore factors influencing end-of-life care after stroke. The TDF is a synthesis theory which aims to identify influences on health professional behaviour and determinants of behaviour change. related to implementation of evidence-based recommendations The topics covered included staff experiences, decision-making, barriers and facilitators, care models, communication, patient and family involvement, education, staff support, and readiness for change. The interviews were conducted by telephone or online by experienced qualitative interviewers. All interviews were recorded and then transcribed verbatim and de-identified. Demographic data were collected to describe the sample.

3.3. Data Analysis

Survey data were analysed using descriptive statistics and reported as counts and percentages using STATA SE version 17.

All interview transcripts were checked for accuracy and imported into NVivo. A coding framework was developed deductively using the TDF. The TDF is an integrative framework of 14 domains which can facilitate comprehensive assessment of the determinants of current and desired behaviours. At least two researchers undertook content analysis [27] on each transcript independently using the Framework method [28]. The stages of the analysis were: (1) familiarisation of the data, (2) coding (coding anything that might be relevant, line-by-line) by at least two researchers, and (3) interpreting the data by at least two researchers. Where text mapped onto more than one TDF domain, it was coded in both; otherwise, it was coded under the domain that best matched the content. The researchers (C.D., C.G., and C.T.) met to discuss the codes against the initial coding framework and refined it until they all felt that their codes were reflected. Minor differences arose in relation to the mapping of codes, particularly when codes mapped to more than one domain. Conflicts were resolved by a fourth researcher with expertise in using the TDF (C.E.L.).

4. Results

4.1. Survey

Stroke units were approached between January 2021–September 2022. One hundred and twenty-four hospitals agreed to participate (67% of eligible hospitals) and were sent the questionnaires. One hundred and eight hospitals engaged in the survey across 83 NHS Health Boards/hospitals, serving a geographical area (regional variation 50–100%); 317 survey responses were received, with a site response rate of 87% (i.e., a site completed at least one questionnaire) and 72% of sites providing >=3 responses. Key issues with/reasons for non-participation were: backlogs within R&D that prevented governance; staffing shortages in stroke units, and an inability to identify a suitable principal investigator.

The findings of the survey are presented below, in relation to each of the sections of the survey.

1. Demographics and characteristics of person completing the survey

Survey respondents were stroke nurse consultants, stroke specialist nurses, ward sisters or charge nurses, or physicians. Of the respondents, 39% were nurses, 26% physicians, 25% AHPs, 8% stroke unit palliative care champions/leads, and 2% palliative care specialists. The majority were female (71%), with 182 (57%) having over 5 years' experience in their current role, and 112 (35%) were between the ages of 41 and 50 years.

2. Hospital and stroke service characteristics

The majority 293 (92%) described their hospital setting as acute. The number of stroke-specific beds on the wards varied, with a majority (40%) having between 21–30 beds.

3. The use of end-of-life guidance and tools in acute stroke care

The majority of units (69%) used a general end-of-life care protocol for all patients, with only 22 (7%) having a stroke specific end-of-life care protocol and 63 (20%) respondents either being unaware of a protocol or saying they did not have one. Responses indicated that decisions around end-of-life care were frequently supported using multi-disciplinary meetings; unscheduled discussions with ward colleagues; and referral to specialist palliative and end-of-life care teams. A minority of wards used standardised tools to support decision-making, including the Gold Standards Framework, AMBER Care Bundle, and Supportive and Palliative Care Indicators tool (SPICT) (Figure 1)

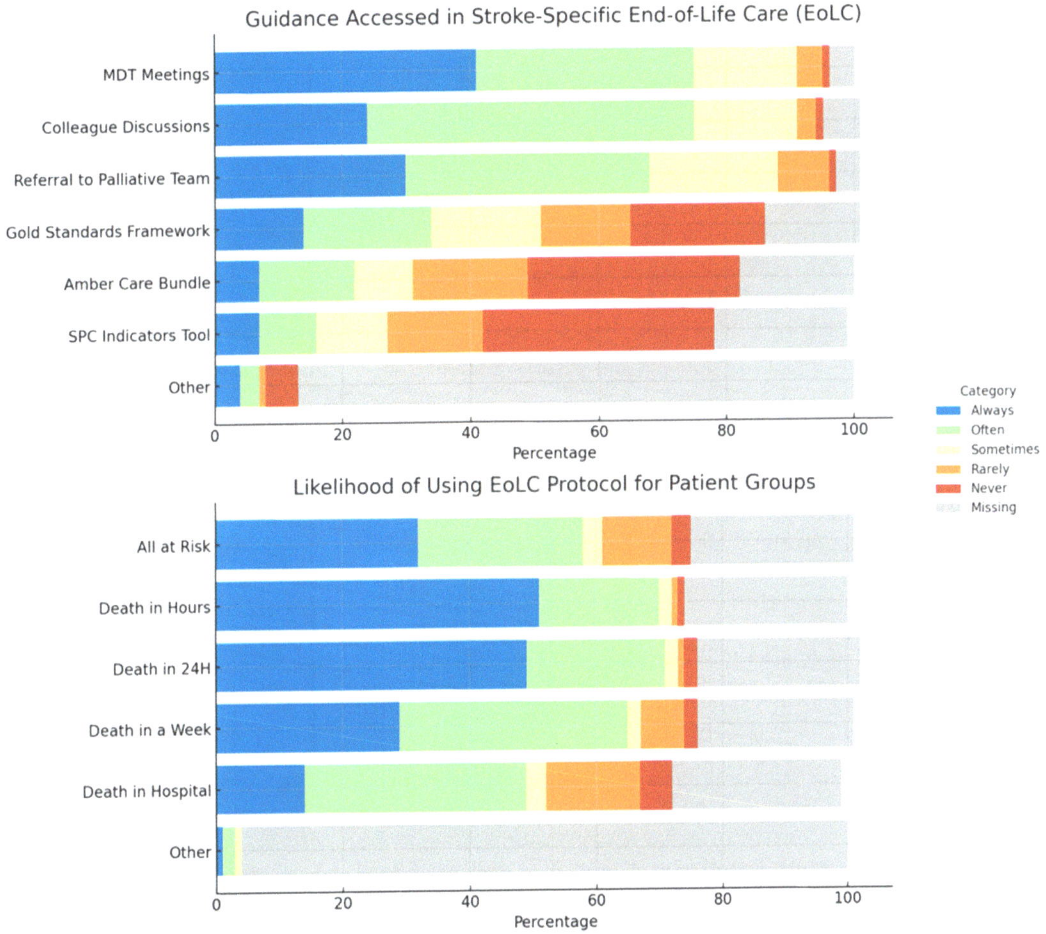

Figure 1. Stacked bar chart depicting use of end-of life care guidance and which patient groups are likely to be managed by an end-of-life care protocol/palliative care team.

Overall, use of end-of-life care protocols were initiated mainly when patients were identified as being at risk of dying imminently, with 163 (51%) of respondents reporting they were highly likely initiated protocols when patients expected to die within the coming few hours, and 154 (49%) when patients were expected to die within 24 h. Those identified as being at risk of dying within a week (n = 91, 29%) or expected to die during this hospital admission but after one week (44, 14%) were less likely to have care supported in this way (Figure 1).

Patients most likely to be referred to the palliative care team were those deemed to require specialist palliative care or complex decision making (Table 1).

Table 1. Patients referred to specialist palliative and end-of-life care teams.

Which Patients Do You Refer to the Specialist Palliative and End-of-Life Care (EoLC) Team?	Yes %	No %	Missing %
None	7	85	8
All patients transitioning to end-of-life care	44	48	8
Patients who require specialist palliative and/or end-of-life care input	65	27	8
Patients who require complex decision making	54	38	8
Patients who require specialist advice on symptoms	64	28	8
Patients who wish to die in their usual place of residence	47	45	8
Patients who wish to die in a hospice	50	42	8
Other	5	87	8

4. People Responsible for Acute Stroke End-of-Life Care

A total of 41% of respondents had an end-of-life care champion/clinical lead and the majority (n = 277, 87%) had access to a specialist palliative/end-of-life care team. Over half (n = 175, 55%) had out-of-hours specialist palliative/end-of-life care support; however, about a fifth (n = 68, 22%) of respondents were unsure if they had out-of-hours access.

Regarding the members of the MDT most likely to participate in decision-making for end-of-life care in acute stroke patients, involvement varied significantly. Stroke consultants and family members were the most frequently involved, followed by nurses and mid-grade doctors (Table S1). Key decision makers around end-of-life care tended to be all grades of doctors (stroke consultant (89%), junior doctor—foundation and core (64%) mid-grade doctor/specialist registrar (52%)), and the family/carer (61%), with the patient only being involved 38% of the time (see Table S1). The stroke consultant (n = 260, 82%) or mid-grade doctor (n = 171, 54%) were highly likely to communicate decisions around prognosis and end-of-life care to the patient and their significant others. Nurses were the other team members likely to be involved.

5. Where Acute Stroke Patients at the End-of-Life Are Cared for

Patients were most likely to receive end-of-life care in the stroke units (hyper-acute, acute, and rehab), whilst some patients received end-of-life care in their own home or a care home. Generally, respondents felt their ward provided a suitable environment, with adequate peace and privacy for the dying patient (usually n = 186, 59%, sometimes n = 90, 28%), with similar figures reported for family members (usually n = 149, 47%, sometimes n = 110, 34%). About 63% felt they were usually or sometimes able to provide a suitable environment for the family members to stay overnight. Most respondents (n = 222, 70%) could arrange discharge in time for patients who were expected to die within the coming days/weeks and preferred to die at home.

End-of-life care discussions were mainly face-to-face, with some by phone and a few online. Face-to-face conversations usually took place in the relatives' room or ward office, with some at the patient's bedside.

6. End-of-Life Care Education and Components of End-of-Life Care

Only 27 (9%) of respondents felt that all staff had the knowledge and skills to provide high quality end-of-life care, and 147 (46%) felt most staff had the knowledge and skills.

The stroke team generally handles direct personal care, MDT communication, and hydration/nutrition management, while symptom assessment, anticipatory prescribing, and psychosocial and spiritual support are shared with the specialist palliative care team. Most respondents (n = 178, 56%) felt there was a procedure for "comfort" or "risk" feeding acute stroke patients receiving end-of-life care, though 20% (n = 62) were unsure (see Table 2). Only a third (n = 97, 31%) reported that stroke patients with end-of-life care needs always or often had an advance care plan. Stroke teams were more likely to discuss end-of-life care and advance care planning with family than the patient. Approximately a third of stroke patients who are conscious, have mental capacity and can communicate (with or without support) are given the opportunity to contribute to an advance care plan, but when the patient is unconscious or lacks mental capacity, 184 (58%) said that they would try to assess the patient's best interests or preferences in the absence of an advanced decision.

Table 2. Who provides different elements of end-of-life care.

Who Provides the Following Elements of Care to Acute Stroke Patients Receiving End-of-Life Care?				
	Stroke Team %	**Specialist Palliative and/or End-of-Life Care Team** %	**Both** %	**Missing** %
Personal care	87	0	3	10
Symptom assessment	36	4	51	10
Symptom management	31	5	54	10
Communicating uncertainty of prognosis	51	3	36	10
Communicating information to the MDT	62	1	27	10
Communicating information to patients	37	1	53	10
Communicating information to those important to the patient	39	1	50	10
Management of hydration and nutrition	63	1	26	10
Anticipatory prescribing	41	4	45	10
Psychosocial support for the patient	34	9	44	12
Psychosocial support for those important to the patient	34	9	45	11
Spiritual support for the patient	32	16	36	16
Spiritual support for those important to the patient	32	18	33	17
Other	3	0	1	96

7. Factors Influencing the Provision of End-of-Life Care in Acute Stroke

Staff, organisational, and patient factors influencing end-of-life care provision are presented in Figure 2. Respondents were divided on whether staff had enough time to provide end-of-life care, with most agreeing that staff shortages affected care quality. The majority felt end-of-life care should remain the stroke team's responsibility, not solely specialist palliative teams.

Organisationally, staff reported good access to specialist palliative/end-of-life care, tools and guidance, but despite this there was reported variability and inconsistency in end-of-life care provision. There was uncertainty about whether pre- and post-registration training for nurses in end-of-life care was sufficient.

Patient factors, such as communication difficulties, cognitive impairment, and consciousness levels, were seen as barriers to quality care. This variability was more pronounced with uncertainty around prognosis, delirium, and communication challenges/disagreements with family and carers.

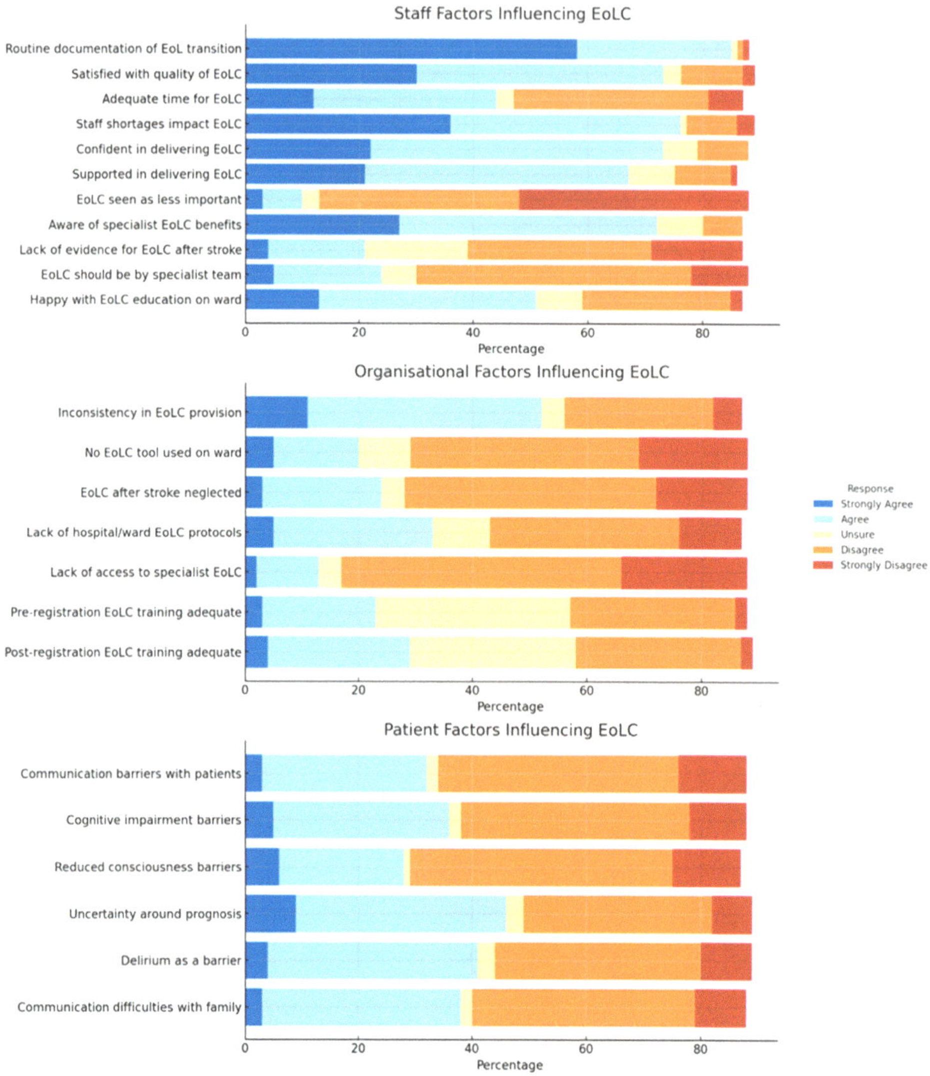

Figure 2. Stacked bar chart depicting staff, organizational, and patient factors influencing provision of end-of-life care in acute stroke.

4.2. Interview

Fourteen staff were approached to take part in an interview across five NHS hospitals. A total of 13 participants were interviewed, and one staff member did not respond. In terms of purposive sampling, we achieved a range in terms of stroke unit typology and job role, but all staff interviewed were relatively senior, reflecting those who had agreed to be interviewed. Table 3 presents a description of the interview participants employing hospital. One researcher (AR) interviewed ten participants and a second interviewed three (CT), two of whom took part in a joint interview. Participant characteristics are described in Table 4.

Table 3. Description of the interview participants employing hospital.

Site	Location	Number of Beds in the Unit	EoLC Lead	Specialist EoLC in Hours	Specialist EoLC out of Hours
Acute stroke unit with hyper-acute beds	Urban	21–30 beds	No	Yes	unsure
Comprehensive Stroke Centre (CSC)	City hospital	40+ beds	Yes	Yes	Yes
Acute stroke unit	Rural	1–10 beds	No	Yes	No
Rehabilitation unit	Rural	11–20 beds	Yes	No	No
Integrated acute and rehabilitation unit	Urban	21–30 beds	No	Yes	Yes

Table 4. Characteristics of interview participants.

Participant Code	Current Role/s	Length of Current Role (Years)
PRE001	Stroke nurse consultant	10
PRE002	Ward manager	Unknown
PRE003	Occupational therapy team leader in a hyper-acute/acute stroke unit	2
PRE004	Stroke physician	12
PRE005	Stroke nurse consultant	5
PRE006	Speech and language therapist	6
PRE007	Ward sister	16
PRE008	Stroke nurse practitioner	10
PRE009	Stroke physician	2
PRE010	Stroke nurse practitioner	Unknown
PRE011	Occupational therapy team leader	4
PRE012	Occupational therapist in acute stroke and AHP team lead for acute stroke services	2
PRE013	Stroke specialist nurse—integrated unit with HASU beds, acute beds and rehab beds in one site	1

Within these interviews the TDF domains of "Environmental Context and Resources", "Social/Professional Role and Identity" and "Memory, Attention and Decision Process" were coded most frequently, accounting for 54% of all references between them. Figure 3 presents the eight most frequently coded domains with illustrative quotes. Themes within the TDF domains and supporting quotes can be found in Table S2.

4.2.1. Environmental Context and Resources

Managing both recovering and end-of-life care patients on the same ward was emotionally challenging for families and staff, as they were antithetical experiences in the same space. Limited space, time, and training hindered patient-centred care. Stroke-specific end-of-life care occurred in stroke or palliative care wards, depending on the Trust, with the ideal setting debated, and dependent on bed availability. Individual rooms offered more dignity but were scarce commodity and usually prioritised for those patients who were imminently going to die.

It was deemed that better and consistent staffing improved support, as interactions with patients/family were more likely to be adequately documented. The involvement of bereavement and palliative care teams were valued and helped free up staff time. Some participants felt experiencing empathy could help prioritise end-of-life care with competing clinical demands.

"If you don't have empathy you won't prioritise" (PRE002)

Discharge delays upset families when patients wished to die at home. Staff supported home deaths but faced logistical barriers. End-of-life care discharge processes varied, often delayed by documentation and equipment issues, which meant it was not always achieved. Balancing what feels right with practical needs was difficult.

One hospital had an 'Emergency Healthcare Plan' to facilitate patient readmission if home care failed.

"we have had people that were desperate to get home and we have done everything we could to get everything in place, but unfortunately they passed away before we even got a chance of taking them." (PRE013)

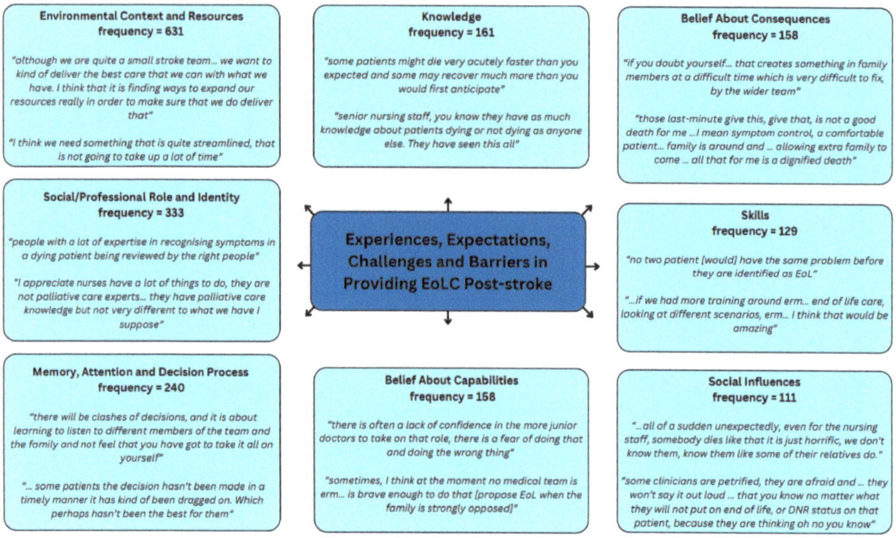

Figure 3. Most frequently coded TDF domains with illustrative quotes.

4.2.2. Social/Professional Role and Identity

End-of-life care was delivered by a multidisciplinary team, including specialist palliative care and bereavement staff. Generally, specialist palliative care teams, consultants, and stroke teams worked closely together. However, multidisciplinary engagement varied, with some hospitals lacking a clear process.

"within this trust there is no proper process of multidisciplinary engagement for end-of-life-care" (PRE004)

Speech and language therapists advised on maintaining patient comfort while eating and drinking.

"advising on what is the least distressing consistency and educating the family and the staff on the ward" (PRE006)

Nursing assistants provided hands-on care but lacked palliative training despite strong interest.

"they (nursing assistants) are showing such an interest in palliative care, and I think they feel quite frustrated that they can't act on that interest there" (PRE008)

Occupational therapists supported functional needs, decision-making, and discharge facilitation before specialist palliative care took over, though some felt their role in stroke end-of-life care needed better understanding.

> *"because someone is end-of-life, doesn't mean that ... the person could not be more comfortable ... be able to gain more connection with people, or more joy in eating and drinking"* (PRE011)

In some wards, experienced nurses led end-of-life care due to limited consultant availability. Nurses often wanted more consultant involvement, particularly in family communication, with a liaison role suggested to improve family communication. However, one nurse considered that nurses are experts in palliative care and always at the forefront.

> *"we are relatively self-sufficient in that care is quite nurse-led a lot of the time because we don't have that senior consultant around 5 days a week".* (PRE007 and PRE008)

Consultants' views on their role in end-of-life care varied. Some consultants admitted minimal involvement choosing instead to focus more on acute care, reassured by the skills of their team, especially nurses.

> *"I don't usually talk to families if I think the patient is not going to die within 6 months, I should be but I don't"* (PRE009)

4.2.3. Memory, Attention, and Decision Process

Decisions are usually made by a consultant-led MDT. This approach is valued as it helps manage disagreements within the team and encourages listening to team members and families, although some felt a consultant was not always needed.

> *"If those conversations are had, and it is clear, then I don't think it has to be a consultant"* (PRE007 and PRE008)

Nurses were frustrated when decision-making was unnecessarily protracted or disagreement amongst clinicians or family members prevented the decision from going ahead, resulting in some patients being 'over-treated'. This was not deemed to be in the patient's best interest. Staff occasionally made "difficult calls" moving patients against family wishes, believing families should be informed that it is not their decision to make to avoid delays. End-of-life care could overwhelm staff, but teamwork ensured patient and family needs were met.

> *"often times the consultants will delay end-of-life-care until all the family are in agreement".* (PRE002)

Early end-of-life care discussions were seen as essential, helping meet "spiritual, emotional, and religious" needs. Patients with capacity could be involved in end-of-life care decisions, but often stroke patients are not able to make decisions. One participant shared their timing approach:

> *"I don't do it when they are extremely unwell. When they are stable, when I still do think they are very high risk of having a problem I do discuss it with them"* (PRE009)

Experienced staff felt more comfortable having end-of-life care discussions, while junior doctors often lacked confidence. Triggers for end-of-life care discussions included airway issues, patient not 'doing well', or lack of treatment options. Stroke-related end-of-life care decisions were challenging due to unpredictable outcomes.

> *"in stroke the challenge is that sometimes that the suddenness or the acuteness of the stroke makes it a lot more difficult. [...] probably patient was not dying last week or when the stroke happened but now that the patient has changed, identifying that probably is one of the, you know something can be improved actually"* (PRE005)

There was variability in the use of tools to support decision making. Tools reported included the ICARE plan, which was seen as comprehensive covering patient care, family needs, medical review, decision-making, and patient wishes, the NIHSS for measuring severity, and the ICH score to measure blood volume in intracerebral haemorrhage. These scores were considered alongside comorbidities and stroke history. Those who used tools generally felt they had utility.

> *"it encourages you each day to identify any issues that you, any needs that you are not meeting ... and put a care plan in place for that. And, then it asks you to reflect on the outcome of that as well, how successful that's been."* (PRE007 and PRE008)

However, others noted a lack of tools. One participant felt a tool to predict stroke patient mortality within a certain period would be valuable. The importance of documenting decision-making was also referenced to avoid confusion amongst staff.

4.2.4. Knowledge

Stroke end-of-life care is complex due to unpredictable prognoses. Staff highlighted the need to explain how stroke differs from typical end-of-life care trajectories. More palliative care training was desired but limited by time. Learning was often described as opportunistic.

> *"it is the cascade of that information isn't it, it is like who is at that meeting, and who else learns from it."* (PRE006)

Teaching and training are important, but only part of the solution; experience helps with understanding patients' needs and increases competence.

> *"I don't usually ask my junior doctors to do this discussion, I usually ask them to come to see how I discuss it."* (PRE009)

One Trust required all stroke unit staff to complete e-learning resource STARS (Stroke Training and Awareness Resources) competencies, including advanced training for doctors and nurses. Over time, experienced staff found end-of-life care management became 'second nature.'

> *"it comes with experience [....] a lot of what we do nursing wise on the job is from peer learning..."* (PRE010)

4.2.5. Belief About Capabilities

Staff believed they provided dignified, respectful care and valued the specialist palliative care team. However, care quality varied by staff experience.

> *"we do a good job at treating these patients,...providing the dignity and respect that they need and the comfort to the family"* (PRE003)

Nurses are used to death and felt they had confidence and competence to advocate on behalf of families. However, they felt less confident in having discussions about end-of-life care and wishes.

> *"the discussion about where the patient would want to die... that is something we are not good at"* (PRE009)

Junior doctors lacked confidence due to fear of mistakes (PRE007 and PRE008). It was felt that clear guidance would help raise confidence in making end-of-life care decisions and discussions. Better MDT support and staffing levels could facilitate collaborative end-of-life care decision-making. Stroke's sudden onset was hard for families to accept, especially when the patient was younger, which led to more family disagreements. Staff reported balancing medical care with family wishes as difficult and best interest meetings were reported as supporting complex decisions, helping to resolve disagreements.

> *"no medical team is brave enough to do that" (propose end-of-life-care when the family is strongly opposed)* (PRE002)

4.2.6. Belief About Consequences

Varying capabilities of individual staff were reported, with junior staff lacking the confidence in communicating with families and making decisions due to fear of getting it wrong. Staff felt that lack of confidence in decision-making could delay end-of-life care, causing distress for families and frustration for nurses, as clinicians are just delaying the inevitable. There were reports that some clinicians may lengthen or change end-of-life care decisions out of fear of making the wrong decision, which was deemed to be emotional for the family, and not in the patient's best interest.

> *"I do feel that I know for sure that some patients the decision hasn't been made in a timely manner it has kind of been dragged on. Which perhaps hasn't been the best for them."* (PRE006)

> *"So those last-minute give this, give that, is not a good death"* (PRE002)

Doctors were uneasy about communicating end-of-life care decisions, fearing they would upset families further. Wording was key. Fear and lack of confidence of being direct with families affected communication quality, with doubt creating issues that require multiple meetings to resolve.

> *"Saying "I'm putting your mum on a pathway" sounds horrible and inhumane"* (PRE004)

Despite staff hesitations, respondents felt families appreciated honesty. However, families were distressed when end-of-life care decisions were reversed; communication was tricky when end-of-life tools were not used and patients recovered after end-of-life care discussions. It was felt that the Liverpool Care Pathway controversy still affects end-of-life care decisions. Staff reported moving a patient to a 'bounty bed' which is a hospital bed that is temporarily made available to accommodate patients, could feel like taking their life. Staff considered that there was a 'label' attached to the end-of-life care and felt they had to reassure worried families about hospital tools being used.

> *"End-of-life-care or DNR, thinking, oh no, I can't do that"* (PRE005)

> *"it is more of a tool to make sure that when you come into hospital, we have been doing your observations routinely to make sure that if something goes wrong we can act on it."* (PRE004)

There was a feeling that better understanding of end-of-life care would support high-quality care and that training, combined with experiential knowledge will help the MDT understand palliative care.

4.2.7. Skills

Identifying end-of-life care patients relied on highly-skilled staff with experience and MDT input, as there is no universal approach. Some nurses felt skilled enough to manage final stages, especially for elderly patients and where the family were in agreement. Senior staff were recognised for their experience which led to good communication skills. However, it was felt some consultants, registrars, and nurses lacked end-of-life care skills due to low confidence and time constraints.

> *"you often have to do it to get it right. And you can listen to someone else doing it. . .but it is slightly different"* (PRE004)

Building a rapport with the family and using lay language supported family understanding. Staff emphasised the need for education and experiential learning, as end-of-life care discussions required skill, emotion, and energy

> *"a lot of skill... a lot of emotion... a lot of energy' and that 'you have got to have the right people who are able to deliver that message"* (PRE006)

4.2.8. Social Influences

Staff prioritised patient and family wishes for a 'good death'. However, families could sometimes pressure staff to continue with treatment even though it was not in the patient's best interest, and staff went along with it to appease them.

> *"we have had consultants go, oh well just keep the fluids going because the relative wants them."* (PRE010)

Some staff felt that documentation and communication were reinforced through daily safety briefs, ensuring senior nurses and the wider team were aware of and addressed issues, ensuring better MDT collaboration and improved patient care, but this required collective action to implement.

> *"we need collective work to improve patient care but often that is difficult. We need to set it all up."* (PRE004)

However, one participant noted a hospital culture where death was an unmentionable topic.

> *"it is still you know it has got to be the most taboo subjects in hospital still [....] we can't talk about somebody dying"* (PRE008)

4.2.9. Emotion

Managing end-of-life care was emotionally challenging, especially when staff had to support both the patient and their family. Staff acknowledged the challenge of managing family's emotions but felt engaging multiple family members helped.

> *"if there is more than one family member...there are different emotions in the room...it just helps manage the situation more effectively."* (PRE011)

The busy nature of acute wards and bed shortages often led to staff feeling overwhelmed and conflicted. Patient distress affected staff deeply, with one nurse stating,

> *"I hate it when patients are distressed in a bay, sometimes I feel when they know that they are dying I don't want them to even have any awareness sometimes."* (PRE001)

The emotional impact could be long-lasting, especially when care was deemed to have gone "wrong". Sudden deaths were described as "horrific" and "very emotional" for nursing staff, yet nurses felt compelled to continue working despite the recent loss.

> *"we still talk about it now... that case will always stick with me"* (PRE001)

Most stroke end-of-life care teams lacked official psychological support; instead, support often came from peers or hospital well-being services. One Trust had a psychological support team offering group sessions, initially seen as 'awkward' but later as 'amazing' and highly valued, though not often used. Another participant mentioned a rare one-off reflection session following a traumatic case, with deaths usually discussed in monthly mortality meetings. Some felt showing emotion demonstrated empathy and improved care.

> *"I've never had the conversation without crying... it shows you care ...I think it makes them feel better"* (PRE007 and PRE008)

5. Discussion

This study has enhanced our understanding of what current end-of-life care post-stroke looks like and the significant challenges that health professionals face in providing compassionate and dignified care. These challenges stem from the uncertain prognosis, complex decision-making process, varying skill levels, staffing levels, the hospital environment, emotional strain on both families and staff, inequitable access to specialist palliative care; and difficulties associated with different models of care.

The multidisciplinary nature of end-of-life care delivery is a crucial finding in this study. Although there was a strong collaboration between stroke and specialist palliative care teams, the lack of clear processes in some hospitals led to inconsistencies in care. These findings align with previous studies that have identified the need for standardised processes and better communication within multidisciplinary teams to ensure consistent and holistic care [29].

Honest, clear, and timely communication around end-of-life care and the potential of death is required to ensure quality care and more informed decisions for patients. Conversations about death and end-of-life care should be started early, but uncertainty about when to initiate end-of-life care after a stroke remains a significant challenge for clinicians. Prognostication in the acute phase is often difficult due to the variable trajectory of stroke recovery, making it hard to determine whether a patient will survive with severe disability or experience further deterioration [30].

Different healthcare professionals faced distinct barriers in making end-of-life decisions for patients following a stroke, with consultants navigating prognostic uncertainty and complex medical decision-making, nurses struggling with prolonged decision processes and emotional burdens, and junior staff lacking confidence due to limited training and experience in end-of-life care. While decisions are generally led by consultants, the role of nurses and other staff in making difficult decisions and communicating with families was also significant. Nurses were often at the forefront of providing care but expressed frustration with prolonged decision-making processes. The emotional and social pressures exerted by family members often complicated decisions, with some staff members feeling compelled to extend treatment to appease families. This often arose when there was a misunderstanding, differences in beliefs or families struggling with the emotional burden of uncertainty [31] or when communication was fractured. For example, it was difficult when families had not accepted their relatives' imminent death and did not agree with treatment withdrawal or their relative being placed on end-of-life care. This tension between medical recommendations and familial expectations meant that staff sometimes felt they were prioritising relatives wishes over patient wishes. This may stem from debates around the Liverpool Care Pathway where the media portrayed it as "a pathway to euthanasia", compounded by a deep-rooted reluctance within the UK to address issues around mortality, with hospitals seen as places to heal and prolong life. This aligns with previous research indicating that communication breakdowns, which operate in a complex social context about death and dying, can lead to delays in care and sometimes unnecessary treatment, which may not be in the best interest of the patient [32] and can lead to moral distress among healthcare providers [33]. Better communication about the realities of end-of-life care could help mitigate these tensions and support a more patient-centred approach. One strategy suggested by staff was the use of a liaison role to improve communication with families, which could help bridge the gap between clinical decisions and familial expectations, ensuring that patients receive care that aligns with their best interests.

There was also a lack of consistency and variable quality in the documentation of any conversations had with families' or patients, meaning that information sometimes did not get effectively communicated. Limited staffing compounded the problem, contributing to delayed decision making, inadequate documentation of patient-family discussions and delayed discharge processes for patients wishing to die at home. Staffing shortages have previously been reported as negatively affecting the quality of communication and the timeliness of end-of-life care decisions [34]. However, the support from specialist palliative care and bereavement teams was viewed as invaluable, assisting in both the logistical aspects of care and providing emotional support for families and staff.

In terms of knowledge and training, this study highlighted training needs across a range of healthcare roles and levels of seniority, including non-professional staff. Staff recognised that stroke end-of-life care requires specific knowledge due to the unpredictable trajectory of the disease, which is often complicated by comorbidities. Consequently, many staff described a need for training around how best to have difficult conversations around end-of-life care with patients and families. Although staff could be taught to have effective discussions with families, this was regarded as a skill learned through experience, so opportunities to learn from more experienced staff should be available. The desire for more formal training, alongside experiential learning, reflects the current understanding in the literature that end-of-life care training must be ongoing, incorporating both theoretical knowledge and practical experience [35].

Additionally, tools such as the ICARE plan, Amber Care, NIHSS, and ICH score, while helpful, were not universally used, indicating a lack of standardised tools to guide decision-making in stroke end-of-life care. Locally developed generic end-of-life care policies and guidance were commonly used. There is evidence to suggest that clinical tools and guidelines can improve the consistency and quality of care, especially in the management of complex, unpredictable cases like stroke [36]. In addition to revealing a lack of use of structured tools and approaches, and an absence of stroke-specific guidance or tools, this work has highlighted huge variation in how end-of-life care is delivered after stroke.

Quality end-of-life care involves multiple components. It is important to ensure that patient needs are met, including symptom control and that patients are treated with dignity. However, this can be challenging in open wards where privacy may not always be provided, and where staff are managing both recovering and end-of-life care patients in the same space. The lack of individualised rooms for end-of-life care patients means that some die in less-than-ideal conditions, with privacy often being sacrificed due to limited bed availability. These observations are consistent with the existing literature that highlights the importance of a dignified death, which can be compromised when patient care spaces are not optimised for end-of-life care [37]. Furthermore, navigating both clinical demands and familial expectations within the same environment often places staff in difficult emotional positions.

The emotional impact on staff, which was especially evident in difficult cases, deeply affected staff, particularly when things were perceived to have gone wrong. However, staff described how there were no formal well-being or psychological support procedures. Support was often provided informally between staff members. A lack of formal debrief or reflection opportunities for staff after patient deaths was also highlighted. The lack of formal psychological support, alongside the emotional demands of the work, reflects a broader issue in healthcare where staff well-being is often overlooked. Peer support, reflective sessions, and institutional programs for staff well-being are critical to maintaining morale and preventing burnout. Moreover, fostering an organisational culture that allows staff to express emotions and seek help when needed is essential for maintaining the quality of care provided [38].

The findings highlight the need for structured policies and systematic training to improve end-of-life care for patients following a stroke. There is a clear need to develop stroke-specific end-of-life care guidelines to address the unique challenges of prognostication, communication, and decision-making, ensuring a more consistent, patient-centred approach that aligns with the complexities of stroke trajectories. Enhanced palliative care training, particularly for nursing assistants and junior doctors, could improve confidence in end-of-life care discussions and prevent unnecessary treatment prolongation. Cultural shifts in hospital settings are needed to normalise conversations around death, ensuring that families receive honest, compassionate communication while prioritising patient dignity and comfort. Addressing these policy and practice gaps could lead to more consistent, timely, and patient-centred stroke end-of-life care. The survey used a self-reporting questionnaire, the assumption being that the responses submitted accurately reflect practice. We tried to mitigate against recall and response bias by having several respondents with different professional backgrounds returning the questionnaire at each hospital. As the survey was not able to provide meaning or context behind responses, we also undertook semi-structured interviews; however, participants self-selected to participate, so there could have been a degree of selection bias. Furthermore, methods to enhance the trustworthiness of the interpretation of the data such as member checking, use of memos, or reflective journaling was not undertaken; however, at least two researchers analysed each transcript, making misinterpretations less likely.

6. Conclusions

Despite stroke's high mortality, there is limited guidance on delivering end-of-life care post-stroke. Variability exists in decision-making, care delivery, and patient/family involvement. End-of-life care after stroke is complex, with challenges like uncertain prognosis, decision-making complexities, inadequate training, emotional distress, and limited staffing. Addressing these challenges requires a multifaceted approach including better training on communication and standardised tools and processes to guide decision-making, while accounting for unique and individual needs of different patients to ensure that patient and family wishes are respected. Prioritising emotional well-being and collaborative multidisciplinary care will improve stroke end-of-life care, ensuring care is compassionate, dignified, and patient-centred. Future research needs to explore the work which needs to be done to implement, embed, and integrate an end-of-life care intervention into everyday practice, providing insight into improving consistency across different healthcare settings.

Supplementary Materials: The following supporting information can be downloaded at: https://www.mdpi.com/article/10.3390/healthcare13080848/s1, Table S1: How likely are the following groups to be involved in the decision-making process around end-of-life care for acute stroke patients? Table S2: TDF domains and supporting quotes.

Author Contributions: C.E.L., C.L.W., D.J., N.S., C.B. and C.T. conceptualised the study. C.E.L., C.L.W., D.J., N.S., C.B., C.T. and C.G. designed the study. C.G., C.D., F.J.P., A.S.P., A.R.-S., C.T. and C.E.L. were all involved in the analysis. The paper was jointly written and reviewed by all authors. All authors have read and agreed to the published version of the manuscript.

Funding: This project is funded by the National Institute for Health and Care Research (NIHR) Programme Development Grant (Grant Reference Number NIHR202049). The views expressed are those of the authors and not necessarily those of the NIHR or the Department of Health and Social Care. C.L.W contributed to this publication in her capacity as NIHR ARC NWC implementation lead but this publication is not NIHR ARC NWC funded.

Institutional Review Board Statement: The study was reviewed by the NRES Committee North West—Greater Manchester South Research Ethics Committee for Study title: PREPARE: imPRoving End of life care Practice in stroke cARE REC reference: 21/NW/0185 IRAS project ID: 289430, 16 August 2021) and received a favourable opinion.

Informed Consent Statement: Informed consent was obtained from all subjects involved in the study.

Data Availability Statement: The original contributions presented in this study are included in the article/Supplementary Material. Further inquiries can be directed to the corresponding author.

Acknowledgments: PREPARE Study Research Team Members: Margaret Ogden (patient and public involvement lead), Irene Carey, Naomi Lynden, Andrew Clegg, Bee Wee and Ailsa Brotherton.

Conflicts of Interest: The authors declare no conflicts of interest.

References

1. Intercollegiate Stroke Working Party. *SSNAP Acute Organisational Audit Report for April 2023–March 2024 Admissions and Discharges*; King's College London: London, UK, 2024.
2. Katzan, I.L.; Spertus, J.; Bettger, J.P.; Bravata, D.M.; Reeves, M.J.; Smith, E.E.; Bushnell, C.; Higashida, R.T.; Hinchey, J.A.; Holloway, R.G.; et al. Risk adjustment of ischemic stroke outcomes for comparing hospital performance. *Stroke* **2014**, *45*, 918–944. [CrossRef] [PubMed]
3. Public Health England and Brine, S. New Figures Show Larger Proportion of Strokes in the Middle Aged (Press Release). 2018. Available online: https://www.gov.uk/government/news/new-figures-show-larger-proportion-of-strokes-in-the-middle-aged#:~:text=While%20the%20majority%20(59%25),compared%20to%20a%20decade%20ago (accessed on 19 November 2024).
4. Connolly, T.; Coats, H.; DeSanto, K.; Jones, J. The experience of uncertainty for patients, families and healthcare providers in post-stroke palliative and end-of-life care: A qualitative meta-synthesis. *Age Ageing* **2021**, *50*, 534–545. [CrossRef] [PubMed]
5. Burton, C.R.; Payne, S.; Turner, M.; Bucknall, T.; Rycroft-Malone, J.; Tyrrell, P.; Horne, M.; Ntambwe, L.I.; Tyson, S.; Mitchell, H.; et al. The study protocol of: "Initiating end of life care in stroke: Clinical decision-making around prognosis". *BMC Palliat. Care* **2014**, *13*, 55. [CrossRef] [PubMed]
6. Holloway, R.G.; Arnold, R.M.; Creutzfeldt, C.J.; Lewis, E.F.; Lutz, B.J.; McCann, R.M.; Rabinstein, A.A.; Saposnik, G.; Sheth, K.N.; Zahuranec, D.B.; et al. Palliative and end-of-life care in stroke: A statement for healthcare professionals from the American Heart Association/American Stroke Association. *Stroke* **2014**, *45*, 1887–1916. [CrossRef]
7. Ramsburg, H.; Moriarty, H.J.; MacKenzie Greenle, M. End-of-life symptoms in adult patients with stroke in the last two years of life: An integrative review. *Am. J. Hosp. Palliat. Care* **2024**, *41*, 831–839. [CrossRef]
8. Payne, S.; Burton, C.; Addington-Hall, J.; Jones, A. End-of-life issues in acute stroke care: A qualitative study of the experiences and preferences of patients and families. *Palliat. Med.* **2010**, *24*, 146–153. [CrossRef]
9. Etkind, S.N.; Bristowe, K.; Bailey, K.; Selman, L.E.; Murtagh, F.E. How does uncertainty shape patient experience in advanced illness? A secondary analysis of qualitative data. *Palliat. Med.* **2017**, *31*, 171–180. [CrossRef] [PubMed] [PubMed Central]
10. General Medical Council. Treatment and Care Towards the End of Life: Good Practice in Decision Making. 2010 19.11.24. Available online: https://www.gmc-uk.org/professional-standards/professional-standards-for-doctors/treatment-and-care-towards-the-end-of-life (accessed on 15 February 2025).
11. National Health Service (NHS). What to Expect from End of Life Care. 2018. Available online: https://www.nhs.uk/conditions/end-of-life-care/what-to-expect-from-care/ (accessed on 19 November 2024).
12. National Institute for Health and Care Excellence (NICE). Care of Dying Adults in the Last Days of Life NICE Guideline (NG31). 2015. Available online: https://www.nice.org.uk/guidance/ng31 (accessed on 15 February 2025).
13. National Institute for Health and Care Excellence (NICE). *Care of Dying Adults in the Last Days of Life. Quality standard (QS144)*. Available online: https://www.nice.org.uk/guidance/qs144 (accessed on 15 February 2025).
14. National Palliative and End of Life Care Partnership. *Ambitions for Palliative and End of life Care: A National Framework for Local action 2021–2026*; National Palliative and End of Life Care Partnership: London, UK, 2021.
15. Intercollegiate Stroke Working Party. *National Clinical Guideline for Stroke*; Intercollegiate Stroke Working Party: London, UK, 2023.
16. Cowey, E.; Smith, L.N.; Stott, D.J.; McAlpine, C.H.; E Mead, G.; Barber, M.; Walters, M. Impact of a clinical pathway on end-of-life care following stroke: A mixed methods study. *Palliat. Med.* **2015**, *29*, 249–259. [CrossRef]
17. Markovitz, N.; Morgenstern, L.B.; Shafie-Khorassani, F.; Cornett, B.A.; Kim, S.; Ortiz, C.; Lank, R.J.; Case, E.; Zahuranec, D.B. Family Perceptions of Quality of End-of-Life Care in Stroke. *Palliat. Med. Rep.* **2020**, *1*, 129–134. [CrossRef] [PubMed] [PubMed Central]
18. Reinink, H.; Geurts, M.; Melis-Riemens, C.; Hollander, A.; Kappelle, J.; van der Worp, B. Quality of dying after acute stroke. *Eur. Stroke J.* **2021**, *6*, 268–275. [CrossRef] [PubMed] [PubMed Central]
19. Su, J.J.; Lin, R.S.Y.; Paguio, J.; Leung, A.Y.M.; Molassiotis, A. Palliative care for older adults hospitalized for stroke from the informal caregivers' perspectives: A qualitative study. *J. Cardiovasc. Nurs.* **2023**, *38*, E110–E119. [CrossRef]
20. Kendall, M.; Cowey, E.; Mead, G.; Barber, M.; McAlpine, C.; Stott, D.J.; Boyd, K.; Murray, S.A. Outcomes, experiences and palliative care in major stroke: A multicentre, mixed-method, longitudinal study. *Cmaj* **2018**, *190*, E238–E246. [CrossRef] [PubMed]

21. Stevens, T.; Payne, S.; Burton, C.; Addington-Hall, J.; Jones, A. Palliative care in stroke: A critical review of the literature. *Palliat. Med.* **2007**, *21*, 323–331. [CrossRef] [PubMed]
22. Department of Health. *End of Life Care Strategy: Promoting High Quality Care for all Adults at the End of Life 2008; Department of Health: 2008*. Available online: https://assets.publishing.service.gov.uk/media/5a7ae925ed915d71db8b35aa/End_of_life_strategy.pdf (accessed on 15 February 2025).
23. The National Council for Palliative Care. *End of life Care Strategy: The National Council for Palliative Care Submission*; The National Council for Palliative Care: London, UK, 2006.
24. General Medical Council. Guidance: Treatment and Care Towards the End of Life Updated on 13 December 2024. Available online: https://www.gmc-uk.org/-/media/documents/Treatment_and_care_towards_the_end_of_life___English_1015.pdf_48902105.pdf (accessed on 15 February 2025).
25. OECD Health Quality Indicators: Acute Care. Organisation for Economic Co-operation and Development. Available online: https://stats.oecd.org (accessed on 15 February 2025).
26. Michie, S.; Johnston, M.; Abraham, C.; Lawton, R.; Parker, D.; Walker, A. Making psychological theory useful for implementing evidence based practice: A consensus approach. *Qual. Saf. Heal. Care* **2005**, *14*, 26–33.
27. Elo, S.; Kyngäs, H. The qualitative content analysis process. *J. Adv. Nurs.* **2008**, *62*, 107–115. [CrossRef]
28. Ritchie, J.; Lewis, J. *Qualitative Research Practice: A Guide for Social Science Students and Researchers*; Sage: London, UK, 2003.
29. Zago, S.; Roberts, S.; Jones, P. Effective communication and decision-making in multidisciplinary teams in palliative care settings. *J. Clin. Palliat. Care* **2019**, *30*, 15–22.
30. Claire, J.; Creutzfeldt; Julia, B.; Amber, C.; Susan, E.; Barbara, L.; Maisha, T.R.; Darin, B.Z.; Robert, G. Holloway, Palliative and End-of-Life Care in Stroke: A Scientific Statement from the American Heart Association. *Stroke* **2024**, *56*, 2. [CrossRef]
31. Kiker, W.A.; Rutz Voumard, R.; Andrews, L.I.B.; Holloway, R.G.; Brumback, L.C.; Engelberg, R.A.; Curtis, J.R.; Creutzfeldt, C.J. Assessment of discordance between physicians and family members regarding prognosis in patients with severe acute brain injury. *JAMA Netw. Open* **2021**, *4*, e2128991. [CrossRef]
32. Foster, M.; Patterson, M.; Jackson, J. Family involvement in palliative care decision-making: Impact on patient and family outcomes. *Palliat. Care J.* **2017**, *21*, 312–321.
33. Whitehead, J.; Cooper, R.; Stone, B. Managing ethical dilemmas in end-of-life care: A survey of healthcare providers. *J. Ethics Med.* **2015**, *33*, 128–134.
34. Harrison, K.; Tilley, C.; Jacob, A. The impact of staffing shortages on palliative care delivery in hospitals. *J. Palliat. Care* **2016**, *32*, 5–12.
35. Kerr, D.; Jones, A.; Bailey, J. Palliative care education for healthcare professionals: A review of current practices. *Palliat. Care Int.* **2016**, *19*, 201–210.
36. Lam, S.; Leung, K.; Tan, S. Decision support tools in stroke end-of-life care. *Stroke Res. Ther. J.* **2020**, *15*, 56–62.
37. Groot, M.; Stijn, B.; Dijkstra, H. Improving dignity in end-of-life care: Insights from patients and families. *Eur. J. Palliat. Care* **2015**, *22*, 354–359.
38. McClelland, L.E.; Gabriel, A.S.; DePuccio, M.J. Compassion practices, nurse well-being, and ambulatory patient experience rating. *Med. Care.* **2018**, *56*, 4–10. [CrossRef]

MDPI AG
Grosspeteranlage 5
4052 Basel
Switzerland
Tel.: +41 61 683 77 34

Healthcare Editorial Office
E-mail: healthcare@mdpi.com
www.mdpi.com/journal/healthcare

www.ingramcontent.com/pod-product-compliance
Lightning Source LLC
Chambersburg PA
CBHW041346210926
51850CB00013B/3008